Certification Exam Review
for Pharmacy Technicians

Third Edition

Cheryl Aiken, BS, PharmD, RPh
Robert J. Anderson, PharmD

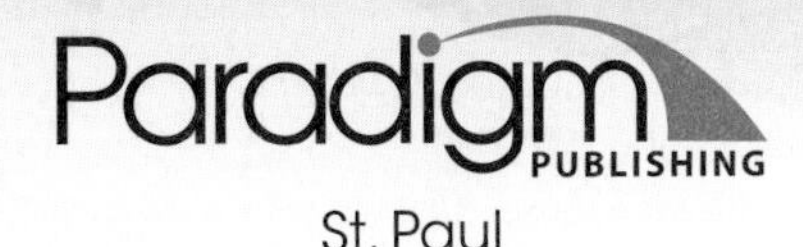

St. Paul

Managing Editor	Brenda M. Palo
Developmental Editors	J. Trout Lowen and Grant E. Mabie
Production Editor	Lori Michelle Ryan
Cover and Text Designer	Jaana Bykonich
Copy Editor	Susan Giniger
Proofreader	Susan E. K. Foster
Indexer	Ina Gravitz
Cover Images	© iStock/kimeveruss (upper left); © Pharmacy Technician Certification Board (upper right); © Paradigm Publishing, by George Brainard (bottom left)

Photo Credits: Chapter and appendices title pages iii, iv, vii, 1, 19, 57, 83, 97, 117, 133, 143, 163, 179, 185, 191, 199, 215, 245 © iStock/kimeveruss; **75** © Paradigm Publishing; **88** © Paradigm Publishing (top & bottom); **99** © Paradigm Publishing, by George Brainard; **100** © Paradigm Publishing, by George Brainard; **107** © Paradigm Publishing; **108** © George Brainard; **113** © Paradigm Publishing; **120** Reprinted with permission of Mylan Pharmaceuticals Inc. All rights reserved (top left); Images used with permission from Fresenius Kabi USA, LLC (top, right); © Eli Lilly and Company. All Rights Reserved. Used with Permission. Cymbalta is a trademark of Eli Lilly and Company (bottom left & right); **125** © Paradigm Publishing; **135** With permission, courtesy of Terurmo Medical Corporation; **145** © Paradigm Publishing; **146** © Paradigm Publishing; **147** © Paradigm Publishing; **148** © Paradigm Publishing; **149** © Paradigm Publishing; **150** © Paradigm Publishing; **151** © Paradigm Publishing; **155** © George Brainard (top), with permission, courtesy of McKesson Provider Technologies, Inc. (bottom); **156** © Paradigm Publishing; **157** © Paradigm Publishing; **171** With permission, courtesy of McKesson Provider Technologies, Inc.; **172** Image courtesy of Sanofi-Aventis; **181** © Paradigm Publishing; **187** Courtesy of Tova Weigand Green; **188** With permission, courtesy of McKesson Provider Technologies, Inc.

ISBN 978-0-76385-215-3 (Text)
ISBN 978-0-76385-217-7 (Text and CD)

875 Montreal Way
St. Paul, MN 55102
E-mail: educate@emcp.com
Web site: www.emcp.com

Printed in the United States of America

22 21 20 19 18 17 16 15 14 13   1 2 3 4 5 6 7 8 9 10

Brief Contents

Contents

Preface

Certification Exam Review for Pharmacy Technicians, Third Edition, and the companion Study Partner CD offer a comprehensive review of the key concepts, skills, and information that students need to know to successfully pass a national certification exam, and to work successfully as a certified pharmacy technician (CPhT) in a community, institutional, or other pharmacy setting.

The third edition of *Certification Exam Review for Pharmacy Technicians* has been substantially restructured to focus on the skills and competencies that are central to the newly revised Pharmacy Technician Certification Exam (PTCE). The revised exam is one of several changes announced by the Pharmacy Technician Certification Board in early 2013. For more information on when and how those changes will affect certification and recertification requirements, consult your instructor. Additional information is also available at www.paradigmcollege.net/certexam review3e/ptcbchanges. This textbook also provides a comprehensive review for students taking the Exam for Certification of Pharmacy Technicians (ExCPT).

In *Certification Exam Review for Pharmacy Technicians, Third Edition*, chapter titles, structure, and content are aligned with the nine knowledge domains identified by the PTCB in its blueprint for the exam. Changes to the PTCE are part of a broader initiative by the PTCB to elevate the qualifications and standards for national certification and recertification as a pharmacy technician. By the end of the decade, the PTCB will require all pharmacy technicians to complete an education program accredited by the American Society of Health-System Pharmacists (ASHP) as a prerequisite to national certification.

The healthcare environment is evolving rapidly, and qualified and credentialed pharmacy technicians are integral to the delivery of high-quality patient care. Certification demonstrates an individual's commitment to the profession and to the patients he or she serves.

Certification Exam Review for Pharmacy Technicians, Third Edition, and the Study Partner CD include expanded content in each of the nine domains identified as essential knowledge for pharmacy technicians practicing in a modern healthcare environment, including:

- up-to-date information on the most commonly prescribed pharmaceuticals
- a chapter completely dedicated to pharmacy laws and regulations
- a new 50-question practice test designed to strengthen students' skills in pharmacy calculation
- more in-depth information on sterile and nonsterile compounding regulations and procedures
- expanded information on infection control and the proper handling and disposal of pharmaceutical and hazardous wastes
- new sections on professional standards, electronic medical records and e-prescribing, new technologies, and information management in the pharmacy
- an increased focus on medication errors and prevention strategies
- the application of quality-assurance procedures in pharmacy settings

- expanded information on pharmacy ordering and receiving, and management of outdated and recalled pharmaceuticals
- up-to-date information on billing, reimbursement, and healthcare reform as it relates to pharmacy

As in the previous edition, *Certification Exam Review for Pharmacy Technicians, Third Edition* includes helpful instructions for students preparing to take a high-stakes exam, as well as study and test-taking tips.

The Skills Quiz and Thinking Beyond the Exam features at the end of each chapter reinforce key concepts in each knowledge area.

Practice Tests

Practice tests provide students with an opportunity to gauge their knowledge, identify areas for additional study, and hone their test-taking skills.

- A 90-question pretest at the end of Chapter 1 allows students to assess current knowledge and identify areas for additional study.
- New! A 50-question calculations test includes problems on weights and measures, dosage, dilution, alligation, mark-up, Drug Enforcement Administration (DEA) verification, and more.
- New! A 25-question pharmacology test covers brand and generic drugs, adverse reactions and drug interactions, auxiliary labeling, over-the-counter medications, and dietary supplements.

Chapter Features

1

LEARNING OBJECTIVES establish clear goals for pharmacy technician students as they begin their chapter study.

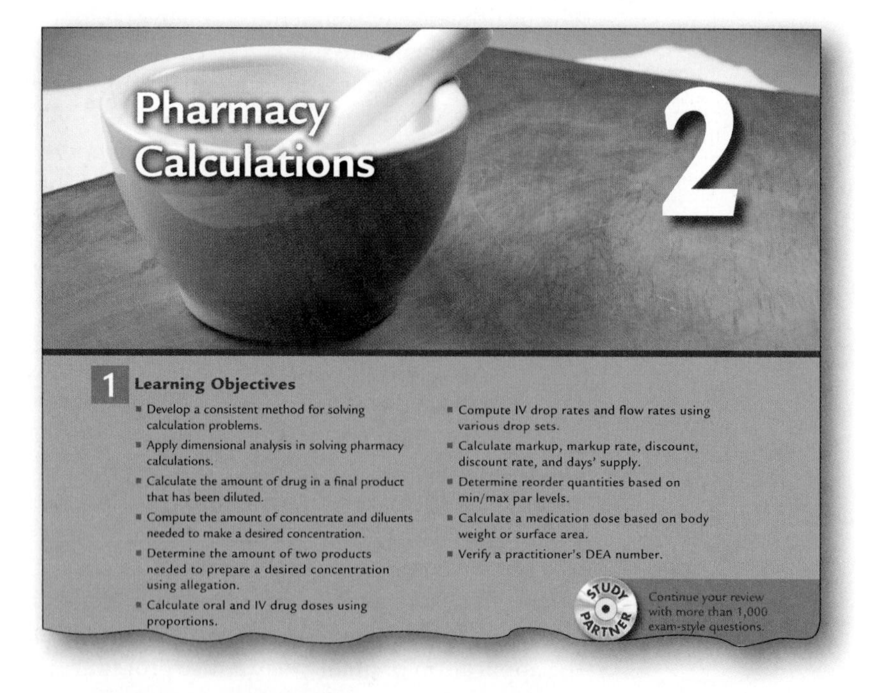

Pharmacy Calculations

2

1 **Learning Objectives**

- Develop a consistent method for solving calculation problems.
- Apply dimensional analysis in solving pharmacy calculations.
- Calculate the amount of drug in a final product that has been diluted.
- Compute the amount of concentrate and diluents needed to make a desired concentration.
- Determine the amount of two products needed to prepare a desired concentration using allegation.
- Calculate oral and IV drug doses using proportions.
- Compute IV drop rates and flow rates using various drop sets.
- Calculate markup, markup rate, discount, discount rate, and days' supply.
- Determine reorder quantities based on min/max par levels.
- Calculate a medication dose based on body weight or surface area.
- Verify a practitioner's DEA number.

Continue your review with more than 1,000 exam-style questions.

2

TABLES highlight important information related to the chapter topics and serve as a study aid.

2 TABLE 5.1 USP Good Compounding Practices

Component Standards	
Facility	designated area with low traffic flow and adequate space for working and equipment storage
Personnel	compounding staff trained and proficient in the skills necessary to compound drugs and maintain equipment
Equipment	must be maintained and calibrated for accurate compounding and adequate for the products being compounded
Ingredient selection	USP/National Formulary-quality ingredients stored and used appropriately
Compounding	periodic and final check by the pharmacist process
Packaging and storage	product-appropriate containers that meet storage requirements for the product
Beyond-use dating	stability of preparation after compounding calculated by ingredients and dosage form
Controls	quality assurance programs established to guarantee equipment, staff, and product quality
Labeling of excess product	ingredients, lot, compound date, beyond-use date, and compounder information
Records and reports	records of ingredients, personnel, and equipment for compounding an individual product as well as for all the ingredients and equipment used

3

FIGURES provide additional detail and visual reinforcement of chapter topics.

labels are commonly affixed to the container by the pharmacist or an experienced technician.

3 FIGURE 8.4

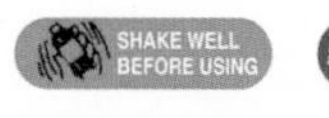

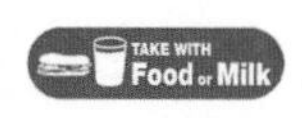

REFRIGERATE

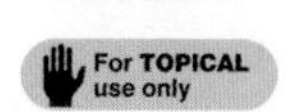

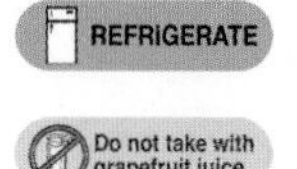

For TOPICAL use only

Auxiliary labels are placed on dispensed medications to help inform patients about how to take and store their medications safely and effectively.

A medication information sheet is a computerized printout that provides details on how to safely take the prescribed medication. The information sheet is automatically printed after the pharmacist has verified the prescription. After the pharmacist conducts a final check of the prescription and medication, the information sheet is attached to the bag containing the medication, which then is ready for patient pick-up.

The MedGuide (discussed in Chapter 6) is basically a black box warning advising consumers about potential adverse reactions or the proper use of selected high-risk medications. Birth control pills are commonly packaged with a MedGuide; other MedGuides are printed for the patient at the time of the pharmacist's final check.

Finally, by law, the technician must offer the patient counseling by the pharmacist. In some cases, especially with first-time medications or potential drug interactions,

4

SKILLS QUIZ questions at the end of every chapter focus student review on key concepts included in the exam.

4 Skills Quiz

Reflect on the information presented in this chapter and answer the following questions.

1. Who should take the PTCE?
   a. pharmacists
   b. physicians
   c. pharmacy technicians
   d. registered nurses
2. Licensure may require a(n)
   a. college degree.
   b. application.
   c. certification.
   d. all of the above
3. Certification provides
   a. autonomy.
   b. vocational identity.
   c. job security.
   d. career satisfaction.
6. Studying for the certification exam should happen
   a. over time at a steady pace.
   b. by cramming the week before the exam.
   c. only if you do not work in a pharmacy.
   d. if you have previously failed the test.
7. Questions and answers that contain absolutes are
   a. always incorrect.
   b. never correct.
   c. may be incorrect.
   d. none of the above
8. When you are unsure of the answer to an exam question, you should
   a. skip the question entirely.

5

THINKING BEYOND THE EXAM scenario-based questions challenge students to think critically about the role of the pharmacy technician in real-world environments.

5 Thinking Beyond the Exam

Medication errors can happen even in the best circumstances. From your experience, write a list of all the steps a prescription or medication order goes through before dispensing the final drug. Identify where potential medication errors might occur and what should be done to prevent errors from happening. Discuss whether these changes could be implemented at your work site and what barriers exist to making changes that may reduce errors.

Additional Resources for the Student

Appendices

The appendices provide important reference material for pharmacy technician students:

- **Appendix A:** Most Commonly Prescribed Drugs
- **Appendix B:** Practice Exams
- **Appendix C:** Answer Keys (Includes step-by-step instruction for calculations problems.)

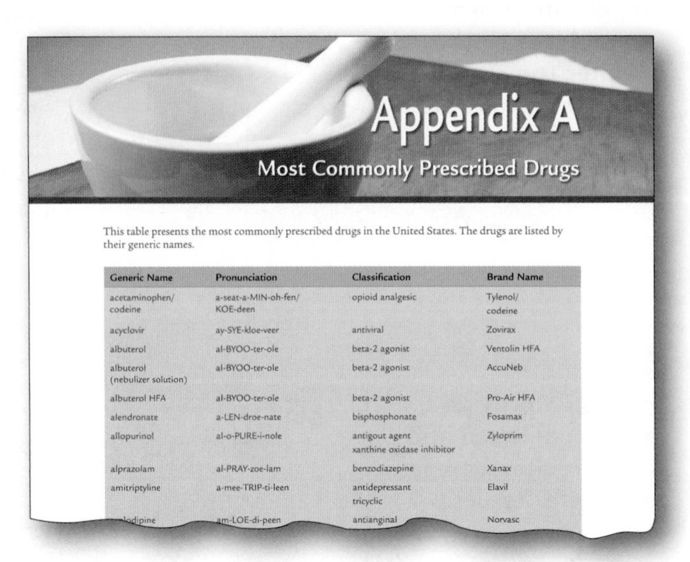

Appendix A

Most Commonly Prescribed Drugs

This table presents the most commonly prescribed drugs in the United States. The drugs are listed by their generic names.

Generic Name	Pronunciation	Classification	Brand Name
acetaminophen/ codeine	a-seat-a-MIN-oh-fen/ KOE-deen	opioid analgesic	Tylenol/ codeine
acyclovir	ay-SYE-kloe-veer	antiviral	Zovirax
albuterol	al-BYOO-ter-ole	beta-2 agonist	Ventolin HFA
albuterol (nebulizer solution)	al-BYOO-ter-ole	beta-2 agonist	AccuNeb
albuterol HFA	al-BYOO-ter-ole	beta-2 agonist	Pro-Air HFA
alendronate	a-LEN-droe-nate	bisphosphonate	Fosamax
allopurinol	al-o-PURE-i-nole	antigout agent xanthine oxidase inhibitor	Zyloprim
alprazolam	al-PRAY-zoe-lam	benzodiazepine	Xanax
amitriptyline	a-mee-TRIP-ti-leen	antidepressant tricyclic	Elavil
lodipine	am-LOE-di-peen	antianginal	Norvasc

Study Partner CD

The Study Partner CD included with this textbook contains the following tools to support and enhance student learning:

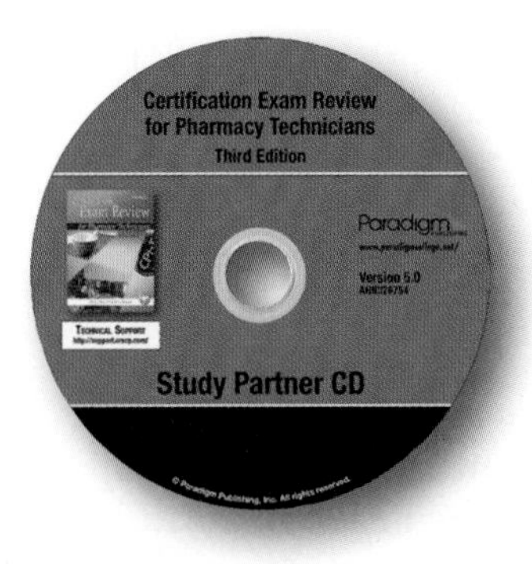

- **Pretest** Students can assess their strengths and identify areas for further study.
- **Practice Exams** A bank of more than 1,000 exam-style questions allows students to generate a nearly unlimited number of unique, randomized 90-question exams in Practice and Reported modes.
- **Flashcards** for the top 200 generic and brand name drugs.

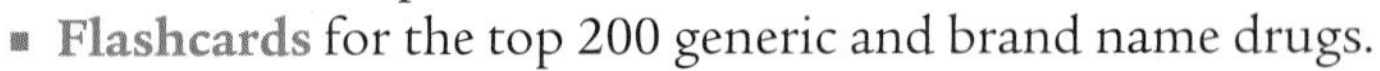

EBook and Online Resources

eBook

For students who prefer studying with an eBook, this text is available in electronic format. The Web-based, password-protected eBook features dynamic navigation tools, including bookmarking, a linked table of contents, and page-by-page navigation. The eBook format also supports helpful study tools, such as highlighting and note taking.

Student Internet Resource Center

The Internet Resource Center for this title, www.paradigmcollege.net/certexamreview3e, provides additional reference information and resources for students, including:

- common pharmacy abbreviations
- medical abbreviations and acronyms
- glossary of terms
- ISMP List of Confused Drug Names
- pharmacy organizations and resource links

Additional Resources for the Instructor

Certification Exam Review for Pharmacy Technicians, Third Edition is supported by several tools to help instructors plan their courses and assess student learning. The password-protected instructor's section of the Internet Resource Center, which includes additional support materials and the answers to all end-of-chapter Skills Quiz questions, is available at www.paradigmcollege.net/certexamreview3e.

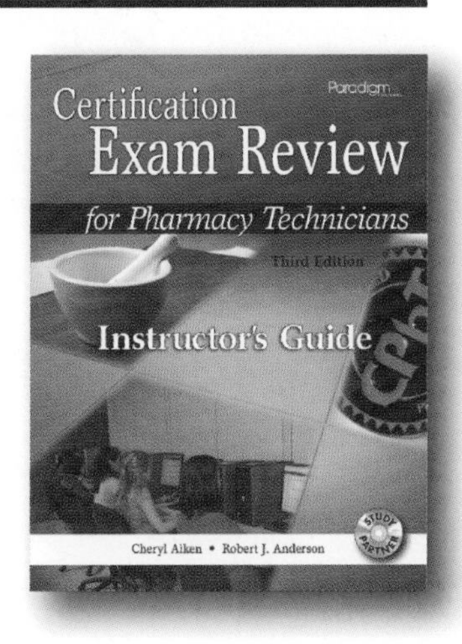

Textbooks in the Pharmacy Technician Series

Certification Exam Review for Pharmacy Technicians, Third Edition is intended to help students efficiently and effectively review for the pharmacy certification exam. This text builds on the work of the other books in the pharmacy technician series published by Paradigm Publishing, Inc.

- *Pharmacology for Technicians, Fifth Edition*
- *Pharmacology for Technicians Workbook, Fifth Edition*
- *Pharmacy Labs for Technicians, Second Edition*
- *Pharmacy Practice for Technicians, Fifth Edition*
- *Pharmacy Calculations for Technicians, Fifth Edition*
- *Sterile Compounding and Aseptic Technique*
- *Pharmacology Essentials for Technicians*

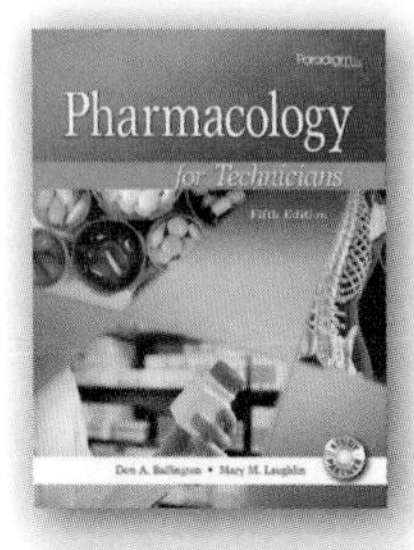

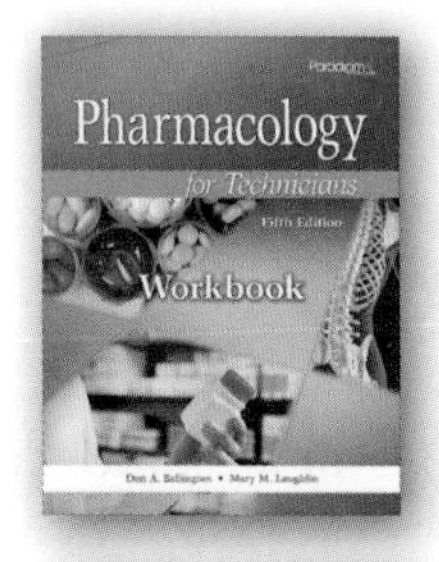

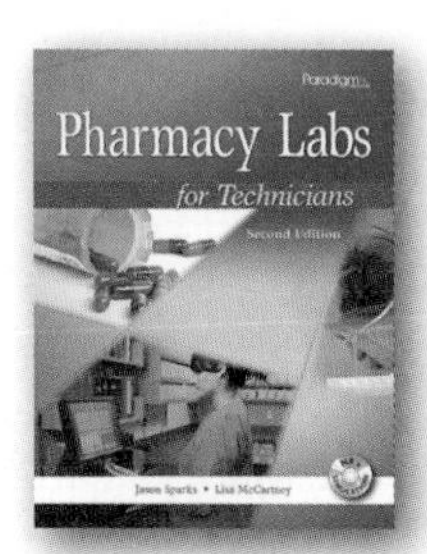

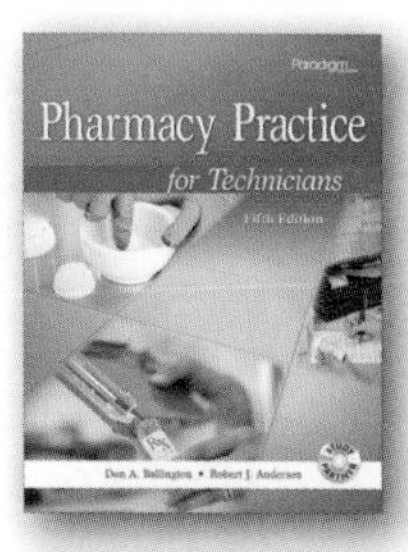

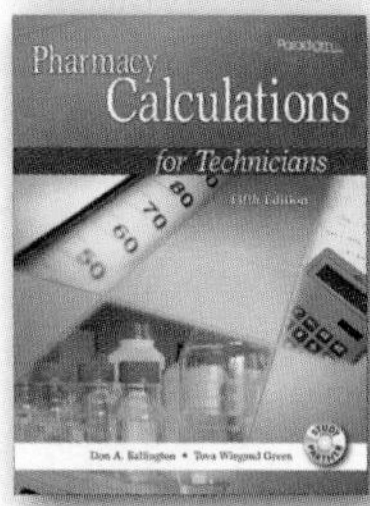

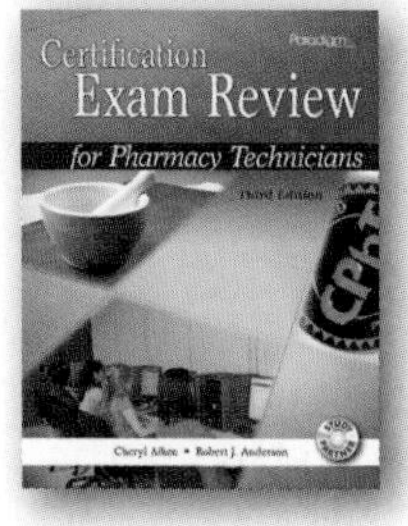

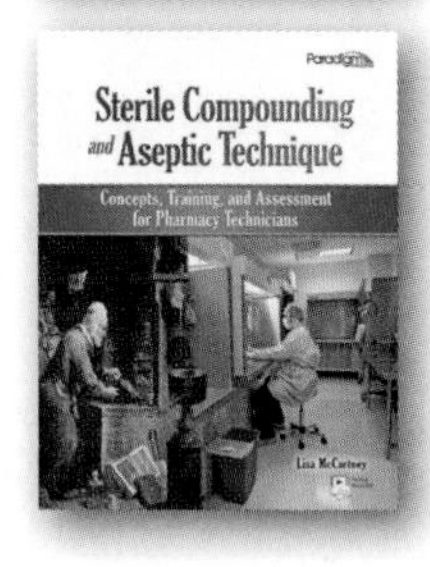

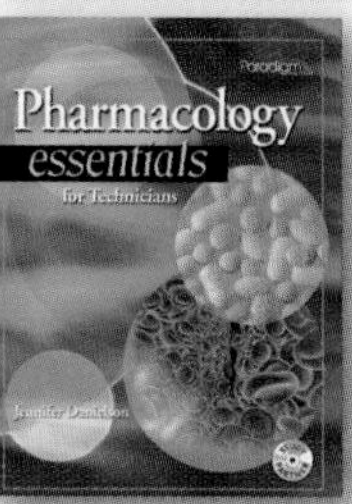

About the Authors

Cheryl Aiken, BS, PharmD, RPh, is a staff pharmacist at the Brattleboro Retreat, a private psychiatric hospital in Brattleboro, Vermont. In addition to her work in the psychiatric field, she has served as a community pharmacist for independent and chain pharmacies, and as a staff pharmacist at the Brattleboro Memorial Hospital. In 2002, she helped establish an associate's degree and the Pharmacy Technician Training Program certificate at Vermont Technical College. She lives in Vermont with her husband and three dogs.

Robert J. Anderson, PharmD, has more than 40 years of experience in academia and pharmacy practice, having worked in both independent and chain community pharmacies. Dr. Anderson is a professor emeritus at the Southern School of Pharmacy at Mercer University in Atlanta, Georgia, and is currently a part-time community pharmacist. He is also president of RJA Consultants, LLC for legal consulting. He has been a guest lecturer in clinical pharmacology at several state nurse practitioner programs, as well as a clinical pharmacy specialist at Kaiser Permanente, Southeast Region, in Atlanta. Dr. Anderson has served as an associate director for the Department of Pharmaceutical Services at the University of Nebraska Medical Center in Omaha, Nebraska, and is a past member of the United States Pharmacopeia (USP) Expert Committee. He is co-author on the third, fourth, and fifth editions of *Pharmacy Practice for Technicians*, as well as the second and third editions of *Certification Exam Review for Pharmacy Technicians*. In addition, he has written chapters in *Clinical Pharmacology and Therapeutics* and *Handbook of Nonprescription Drugs* and has served on the editorial boards of *Family Practice Recertification* and *American Journal of Managed Care Pharmacy*.

Author Acknowledgements

I want to thank my husband for all of his understanding during the editing process and the time commitment it required. J. Trout Lowen has been super in providing the guidance and commitment needed to bring the third edition to completion.

Cheryl Aiken

I would like to offer a special thank you to the entire staff at Walgreen's Pharmacy in Jasper, Georgia, and the staff at Ball Ground Pharmacy in Ball Ground, Georgia, for their support and valuable insights into the practice of retail and independent community pharmacy, and to thank the staff at Cherokee Custom Scripts for their support and help in understanding the day-to-day operation of an accredited compounding pharmacy.

Robert J. Anderson

Acknowledgments

The quality of this body of work is a testament to the support and assistance provided by the contributors and reviewers who participated in *Certification Exam Review for Pharmacy Technicians, Third Edition*. We appreciate their contributions.

Robert W. Aanonsen, CPhT
Platt College
Tulsa, Oklahoma

Harold S. Bender, PharmD, RPh
National College of Business and Technology
Spring Hill, Tennessee

Diana V. Broome, AS, AA, CPhT, PhTR
Lone Star College
Tomball, Texas

Christina Cox, BS, CPhT
Heald College
Honolulu, Hawaii

Erika D'Arezzo, BS, CPhT
Sanford-Brown
Cranston, Rhode Island

Elizabeth Garcia, AA, CPhT
San Joaquin Valley College
Visalia, California

Aldo Gatti, BSc Pharm, RPh
Centennial College
Toronto, Ontario, Canada

Joseph P. Gee, PharmD
Cosumnes River College
Sacramento, California

Mary Good, AA, CPhT
National College
Harrisonburg, Virginia

Jeff Gricar, MEd, CPhT, PhTR
HCC Coleman College
Houston, Texas

Lisa Homburg, RPh
College of the Mainland
Texas City, Texas

Susan Howell, BS, CPhT
Ivy Tech Community College
Muncie, Indiana

Kent LaFary, CPhT

Belva J. Matherly, BA, BA, CPhT
National College
Salem, Virginia

Lisa McCartney, BAAS, CPhT, PhTR
Austin Community College
Austin, Texas

Shawn McPartland, MD, JD
Harrison College
Indianapolis, Indiana

Lynda Melendez, AS, CPhT, PhTR
Texas State Technical College
Waco, Texas

Mary Stende Miller, BS, RPh
Minnesota State Community & Technical College
Wadena, Minnesota

Michael T. Mockler, MBA, RPh
Heald College
Portland, Oregon

Jody Myhre-Oechsle, MS, CPhT
Chippewa Valley Technical College
Eau Claire, Wisconsin

Elina Pierce, MS, CPhT
Southeast Community College
Beatrice, Nebraska

Vickey L. Rose, CPhT

Becky Schonscheck, BS
Maricopa, Arizona

Julia B. Sherwood, AA, CPhT
Spartanburg Community College
Spartanburg, South Carolina

Shahriar Siddiq, MBBS (MD), DNM
Algonquin Careers Academy
Ottawa, Ontario, Canada

Jacqueline T. Smith, RN, CPhT
National College
Princeton, West Virginia

Maureen Simmons Sparks, CPhT
Clover Park Technical College
Lakewood, Washington

Bobbi Steelman, MEd, CPhT
Daymar College
Bowling Green, Kentucky

Cynthia J. Steffen, MS, RPh
Milwaukee Area Technical College
Milwaukee, Wisconsin

Dawn M. Tesner, DHEd, MSHA, CPhT
Mid Michigan Community College
Mt. Pleasant, Michigan

Traci Tonhofer, CPhT
Davis Applied Technology College
Kaysville, Utah

Sandi Tschritter, MEd, CPhT
Spokane Community College
Spokane, Washington

Terry Walker, RN (retired)
Selkirk College
Castlegar, British Columbia, Canada

Jeremy Watson, BS, CPhT, RT
National College
Knoxville, Tennessee

Elaine Young, MEd, CPhT
Angelina College
Lufkin, Texas

We offer a special thank you to Lisa McCartney for her valuable input on chapter content and to Shawn McPartland and Traci Tonhofer for their expert chapter reviews.

The authors and editorial staff invite your feedback on the text and its supplements. Please reach us by clicking the “Contact us” button at www.emcp.com.

The Importance of Certification and Taking a High-Stakes Test

1

Learning Objectives

- Discuss the importance of certification for a pharmacy technician.
- Understand the elements of certification, registration, and licensure.
- Describe the major testing components of the PTCB examination.
- Make a study plan for the examination.
- Use techniques for successfully taking a multi-choice examination.

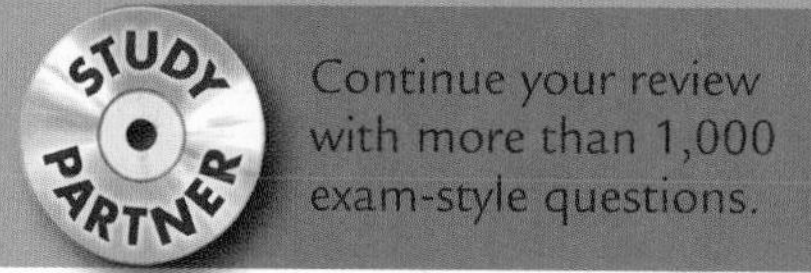

The Purpose of Certification

A certification exam is a nationally recognized test used to measure competency. The purpose of the exam is to protect the public interest by evaluating candidates' knowledge in a specific area, in this case, the knowledge necessary to perform the duties of a pharmacy technician. A nongovernmental agency develops the exam and implements the rules and policies related to certification. State pharmacy boards determine whether pharmacy technicians need to be registered, licensed, or certified. If certification is required, the state board of pharmacy determines which certification exam is offered.

Who should consider taking a pharmacy technician certification exam? Any person already working in a pharmacy or considering a career as a pharmacy technician should plan to study for and take a certification exam.

Some states require certification for anyone working as a pharmacy technician. Many employers encourage pharmacy technicians to become certified, and some offer a monetary incentive. Certification also provides a sense of vocational identity and offers the technician the potential for increased job satisfaction. It demonstrates to prospective employers (as well as the public) that the technician has the necessary skills and knowledge to work in a pharmacy and is committed to the profession. Successful completion of a national certification exam qualifies the technician to work in a variety of pharmacy settings including retail, institutional, mail order, administration, and educational. Employer-specific examinations—such as those offered by some chain pharmacies—may test an individual's ability to work in one specific pharmacy environment, but those exams are not comprehensive enough to demonstrate the skills needed to work in many different pharmacy environments.

Certification, Registration, and Licensure

Board of Pharmacy rules and regulations include terms such as certification, registration, and licensure. State requirements for pharmacy technicians may include one or all of these components.

Certification

Certification recognizes an individual for meeting predetermined qualifications in a specific area of study. For a pharmacy technician, passing a certification exam means he or she has met the qualifications to work in a pharmacy and assist the pharmacist. A technician who successfully passes the exam may use the designation Certified Pharmacy Technician (CPhT) after his or her name.

Registration

Individual states may require that anyone working behind the pharmacy counter be registered as a way to control access to the restricted area of the pharmacy. The state maintains a list of all employees who have access behind the pharmacy counter and are permitted to assist the pharmacist.

There is no test required for registration but the process generally includes an application to the state Board of Pharmacy and payment of appropriate fees. The application process may include a background check. Registration may be denied if the applicant has a history of criminal activity or charges related to drugs or alcohol use. Registration will be denied or revoked for actions that compromise the lawful activities of a pharmacy, and the state may levy fines against pharmacies that allow nonregistered individuals in restricted areas.

Licensure

Some states require pharmacy technicians to be licensed. Licensure is a more rigorous application process than registration. The process varies by state. In addition to passing a licensure exam, applicants need to be a graduate (associate degree or higher) of a certificate accredited college program specializing in pharmacy technology. Individual states also have continuing education requirements for license renewal.

Visit the state Board of Pharmacy website for information on individual state requirements. To learn more about state licensure requirements, visit the National Association of Boards of Pharmacy website at www.paradigmcollege.net/certexamreview3e/napb/pharmacyboards and click on Boards of Pharmacy.

Why Become Certified?

The effective and safe delivery of pharmaceuticals depends on competent and knowledgeable individuals. Pharmacists and employers recognize that certified pharmacy technicians have demonstrated the ability, knowledge, and skills necessary to function effectively in a pharmacy. As a certified pharmacy technician, you may receive increased responsibilities, job opportunities, and promotions, along with increased respect from your peers. In addition, certification offers a sense of accomplishment and the potential for greater job satisfaction. As the profession of pharmacy advances, the need for qualified pharmacy technicians becomes more essential.

Several organizations are currently working to improve training and education for pharmacy technicians. By the end of the decade, the Pharmacy Technician Certification Board (PTCB) will require all candidates seeking initial certification to complete a training program accredited by the American Society of Health-System Pharmacists (ASHP) that includes both didactic coursework and practical experience. The PTCB is also phasing in additional requirements, including mandatory criminal background checks for initial candidates for certification and changes to continuing education requirements for recertification. More information on the PTCB's new requirements is available at www.paradigmcollege.net/ptcb/certification_changes.

ASHP, in partnership with individual state affiliates, is advocating in support of legislation at the state level through its Pharmacy Technician Initiative that would require all pharmacy technicians to complete an ASHP-accredited training program and earn PTCB certification as a prerequisite to licensure by a state board of pharmacy and for practice in a hospital. The intent of the initiative is to improve patient safety and reduce medication errors through enhanced education and training. More information on the Pharmacy Technician Initiative is available at www.paradigmcollege.net/ashp/initiative.

The Exam

Certification Exam Review for Pharmacy Technicians is intended to help you study for and pass a pharmacy technician certification exam. Two exams are offered: the Pharmacy Technician Certification Exam (PTCE) and the Exam for the Certification of Pharmacy Technicians (ExCPT). Individual states may recognize one exam or the other. Check your state's requirements before deciding which exam to take.

Certification Exam Review for Pharmacy Technicians is not designed to support one test over the other. It includes 10 chapters that are based on nine new domains for testing job performance developed by the Pharmacy Technician Certification Board (PTCB). Other exams will test on similar material, though they may be weighted slightly differently.

The Pharmacy Technician Certification Exam (PTCE) is developed by the Pharmacy Technician Certification Board (PTCB). The PTCB is a nongovernmental agency governed by five professional associations: the American Pharmacists Association (APhA), the American Society of Health-System Pharmacists (ASHP), the National Association of Boards of Pharmacy (NABP), the Illinois Council of Health System Pharmacists (ICHP), and the Michigan Pharmacists Association (MPA).

The PTCE is administered by the Pearson Professional Centers, which are located nationwide. The exam is a two-hour multiple-choice test. The exam includes 10 minutes for a tutorial and survey and 1 hour and 50 minutes for the exam. There are 90 questions on the exam; 80 questions are scored. The remaining 10 questions are considered pretest questions. The 10 nonscored questions are placed randomly throughout the test and are not identified. The final score is based on the 80 scored questions. Questions are scaled on the level of difficulty. The minimum score required to pass the exam is 650; possible scores range from 300 to 900.

The current PTCE exam, which will be offered until new testing domains are implemented in the second half of 2013, assesses knowledge in three practice areas:

1. Assisting the pharmacist in serving the patient (66%)
2. Maintaining the medication and inventory system (22%)
3. Participation in the administration and management of pharmacy practice (12%)

The revised test, which will be offered beginning in the second half of 2013, focuses on nine new knowledge domains for job performance:

1. Pharmacology for Technicians (13.75%)
2. Pharmacy Law and Regulations (12.5%)
3. Sterile and Nonsterile Compounding (8.75%)
4. Medication Safety (12.5%)
5. Pharmacy Quality Assurance (7.5%)
6. Medication Order Entry Fill Process (17.5%)
7. Pharmacy Inventory Management (8.75%)
8. Pharmacy Billing and Reimbursement (8.75%)
9. Pharmacy Information System Usage and Application (10%)

Questions from each of these areas are randomly distributed throughout the exam. A complete outline of knowledge requirements in each area can be found at www.paradigmcollege.net/certexamreview3e/ptcb/exam_domains.

The Exam for the Certification of Pharmacy Technicians (ExCPT) is offered by the Institute for the Certification of Pharmacy Technicians, a nongovernmental agency governed by the National Association of Chain Drug Stores (NACDS) and the National Community Pharmacists Association (NCPA). More information concerning the ExCPT exam is available at www.paradigmcollege.net/certexamreview3e/ExCPT/exam_registration.

Eligibility Requirements

Candidates must also meet certain eligibility requirements. Although many of the requirements are the same for both tests, some differences may exist. Check the website for the exam for the most recent requirements. Table 1.1 lists the requirements for the PTCE. Check the website for information about considerations for special circumstances.

TABLE 1.1 PTCE Requirements

PTCE Requirements
High school diploma or GED
No felony convictions
No drug- or pharmacy-related convictions, including misdemeanors (Misdemeanors must be disclosed.)
No denied, suspended, revoked, or restricted registration or licensure, consent order, or other restrictions by any state Board of Pharmacy
No admission of misconduct or violation of regulations of any state Board of Pharmacy

Taking a High-Stakes Exam

A certification exam for pharmacy technicians is a high-stakes, professional exam. Your future as a pharmacy technician will change after successful completion of the exam. To successfully complete the exam, it is important to become proficient in the knowledge and skills necessary to be a pharmacy technician and to practice good test-taking strategies. The exam is similar to other high-stakes tests, such as the standardized tests required in grade school and high school. With a positive attitude and strong study skills, you have the potential to become a certified pharmacy technician.

Test Preparation Strategies

Preparation is an important part of taking a high-stakes exam. This text focuses on two areas of preparation: knowledge in the subject matter and test-taking strategies. This section discusses important test-taking skills and strategies. Chapters 2 through 11 review the knowledge and skills needed by pharmacy technicians.

How and When to Study

Start studying now to become familiar with the skills and concepts on the exam. Do not wait to study until just before the exam. Cramming will not help in a high-stakes professional exam.

There are many ways to study for the exam. Take practice exams, such as those presented in Appendix B and on the Study Partner CD included with this book. Answer the questions at the end of each chapter. In addition to practice tests, the Study Partner CD includes a pretest and flash cards for the top prescription and generic drugs. Use these flash cards to help you study or create your own.

Study groups can be an effective way to review and discuss information. If you work in a pharmacy, ask your colleagues for help. If you do not work in a pharmacy, ask a local pharmacy if you may shadow one of their technicians. (You may have to register with the state Board of Pharmacy to be behind the pharmacy counter.) Getting hands-on experience and observing the work of practicing pharmacists and pharmacy technicians is an excellent way to study for the exam.

Budget Time to Study

Set aside a few hours each day to study uninterrupted by family or friends. Spread your review over a period of weeks. Focused reviews conducted over time are more effective than cramming at the last minute. As a certified pharmacy technician, you will use this information for years to come, not just on the exam. By developing your skills and knowledge slowly over time, you will retain more information and improve your recall in the future.

Talk with Professionals in the Field

After choosing which exam to take, check the organization's website for the most up-to-date knowledge content for that test. Does the testing authority offer a practice exam online? Practice exams can help to determine where to focus your study efforts. Talk to certified pharmacy technicians about their experiences taking the exam. Ask your instructors to identify areas where you need to focus your attention. Ask a pharmacist for help in areas like calculations and pharmacology.

Develop Relaxation Techniques

Taking a high-stakes professional exam can be stressful. Relaxation techniques can help to reduce anxiety and keep your mind clear. Deep breathing, positive thinking, and visualization exercises can help calm the body and mind and allow you to focus on the exam questions. If the testing facility allows it, it may be helpful to visit the test site before the exam to become familiar with the area.

Prepare in Advance for Test Day

Think of preparing for the exam as you would for a trip. You do not wait to pack until it is time to go. The night before the exam, pack all the items needed for the test. Depending on which exam you take, you will need a government-issued photo identification, such as a valid passport, driver's license, U.S. Armed Forces identification card, or nondriver identification issued by your state Department of Motor Vehicles. (Table 1.2 lists approved IDs.) Remember, the name on your identification must be identical to the name provided to the testing center when you registered. The testing center may also require biometric identification, such as a fingerprint scan or a palm vein scan.

TABLE 1.2 Approved Government-Issued Photo IDs*

Driver's license
Learner's permit
Nondriver identification
U.S. passport
U.S. Armed Forces identification

*ID must not be expired.

You are allowed to bring certain items, such as religious apparel and comfort aids, to the PTCE test site, including:

- tissues
- cough drops
- eyeglasses, eye patches, magnifying glasses
- hearing aids, earplugs
- canes, crutches, casts, braces, slings, walkers
- medical devices attached to the body
- wheelchairs and other mobility devices
- pills (unwrapped and not in a container)

Pack only the necessary items. You will not need pencils, paper, calculator, phone, or anything else. Anything needed to take the exam will be provided at the test site. Bring as little as possible. You will be provided with a secure locker to store items not allowed in the exam area.

Follow Good Sleeping and Eating Habits

The night before the exam, do not pull an all-nighter cramming for the exam. Get a good night's sleep. Set the alarm and wake up on time, refreshed and ready. Eat a nutritious meal or snack before the test to help maintain energy. Avoid eating high-fat foods or excessive sugar before the exam as these foods can make you groggy or sleepy in the middle of the test.

TABLE 1.3 The day of the exam
Get enough sleep the night before the test. Also, make sure to get adequate sleep the week before the test.
Arrive at the testing center early and choose a comfortable work area.
Dress casually and comfortably. Take extra time to plan what to wear.
Arrive prepared with the necessary supplies.
Before the test, practice relaxation techniques, such as deep breathing.

Arrive Early

Depending on exam site and type of test, you may be required to arrive at least 30 minutes before the scheduled start time. Check with the website and follow the instructions. Failure to follow instructions may result in cancelation of your appointment and loss of your exam fee. Table 1.3 provides a list of key things do on the day of the exam.

The High-Stakes Test Environment

The certification exam is a secure, computer-based test, given in a comfortable, properly lit, temperature-controlled environment. The PTCE exam is given at a Pearson VUE Testing Center. A list of test sites is available at http://www.paradigmcollege.net/certexamreview3e/PTCE/Pearson_test_centers.

At the exam site, you will be provided with an erasable board to serve as a scratch pad. A calculator will be available on the exam computer. Practice with and become proficient using your computer's calculator so this does not slow you down during the exam.

You are not allowed to ask the exam site staff questions concerning the test content. There are no scheduled breaks. If you must leave the testing area to use the restroom you will not be given additional time to complete the test. You must present identification to re-enter the test area. Cell phones, calculators, recording devices, and photography equipment are not allowed in the test area.

You will be given time to view a tutorial before the exam. You may download the tutorial in advance from the Pearson VUE website (www.paradigmcollege.net/cert examreview3e/Pearson_tutorial). This may help to reduce test anxiety.

Tips for Taking Multiple-Choice Tests

One of the advantages of taking a multiple-choice test is that the correct answer is provided in the list of possible answers. If you are unsure of the correct answer, following some standard test-taking tips will help you choose a response. There is no penalty for guessing. Answer every question if time allows.

- Plan your time. You will have 1 hour and 50 minutes to answer 90 multiple-choice questions. Do not get stuck on one question. Allow enough time to finish the exam. If you are not sure of the answer in 30 to 60 seconds, move on and return to the question later.
- Read the whole item. Make sure you understand what the question is asking. Take the question at face value. Do not waste time looking for trick questions.
- Answer the question in your head before reviewing the choices. This will prevent you from being influenced by the answers provided.
- Remember there is only one correct answer listed, although more than one answer may appear to be correct. When writing multiple-choice questions, one correct answer and three distractors are assigned. The distractors are usually terms you know. By studying the information you will understand their significance.

- In calculation questions, the distractors may use the correct numbers in incorrect ways and include answers you might get if you are not sure how to do the calculation or make a mistake moving a decimal point.
- Anticipating the answer or solving the problem before you look at the choices provided helps eliminate distractors.
- If you do not know the answer, use a process of elimination. Eliminate the most obviously wrong answer first, then the second, and make your best decision from the remaining two choices. This tactic gives you a 50 percent chance of selecting the correct answer.
- Do not look for patterns in the answers. Computerized tests are written without concern for answer placement.
- If you are still unsure of the correct answer, select the longer or more descriptive answer of the remaining choices, although a good test writer will make all of the answers approximately the same length.
- If the answer set presents a range of numbers and you are not sure of the correct answer, eliminate the highest and lowest choices and select from the middle range of numbers.
- Slow down when you see negative words in a question. Be alert for words such as *not* or *except*. These questions ask you to identify the false statement instead of the true statement. Read the question carefully and make sure you understand what is asked.
- Questions and answers that contain absolutes, such as *always*, *never*, *must*, *all*, and *none*, severely limit the meaning of the item. Answer statements that contain absolutes are usually incorrect.
- Become familiar with the computerized testing process and take the online tutorial before beginning the exam. The tutorial is there to help you during the exam process.
- If you feel a question is ambiguous, misleading, or deficient in accuracy or content, fill out the comment section at the end of exam. This may help your grade if the question is found faulty.

Table 1.4 summarizes some key tips to consider while taking the certification exam.

TABLE 1.4 During the Exam
Listen, read, and follow directions carefully.
Make sure to follow the computer screen prompts.
Answer easy questions first and come back to the more difficult questions.
Never leave a question unanswered. There is no penalty for guessing.
Manage your time.
Change your answer only if you are certain you made a mistake. Your first answer is usually correct.
Do not leave the testing area unless you must.

After the Exam

After completing the exam you will receive your results immediately as *pass* or *fail*. Your numerical score will be sent to you or made available online at a later date. Each exam has its own scoring system. Questions for the PTCE are weighted based on level of difficulty. Go to the PTCB website for a description of the scoring process. You need at least 650 points to pass the exam.

Unsuccessful candidates may appeal their scores or a specific testing item by completing an appeal form and submitting a review fee. The review fee may be refunded if the appeal is successful.

Candidates are allowed to retake the PTCE after 60 days. Candidates can take the exam three times. Additional attempts may be allowed on a case-by-case basis pending a review appeal.

Candidates who pass the exam are certified as pharmacy technicians by the PTCB and may use the designation CPhT after their names. Certification is valid for two years. During that time the pharmacy technician must complete 20 hours of continuing education, including at least one hour on pharmacy law. Appropriate paperwork to document this requirement is located on the website for the specific recertification group.

Certification may be revoked if a technician is convicted of a felony or a crime involving moral turpitude (including illegal sale, distribution, or use of controlled substances or prescription drugs), or for making false statements in connection with certification or recertification. Refer to the exam website or the Board of Pharmacy in your state for more information.

Skills Quiz

Reflect on the information presented in this chapter and answer the following questions.

1. Who should take the PTCE?
   a. pharmacists
   b. physicians
   c. pharmacy technicians
   d. registered nurses

2. Licensure may require a(n)
   a. college degree.
   b. application.
   c. certification.
   d. all of the above

3. Certification provides
   a. autonomy.
   b. vocational identity.
   c. job security.
   d. career satisfaction.

4. Registration of pharmacy technicians allows a state Board of Pharmacy to identify
   a. the number of customers entering a pharmacy.
   b. the number of pharmacy technicians working in pharmacy.
   c. emergency contact information for individuals working in pharmacy.
   d. the pharmacist-to-technician ratio.

5. A certification exam for pharmacy technicians is offered by
   a. a governmental agency working for the National Boards of Pharmacy.
   b. nongovernmental agencies governed by professional pharmacy organizations.
   c. individual state Boards of Pharmacy.
   d. the National Institutes of Health in conjunction with Illinois Council of Health-System Pharmacists.

6. Studying for the certification exam should happen
   a. over time at a steady pace.
   b. by cramming the week before the exam.
   c. only if you do not work in a pharmacy.
   d. if you have previously failed the test.

7. Questions and answers that contain absolutes are
   a. always incorrect.
   b. never correct.
   c. may be incorrect.
   d. none of the above

8. When you are unsure of the answer to an exam question, you should
   a. skip the question entirely.
   b. narrow the choices and pick one.
   c. look for a pattern in the answers.
   d. pick the answer with the absolute.

9. Certification exams are given
   a. twice a year at your state Board of Pharmacy location.
   b. in paper format with a computerized answer sheet.
   c. online at home with a certified proctor.
   d. at a certified testing center via computer.

10. Revocation is the process of
    a. submitting an application to take a certification exam.
    b. continuing education to retain certification.
    c. withdrawing your certification due to moral turpitude.
    d. changing career fields to increase job satisfaction.

Thinking Beyond the Exam

1. Your state board of pharmacy is considering adopting rules and regulations concerning the certification, registration, or licensure of pharmacy technicians. You have decided to write a letter to the board explaining your support for one of these processes. Write a brief letter explaining the route you have chosen, and describe why it is the best process to protect the public and ensure pharmacy personnel are well qualified.
2. Why do pharmacy technicians have to take the exam in a secured testing environment? What is the purpose of this type of testing?
3. Why is the pharmacy technician certification exam considered a high-stakes test? (In your answer, consider that at a testing center, many different professions, including pharmacists, physicians, accountants, plumbers, IT professionals, and others, take various exams there. Think about their professional liability.)
4. Why is a chain store's technician exam not adequate to earn the designation CPhT?

Pretest

Complete the following pretest to assess your understanding of the concepts and skills critical to practicing as a safe and effective pharmacy technician. The answer key at the back of this textbook provides answers and chapter references to help you identify which chapters in this text require more thorough study to better prepare for the certification exam.

1. A prescription for a controlled substance must have the prescriber's
   a. DEA number.
   b. NPI number.
   c. state license number.
   d. home address.
2. Which is a sound-alike/look-alike drug pair?
   a. atenolol and acetaminophen
   b. clonidine and Catapres
   c. Celebrex and Celexa
   d. Xanax and Zyrtec
3. On a Friday night, an unknown patient brings in a prescription from an out-of-town physician for a controlled substance. The patient wants the brand name drug dispensed, not the generic drug. The patient has no insurance and is willing to pay cash. What should the pharmacy technician do?
   a. be cautious of a forgery
   b. fill the prescription
   c. call the prescriber
   d. give the prescription back to the patient
4. A secure cabinet for dispensing and tracking patient medication administration in the hospital is called
   a. eMAR.
   b. Pyxis.
   c. CPOE.
   d. ACD.
5. Which of the following is a Schedule II drug?
   a. simvastatin
   b. oxycodone
   c. amlodipine
   d. diazepam

6. A patient on Medicare may purchase a prescription drug plan to supplement her health insurance. This is referred to as
   a. Medicare Part A.
   b. Medicare Part B.
   c. Medicare Part C.
   d. Medicare Part D.

7. A physician can send a prescription to a pharmacy using
   a. eMAR.
   b. email.
   c. e-prescribing.
   d. express scripts.

8. How many capsules will be dispensed for an amoxicillin 500 mg prescription with a quantity of XXX?
   a. 15
   b. 21
   c. 30
   d. 300

9. Online adjudication is the process of
   a. verifying a DEA number.
   b. submitting prescriptions for payment.
   c. submitting a prescription to a pharmacy.
   d. verifying an order from a wholesaler.

10. An Augmentin pediatric suspension prescription has a sig of 1 tsp PO b.i.d. x 7 days. What volume bottle should be dispensed?
    a. 75 mL
    b. 100 mL
    c. 150 mL
    d. 200 mL

11. Which abbreviation is best used to describe the route of administration for ProAir HFA?
    a. PR
    b. AU
    c. PO
    d. SL

12. Which agent is an antiplatelet drug?
    a. Plavix
    b. Coumadin
    c. Pradaxa
    d. Lovenox

13. When a patient has more than one insurance plan to help cover the cost of medications, which insurer is always billed last?
    a. private insurance
    b. state Medicaid
    c. Medicare Part D
    c. health maintenance organization

14. E-prescriptions decrease the potential for
    a. forgeries.
    b. non-compliance.
    c. lawsuits.
    d. over payment.

15. The beyond-use date of a compounded nonsterile ointment without an aqueous phase can be up to
    a. 14 days.
    b. 30 days.
    c. 6 months.
    d. 1 year.

16. Maintenance records of equipment used for compounding should be kept to document
    a. quality control.
    b. appropriate use and storage.
    c. manufacturing requirements.
    d. personnel skills.

17. Pharmacy technicians in a community pharmacy will be in charge of sales and ordering of
    a. EOBs.
    b. DME.
    c. PBM.
    d. COBs.

18. A patient presents a new prescription for azithromycin and asks to pick it up later in the day. After you prepare the prescription, where should the medication be stored?
    a. in the refrigerator
    b. on the pick-up shelf
    c. in the freezer
    d. on the pharmacy counter

19. What should you do if a patient calls and requests a refill on a prescription for Singulair that is out of refills?
    a. ignore the request
    b. add a refill
    c. fax the doctor
    d. rewrite the prescription for another year
20. Verifying insurance information when a patient drops off a new prescription eliminates
    a. customer wait time.
    b. needlessly transmitting the prescription to expired insurance.
    c. customer co-insurance.
    d. needlessly filling a prescription.
21. When entering a prescription and transmitting to the PBM, the technician should not
    a. enter the drug name.
    b. override drug interactions.
    c. forget to counsel the patient.
    d. be involved with new prescriptions.
22. Lower-cost generics help patients with Medicare Part D
    a. pay more out of pocket.
    b. pay less for insurance.
    c. coordinate benefits.
    d. pay less out of pocket.
23. Excessive inventory in the community pharmacy compromises
    a. profit levels.
    b. patient safety.
    c. medication storage.
    d. work space.
24. Of all the steps necessary to prepare a prescription, which one is the technician allowed to perform?
    a. override warnings
    b. final check another technician
    c. call the prescriber to change the dose
    d. label the prescription vial
25. What information is required on a prescription label?
    a. prescriber's address
    b. patient's address
    c. prescription serial number
    d. provider DEA number
26. What type of spatula should be used to transfer iodine salts?
    a. glass
    b. plastic
    c. stainless steel
    d. hard rubber
27. Coordination of benefits (COB) involves
    a. billing more than one insurance plan.
    b. reviewing a patient's medication list.
    c. talking to providers about lower cost generics.
    d. providing hospitalized patients medication.
28. Which is an error-prone abbreviation the ISMP recommends not be used?
    a. gr
    b. BID
    c. mL
    d. stat
29. The barcode on a pharmaceutical is encrypted with which piece of information?
    a. NDC
    b. NABP
    c. chemical name
    d. MSD
30. Approval for participation in an investigational drug trial at a hospital is granted by the
    a. P&T committee.
    b. IRB.
    c. ANDA.
    d. DEA.
31. When reconstituting a sterile vial of cefazolin, it should be
    a. prepared in the pharmacy.
    b. prepared in a LAFW.
    c. placed in an LVP.
    d. administered only through a central line.

32. TPN is used in a hospital to _____ a critically ill patient.
a. nourish
b. hydrate
c. revive
d. treat

33. A patient has knee replacement surgery. He was pretreated with cefazolin but developed a *Staphylococcus* infection in the replaced joint during his recovery in the hospital. This is called a
a. community-acquired infection.
b. hospital error infection.
c. nosocomial infection.
d. nonsterile surgery infection.

34. Healthcare workers should protect themselves from contracting infections from the patients by following
a. hand hygiene.
b. aseptic technique.
c. standards of practice.
d. universal precautions.

35. The Infection Control Committee in a hospital will review the pharmacy's sterile compounding area for
a. proper employee training.
b. cleanliness of environment.
c. security of controlled substances.
d. licensure of pharmacists.

36. In a hospital, medication is dispensed to the
a. patient.
b. physician.
c. nurse.
d. guardian.

37. Medication orders are typically seen in a(n) __________ pharmacy.
a. chain
b. retail
c. institutional
d. mail-order

38. How much medication will be dispensed for a hospitalized patient during a typical cart fill?
a. 1 day supply
b. 30 days' supply
c. 90 days' supply
d. one dose

39. A technician receives a medication order for Protonix, a nonformulary proton pump inhibitor. There is an automatic directive that permits dispensing of a similar product. Which medication might be dispensed?
a. Prilosec
b. Crestor
c. Seroquel
d. Cymbalta

40. Who is responsible for safeguarding the public through review and approval of all prescription and OTC drug products?
a. CDC
b. DHSEA
c. FDA
d. DEA

41. The National Drug Code is used to identify the manufacturer, drug, and
a. package size.
b. schedule.
c. expiration date.
d. barcode.

42. Which medication is considered high risk and must be dispensed with a medication guide?
a. Toprol XL
b. Valtrex
c. Lidoderm
d. Coumadin

43. A prescription is required for Plan B, Next Choice, and Plan B One-Step for patients in what age group?
a. 18 years and older
b. 21 years and older
c. 16 years and younger
d. 18 years and younger

44. When an order is placed by a prescriber into the computer at a hospital, this is referred to as
    a. eMAR.
    b. EHR.
    c. adjudication.
    d. CPOE.

45. Minimum standards for compounding sterile products are found in
    a. the policy and procedure manual.
    b. USP Chapter <797>.
    c. USP Chapter <795>.
    d. the FDA *Orange Book.*

46. The technician dons a gown and washes hands in what part of the sterile compounding pharmacy?
    a. ante area
    b. buffer area
    c. sterile DCA
    d. LAFW

47. Which reconstituted antibiotic must be refrigerated for storage after it is mixed?
    a. azithromycin
    b. clarithromycin
    c. cefdinir
    d. cephalexin

48. How many days after opening a Lantus insulin vial should it be discarded because of loss of potency?
    a. 14 days
    b. 28 days
    c. 30 days
    d. 90 days

49. The stock bottle of amlodipine 10 mg expires in August 2017. When is the last day a 30 days' supply could be dispensed for a patient in the community pharmacy?
    a. August 31, 2017
    b. June 30, 2017
    c. July 31, 2017
    d. May 31, 2017

50. Each month, a patient needs more and more of the hydrocodone and acetaminophen tablets to control his pain. This is an example of
    a. drug seeking.
    b. addiction.
    c. tolerance.
    d. dependence.

51. Computerization of patient health records in a hospital or practitioner's office is called
    a. EHR.
    b. barcoding.
    c. e-prescribing.
    d. CPOE.

52. In the number system for scheduled control substances, the lower the number the
    a. higher the risk of abuse.
    b. lower the risk of abuse.
    c. lower the need for special storage.
    d. higher the cost to the patient.

53. Which schedule of cough medicine may be dispensed without a prescription if state law allows?
    a. none
    b. C-III
    c. C-IV
    d. C-V

54. Traditionally, Schedule II narcotics could only be ordered with a special DEA 222 form, but now they can be ordered electronically via which system?
    a. online adjudication
    b. CSOS
    c. MedWatch
    d. VAERS

55. Federal law requires prescriptions for OxyContin be kept on file for
    a. 1 year.
    b. 2 years.
    c. 5 years.
    d. 7 years.

56. Filled prescriptions for C-III to C-V medications may be stored
    a. with other controlled substances in C-II.
    b. in a separate file from noncontrolled drugs.
    c. with all the other prescriptions.
    d. with other prescriptions as long as stamped with black "N."

57. Computerization in a pharmacy provides better management of data, cost savings, and
    a. errors.
    b. patient compliance.
    c. insurance payments.
    d. infections.

58. What document can a pharmacy technician refer to for information on the correct way to store compounding equipment?
    a. Material Safety Data Sheet
    b. employee handbook
    c. HIPAA notice
    d. policy and procedure manual

59. What agency regulates the registration and licensure of pharmacy technicians?
    a. National Board of Pharmacy
    b. Food and Drug Administration
    c. state boards of pharmacy
    d. Pharmacy Technician Certification Board

60. Errors caused by poor handwriting have been reduced through the use of
    a. barcoding.
    b. automatic dispensing machines.
    c. MTM.
    d. CPOE.

61. What is the term for passing the voluntary survey by the Joint Commission?
    a. registration
    b. licensure
    c. accreditation
    d. certification

62. A patient has prescription insurance coverage that pays 80%, and the patient pays the remaining 20%. This is an example of
    a. a deductible.
    b. a copayment.
    c. a tiered copayment.
    d. coinsurance.

63. The patient has the option of receiving the brand name drug Cozaar or its generic equivalent, losartan. If Cozaar is a nonpreferred brand name, the patient will pay the _____ amount in a tiered program.
    a. lowest
    b. average
    c. highest
    d. entire

64. A PBM is a company that works for the
    a. pharmacy.
    b. insurance company.
    c. physician.
    d. patient.

65. What technology advancement helps ensure the 5 Rs are followed in medication administration?
    a. automatic dispensing machines
    b. computers
    c. barcoding
    d. e-scripting

66. What is the most important thing a technician can do to prevent medication errors?
    a. assume nothing
    b. wash hands
    c. go with your first impulse
    d. assume physicians are never wrong

67. The primary reason to report a medication error is
    a. to punish the person making the error.
    b. to assess the system for problems.
    c. to facilitate legal action by the patient.
    d. to lose accreditation by the state board of pharmacy.

68. What non-profit agency is responsible for assembling a list of abbreviations that should *not* be used in health care?
 a. ASHP
 b. ISMP
 c. MERP
 d. FDA

69. Spills of hazardous chemicals in the pharmacy should be
 a. cleaned when done compounding.
 b. cleaned immediately with a spill kit.
 c. cleaned by housekeeping at the end of the day.
 d. reported to the state EPA.

70. Who must respond to all drug recalls?
 a. prescribers
 b. patients
 c. pharmacies
 d. manufacturers

71. A patient has a prescription for fluoxetine 1 mg PO daily. The liquid formulation on hand is fluoxetine 20 mg/5 mL. What would the dosage volume be?
 a. 1 mL
 b. 0.25 mL
 c. 4 mL
 d. 2.5 mL

72. A patient receives 5% dextrose infusion solution at a rate of 100 mL/hr. How many grams of dextrose will the patient receive in 8 hours?
 a. 5 grams
 b. 120 grams
 c. 40 grams
 d. 100 grams

73. Atropine is a 4:10,000 dilution. How many milligrams is in 1 mL?
 a. 0.00004 mg
 b. 0.004 mg
 c. 0.4 mg
 d. 4 mg

74. To make 1 L of a 0.225% NaCl solution using SWFI and a normal saline intravenous solution, how many milliliters of normal saline will be used?
 a. 250 mL
 b. 333 mL
 c. 667 mL
 d. 750 mL

75. Procrit 3,000 units subcutaneous is ordered and all that is on hand is Procrit 4,000 units/mL. How much will be administered?
 a. 0.075 mL
 b. 0.75 mL
 c. 0.85 mL
 d. 1.3 mL

76. The nurse will use a 60 gtt/mL set to run a pediatric patient's D_5W at a rate of 25 mL/hr. What drip rate will she use?
 a. 1500 gtt/min
 b. 250 gtt/min
 c. 25 gtt/min
 d. 15 gtt/min

77. What is the total markup on 12 boxes of facial tissue if the pharmacy purchases them for $32 and sells each box for $3.25?
 a. $28.75
 b. $39
 c. $6.96
 d. $21.79

78. In the CQI process, after you implement a plan, you must
 a. conduct a team analysis.
 b. measure effectiveness.
 c. discuss alternatives.
 d. discuss how to reduce variations.

79. A prescription for methotrexate 2.5 mg tablets has the sig: 3 tablets weekly. How many tablets will you dispense for a month supply?
 a. 12 tablets
 b. 30 tablets
 c. 90 tablets
 d. 36 tablets

80. What prescription drug should always be taken with food to prevent GI upset?
   a. morphine
   b. naproxen
   c. omeprazole
   d. penicillin

81. Which dietary supplement is used to treat nausea and motion sickness?
   a. garlic
   b. saw palmetto
   c. zinc
   d. ginger

82. Many prescription drugs have more than one use. Gabapentin was originally approved for use in epilepsy but now is commonly used for
   a. pain management.
   b. mood stabilizing.
   c. hypertension.
   d. migraine headaches.

83. Which pharmaceutical should include a patient warning about interaction with grapefruit juice?
   a. lisinopril
   b. simvastatin
   c. metoprolol
   d. furosemide

84. Angiotensin-converting enzyme (ACE) inhibitors are cousins to the angiotensin receptor blocking (ARB) agents. Which of the following is an ARB?
   a. losartan
   b. propranolol
   c. lisinopril
   d. clopidogrel

85. Nitrates can cause a dangerous drop in _____ if taken with Viagra or another erectile dysfunction drug.
   a. performance
   b. heart rate
   c. blood pressure
   d. temperature

86. Which antibiotic has to be dispensed with a medication guide because of the risk of tendon rupture?
   a. nitrofurantoin
   b. tetracycline
   c. Augmentin
   d. Levaquin

87. Alendronate is used to treat osteoporosis and must be taken
   a. on an empty stomach, first thing in the morning.
   b. after a high-fat meal in the evening.
   c. with a full glass of orange juice.
   d. with antacids to protect the stomach.

88. Which medication is used to treat diabetes in which the patient has no islet cell activity?
   a. metformin
   b. insulin
   c. Actos
   d. glipizide

89. Which of the following is a combination drug used to treat the bronchoconstriction and inflammation of asthma?
   a. ProAir HFA
   b. Serevent
   c. Flovent
   d. Advair Diskus

90. ______________ is an over-the-counter agent used to lower triglyceride levels.
   a. melatonin
   b. gemfibrozil
   c. omega-3 fatty acids
   d. ginkgo

Pharmacy Calculations

2

Learning Objectives

- Develop a consistent method for solving calculation problems.
- Apply dimensional analysis in solving pharmacy calculations.
- Calculate the amount of drug in a final product that has been diluted.
- Compute the amount of concentrate and diluents needed to make a desired concentration.
- Determine the amount of two products needed to prepare a desired concentration using allegation.
- Calculate oral and IV drug doses using proportions.
- Compute IV drop rates and flow rates using various drop sets.
- Calculate markup, markup rate, discount, discount rate, and days' supply.
- Determine reorder quantities based on min/max par levels.
- Calculate a medication dose based on body weight or surface area.
- Verify a practitioner's DEA number.

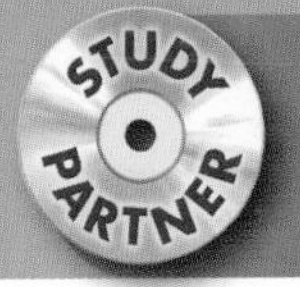

Continue your review with more than 1,000 exam-style questions.

Pharmacy calculations are a major component of any pharmacy technician certification exam. Although some students express apprehension about this part of the exam, with the right preparation and sufficient study, there is no cause for concern. The content covered in this chapter, the practice problems and study questions at the end of the chapter, and the practice exams on the Study Partner CD provide excellent preparation for the exam and for a career as a pharmacy technician.

Test-taking Tips for Calculation Questions

Although there are often numerous ways to approach a pharmacy calculation problem, developing a consistent approach to solving such problems will ensure consistent, correct solutions.

Before taking the practice test at the end of this chapter, in Appendix B, or on the Study Partner CD, study this chapter. It explains many of the math concepts on the exam.

The math portion is arguably the most important aspect of the certification exam. With practice, it can be mastered. Table 2.1 offers helpful tips for answering calculation questions.

TABLE 2.1 Tips for Calculation Questions

- Read the problem carefully. The difficulty with word problems is usually found in the words rather than in the math.
- Make certain you understand exactly what the question is asking.
- Be aware that some questions contain unnecessary information.
- Review the answer choices and eliminate those that do not make sense.
- Approach problems in a methodical way.
- Understand that there may be multiple ways to solve the problem. Choose one method and stick with it.
- Take time to write out the applicable units of measurement when setting up a problem and search for the correct answer in the appropriate units of measurement.
- Make certain the answer is in the correct unit(s) of measure. If the units do not correlate, rework the problem.
- Double check the placement of the decimal in the final answer.
- Do not panic. If you are stumped, take a moment to review. The approach will likely become clear.

Common Measures and Conversions

Before starting any pharmacy calculation, the technician must be familiar with basic units of measure and conversion values. In health care today most products are dosed in metric units, such as milligrams or milliliters. Knowing conversion values makes it possible to convert from household measures to the metric system. Memorize the common conversion values in Table 2.2 before taking the exam.

TABLE 2.2 Common Conversion Values

Volume	Weight
1 tsp = 5 mL	1 oz = 30 g
1 tbsp = 15 mL	1 lb = 454 g
1 fl oz = 30 mL	2.2 lb = 1 kg
1 cup = 240 mL	1000 mcg = 1 mg
1 pt = 480 mL	1000 mg = 1g
1 qt = 960 mL	1000 g = 1 kg
1 gal = 3840 mL	
1000 mL = 1 L	

Example 1

The prescription calls for 1 tsp of an antibiotic suspension three times per day for 10 days. Calculate the amount of antibiotic suspension needed to fill the prescription.

$$1 \text{ tsp} = 5 \text{ mL}$$

$$5 \text{ mL/dose} \times 3 \text{ doses/day} \times 10 \text{ days} = 150 \text{ mL}$$

Based on this calculation, the correct amount is 150 mL of antibiotic.

The calculation on the previous page uses dimensional analysis to solve the problem. The final answer is set up using a ratio in which the given dose units and the units in the denominator cancel out. These are the steps.

Calculate the volume given in 1 day.

The prescribed dose is 1 tsp = 5 mL and the patient will receive 3 doses per day:

$$x \text{ mL/3 doses} = 5 \text{ mL/1 dose}$$

$$x = 15 \text{ mL}$$

Calculate the volume for 10 days.

$$x \text{ mL/10 day} = 15 \text{ mL/1 day}$$

$$x = 150 \text{ mL}$$

Double check the question and be sure the calculation answers what the question asked.

Example 2

A physician writes a prescription for acamprosate 666 mg po t.i.d. The manufacturer makes only 333 mg tablets. How many tablets are needed for a month's supply? Follow these steps.

The unknown is the quantity of tablets for a 30-day supply.

The prescribed dose is 666 mg; the drug is available only as 333 mg.

The daily number of doses is 3.

Set up a ratio using dimensional analysis.

$$\frac{666 \text{ mg}}{1 \text{ dose}} \times \frac{1 \text{ tab}}{333 \text{ mg}} \times \frac{3 \text{ doses}}{1 \text{ day}} \times \frac{30 \text{ day}}{1 \text{ month}} = \frac{180 \text{ tab}}{\text{month}}$$

Re-read the question; does the calculation answer it?

Using dimensional analysis to solve even simple problems is a good way to become proficient with the process.

Concentrations and Dilutions

For medications in liquid dosage forms (e.g., oral solutions, oral suspensions, or parenteral solutions), the concentration or strength of the drug solution may be expressed in a variety of forms.

For example, an oral nutritional supplement that is diluted with an equal amount of water may simply be expressed as half-strength. However, most drug concentrations and dilutions are expressed in different types of mathematical notations, such as fractions, percentages, and ratios.

Fractions Representing Concentration

In general terms, drugs are solids and measured by weight. Liquids, on the other hand, are typically measured by volume, meaning the space they occupy. For example, at the grocery store a pound of sugar (a solid) is sold on the basis of weight, although it has volume as well. Milk (a liquid) is sold on the basis of volume, but anyone who has ever carried a gallon of milk for any distance knows that it also has weight.

When a drug is put into a solution, whether for oral use or a parenteral injection, the drug tends to lose its properties as a solid and becomes one with the liquid. However, it may be necessary to calculate how much of a given drug is contained in a liquid drug solution. For example, amoxicillin oral suspension, a common oral antibiotic in the penicillin family of drugs, is manufactured in different strengths. Two of these strengths are expressed as follows:

200 mg / 5 mL

400 mg / 5 mL

These two fractions represent two different milligram amounts of amoxicillin, both contained in 5 mL of oral drug solution.

When working with concentrations of drugs, keep in mind that if there is a larger or smaller quantity of medication than the amount stated in the concentration, the volume of the medication dispensed will be *proportionally* larger or smaller. By setting up a proportion and using dimensional analysis, problems of this type can be easily solved.

Example 3

Ordered: Amoxicillin 350 mg PO q12h
On hand: Amoxicillin 400 mg/5 mL

Begin by setting up a proportion. On the left side of the equation, write out the strength or concentration of the drug available. On the right side of the equation, write the amount to be dispensed (the amount ordered), with x or some other variable to reflect the quantity to be determined. It is important that the units of measure are the same in both numerators and in both denominators because a proportion is a mathematical comparison of similar things.

Set up the equation.

$$\text{strength on hand} = \text{amount to be dispensed}$$

$$\frac{400 \text{ mg}}{5 \text{ mL}} = \frac{350 \text{ mg}}{x \text{ mL}}$$

Note that both sides of the proportion are expressed in units of milligrams per milliliters.

Cross-multiply, leaving the units of measure alone for now.

$$400x = 350 \times 5$$

$$400x = 1750$$

Divide both sides of the equation by the number that precedes x.

$$\frac{400x}{400} = \frac{1750}{400}$$

$$x = 4.375$$

Attach a unit of measure to the numerical value and round the answer to the closest measureable amount: 4.375 mL of amoxicillin 400 mg/5 mL is dispensed as 4.4 mL of amoxicillin 400 mg/5 mL.

Does the final answer make sense? If the patient needs a dose of 350 mg of amoxicillin, and the pharmacy has 400 mg/5 mL in stock, the volume of antibiotic must be less than 5 mL.

Careful set-up is the key to consistently solving problems that rely on the concept of equivalent fractions. Simply put, equivalent fractions are fractions that are two different expressions for the same amount. Going back to the problem just reviewed, it can be stated as:

$$400 \text{ mg} \div 5 \text{ mL} = 350 \text{ mg} \div 4.375 \text{ mL}$$

This equation solves the problem, and the two terms are equivalent fractions.

Example 4, an order for ceftriaxone, a parenteral antibiotic that is typically dispensed in hospital settings, requires an additional step, the conversion of different units to equivalent fractions.

Example 4

Ordered: Ceftriaxone 125 mg IM now
On hand: Ceftriaxone 1 g/2.5 mL

The ordered amount of ceftriaxone is in milligrams and the concentration on hand is reported in grams. To set up a valid proportion, the units of measure on both sides must match.

First, perform a unit conversion, either by changing the units of the drug concentration from 1 g/2.5 mL to 1000 mg/2.5 mL or changing the ordered amount from 125 mg to 0.125 g. In most circumstances, the ordered amount should be changed to the units reported in the on-hand entry because what is on hand is what is physically available to be dispensed.

Rewrite the problem.

Ordered: Ceftriaxone 0.125 g IM now
On hand: Ceftriaxone 1 g/2.5 mL

Now that the units of measure match, write a proportion.

$$\frac{1\ \text{g}}{2.5\ \text{mL}} = \frac{0.125\ \text{g}}{x\ \text{mL}}$$

Cross-multiply.

$$1x = 0.3125$$

Divide both sides of the equation by the number that precedes the variable x. Round to 0.3 mL for measuring purposes.

$$\frac{1x}{1} = \frac{0.3125}{1}$$

$$x = 0.3125\ \text{mL}$$

$$x = 0.3$$

After determining the numerical value for x, go back to the proportion and look for the unit of measure associated with x (milliliters). The correct answer is 0.3 mL of ceftriaxone 1 g/2.5 mL is needed to prepare a dose of 125 mg of IM ceftriaxone.

Weight-Volume Percent as an Expression of Concentration

Sometimes the strength or concentration of a solution is expressed as a weight-volume percent. This is a shorthand way of expressing the concentration of a solution. For example, the intravenous fluid D_5W is a shorthand notation for a solution of 5% dextrose in water. Essentially, it describes a solution in which a sugar (dextrose) is dissolved in water. Beyond that, it also says something about the strength of the solution. Without knowing more, it is easy to believe that a given volume of a 10% dextrose solution would contain twice as much dextrose as a 5% dextrose solution.

When dealing with weight-volume percent problems, it is important to understand exactly what this notation means. In general terms, weight-volume percent is defined as

$$\frac{\text{grams of dissolved solute or solid}}{\text{100 mL solution}}$$

Keep in mind that this is a weight-volume percent, and the word *percent* literally means *per hundred*. Therefore, a D_5W solution can be expressed mathematically as

$$\frac{\text{5 g dextrose}}{\text{100 mL solution}}$$

A $D_{10}W$ solution, which contains twice as much dextrose, is expressed mathematically as

$$\frac{\text{10 g dextrose}}{\text{100 mL solution}}$$

Use this expression to solve the following problem.

Example 5

How many milligrams of dextrose are in 75 mL of D_5W?

Express D_5W as a fraction.

$$\frac{5 \text{ g dextrose}}{100 \text{ mL solution}}$$

Set up a proportion. Note that the question asks how many milligrams of dextrose are in 75 mL, not how many grams. Although there are various approaches to solving this problem, it is best to use one method consistently. Determine the amount of dextrose in grams, and then convert that amount to milligrams in the final answer.

$$\frac{5 \text{ g dextrose}}{100 \text{ mL solution}} = \frac{x \text{ g dextrose}}{75 \text{ mL solution}}$$

Cross-multiply.

$$100x = 5 \times 75$$

$$100x = 375$$

Divide both sides of the equation by 100, the number that precedes the unknown x.

$$\frac{100x}{100} = \frac{375}{100}$$

$$x = 3.75$$

Attach a unit of measure to the numerical value. According to the original proportion, this is 3.75 g of dextrose. This is not the final answer, however. The question asked how many *milligrams*, not how many *grams*. An intermediate value such as this may show up on the exam as one of four distractor choices. Be careful not to jump at an attractive wrong answer. For the correct answer, convert 3.75 g into milligrams.

$$3.75 \text{ g} = 3750 \text{ mg}$$

There are 3750 mg of dextrose in 75 mL of D_5W.

Ratio as an Expression of Concentration

The certification exam also requires calculating concentrations other than weight-volume percent. Sometimes a concentration of a solid dissolved in a liquid solution will be expressed as a ratio. The approach is the same. Review the example on the next page for epinephrine (adrenaline), which is used to treat serious cases of allergy and asthma. It is also found on hospital crash carts for use in cardiac arrest.

Example 6

How many milligrams of epinephrine are contained in 0.5 mL of a 1:1000 solution?

Express this 1:1000 dilution in mathematical form. A 1:1000 solution is similar to a weight-volume percent. However, instead of the number of grams of solute (solid) in 100 mL of solution, it is *per 1000 mL* of solution. Similarly, a 1:250 dilution expresses the number of grams of solute in 250 mL of solution. Therefore, a 1:1000 epinephrine dilution is expressed as

$$\frac{1 \text{ g epinephrine}}{1000 \text{ mL solution}}$$

Now that the ratio has been rewritten as a fraction, set up a proportion to solve the problem. Note that the question asked for the answer in milligrams. Be sure to convert the value in grams to the equivalent value in milligrams.

$$\frac{1 \text{ g epinephrine}}{1000 \text{ mL solution}} = \frac{x \text{ g epinephrine}}{0.5 \text{ mL solution}}$$

Cross-multiply.

$$1000x = 1 \times 0.5$$

$$1000x = 0.5$$

Solve for the unknown variable by dividing both sides of the equation by 1000, the number that precedes x.

$$\frac{1000x}{1000} = \frac{0.5}{1000}$$

$$x = 0.0005$$

Attach a unit of measure to the numerical answer. Looking back at the proportion, the unit of measure attached to x is grams. Convert 0.0005 g to its equivalent in milligrams, or 0.5 mg. There is 0.5 mg of epinephrine in 0.5 mL of a 1:1000 solution of epinephrine.

An EpiPen, used to treat anaphylactic reaction to a bee sting or food allergy, uses this concentration of epinephrine.

Dilutions

A pharmacy technician is often required to take a stock solution of a liquid and dilute it to a less concentrated solution. Questions of this sort are routinely included on a certification exam.

There is a simple formula for solving this type of problem.

$$\text{initial strength} \times \text{initial volume} = \text{final strength} \times \text{final volume}$$

or

$$\text{is} \times \text{iv} = \text{fs} \times \text{fv}$$

When solving a dilution problem, there are four variables, three from the problem statement and one to be determined. It is advisable to write down the basic formula (is × iv = fs × fv), and plug in the terms from the word problem. There are two important things to remember about a dilution:

- The final volume will always be larger than the initial volume because water (or some other solvent) has been added.
- Because this is a *dilution*, the final strength will always be less than the initial strength.

Remember that when solving word problems, understanding the words may be more difficult than the mathematical computation. Phrases such as "can be made from" will usually refer to an initial solution or a stock solution that is literally taken off the shelf. Also, it is important to use the same units of measure on both sides of the equation. If needed, perform any necessary conversions (e.g., liters to milliliters, ratio to decimals, etc.) before inserting numerical values into the equation.

Example 7

How many milliliters of 10% solution N-acetylcysteine can be made from 30 mL of 20% solution?

Begin by identifying the known values given in the problem statement and the value to be determined.

$$\text{initial strength (is)} = 20\% \text{ (or 0.2)}$$

$$\text{final strength (fs)} = 10\% \text{ (or 0.1)}$$

$$\text{initial volume (iv)} = 30 \text{ mL}$$

$$\text{final volume (fv)} = \text{to be determined}$$

After identifying the known values, enter them into the equation.

$$\text{is} \times \text{iv} = \text{fs} \times \text{fv}$$

$$0.2 \times 30 \text{ mL} = 0.1 = \text{fv}$$

$$6 \text{ mL} = 0.1 \times \text{fv}$$

Calculate the value for the final volume by dividing both sides by 0.1.

$$\frac{6\text{ mL}}{0.1} = \frac{0.1 \times \text{fv}}{0.1}$$

$$60\text{ mL} = \text{fv}$$

According to the calculation, 60 mL of 10% N-acetylcysteine solution can be made from the given volume of 20% solution.

N-acetylcysteine (Mucomyst) is an antidote for acetaminophen overdose. It has the characteristic smell of rotten eggs and must be given by mouth.

Example 8

What quantity of 20% KCl oral solution is needed to make 480 mL of a 10% solution?

Begin by identifying the known values given in the problem statement and the value to be determined.

initial strength (is) = 20% (or 0.2)
final strength (fs) = 10% (or 0.1)
initial volume (iv) = to be determined
final volume (fv) = 480 mL

Enter them into the equation.

$$\text{is} \times \text{iv} = \text{fs} \times \text{fv}$$

$$0.2 \times \text{iv} = 0.1 \times 480\text{ mL}$$

$$0.2 \times \text{iv} = 48\text{ mL}$$

Calculate the value of initial volume by dividing both sides by 0.2.

$$\frac{0.2 \times \text{iv}}{0.2} = \frac{48\text{ mL}}{0.2}$$

$$\text{iv} = 240\text{ mL}$$

It will take 240 mL of 20% KCl oral solution to make 480 mL of 10% solution.

In both examples, the volume increased from the initial solution to final solution, and the strength or concentration decreased. Always make sure the answer makes sense in this context. If it does not, re-examine the question and insert the correct values into the equation.

When working with dilution calculations, a pharmacy technician may also be asked to calculate the volume of diluent that will be needed. For these problems, remember the following equation.

$$\text{final volume} - \text{initial volume} = \text{diluent volume}$$

The following example uses the same formula as the two previous examples but requires one additional step.

Example 9

How much water should be added to 30 mL of dextrose 50% to dilute it to 10% dextrose?

Begin by identifying the known values given in the problem statement and the value to be determined.

initial strength (is) = 50% (or 0.5)
final strength (fs) = 10% (or 0.1)
initial volume (iv) = 30 mL
final volume (fv) = to be determined

Enter the known values into the equation.

$$\text{is} \times \text{iv} = \text{fs} \times \text{fv}$$

$$0.5 \times 30 \text{ mL} = 0.1 \times \text{fv}$$

$$15 \text{ mL} = 0.1 \times \text{fv}$$

Calculate the value for the initial volume by dividing both sides by 0.1.

$$\frac{15 \text{ mL}}{0.1} = \frac{0.1 \times \text{fv}}{0.1}$$

$$150 \text{ mL} = \text{fv}$$

The product, 150 mL, is not the final answer, but it would almost certainly be offered as a distractor on an exam. Reread the question. It did not ask how much 10% dextrose solution would be made, but how much diluent should be added to the initial 50% dextrose solution. The amount of diluent will be the difference between the final volume and the initial volume. Keep in mind that the final volume of 150 mL has two components to it: the initial fluid (30 mL) plus the volume of the diluent added to it to make the final volume of solution.

Calculating the correct answer requires an additional step.

$$\text{final volume} - \text{initial volume} = \text{diluent volume}$$

$$150 \text{ mL} - 30 \text{ mL} = 120 \text{ mL}$$

The final answer is 120 mL of diluent will be added to the initial solution.

Alligation

Alligation is a calculation method used to make a certain amount of a substance of a given concentration by combining a specific amount of a higher concentration with a specific amount of a lower concentration to formulate an intermediate strength. An alligation can be used for solutions, mixtures, creams, ointments, and other products.

The principles used to solve alligation problems remain the same regardless of the media combined (e.g., liquid, semisolid, or even solid). An alligation box, demonstrated in the following examples, is a useful tool to help visualize the process of combining two different stock concentrations to formulate a specific amount of a concentration that is not available in stock.

Example 10

How much 10% and 60% dextrose solutions should be mixed to prepare 1000 mL of 40% dextrose solution?

Before working through the steps to solve this type of problem, it is a good test-taking strategy to look at the answer choices provided. Frequently, one or two choices can be easily eliminated before the problem is solved. Occasionally, three of the four choices may be eliminated, and then working the problem confirms your choice.

In this example, look at the concentration of the final solution (40%). Is 40% closer to the lower concentration solution (10%) or the higher concentration solution (60%)? Because the 40% final solution is closer to the 60% initial solution, more of that will be used. Any answer choice that uses a greater amount of the 10% solution cannot be correct and can be eliminated.

To set up an alligation box, place the final concentration (40%) in the middle of the box. Place the higher concentration (60%) just outside of the box in the upper left corner. Place the lower concentration (10%) just outside the box in the lower left corner.

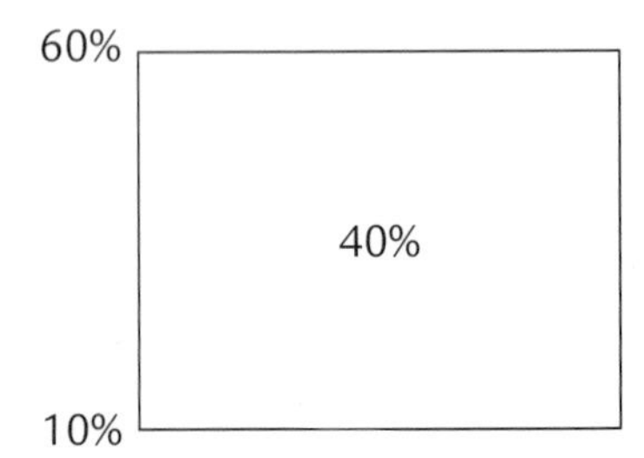

Next, draw a diagonal line from the upper left (higher concentration) through the box (final concentration), to the bottom right. Write the difference (60 − 40) outside the bottom right corner of the box.

Repeat the process for the lower concentration solution, subtracting the lower strength concentration (10%) from the final strength (40%). Write the difference outside the top right corner of the alligation box.

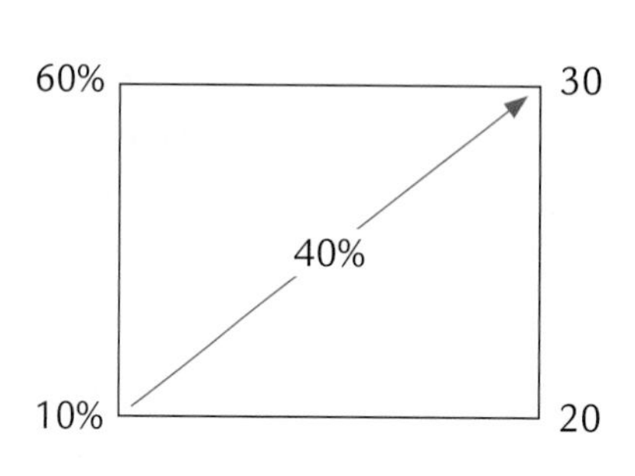

At this point, it is important to note:

- The 30 at the top right side of the box represents the relative contribution of the 60% solution to the final mixture.
- The 20 on the bottom right side of the box represents the relative contribution of the 10% solution to the final mixture.
- The relative contribution of the 60% solution is 30, whereas the relative contribution of the 10% solution is 20, which is less than 30.

Focus on the right side of the box. Imagine that the numbers 30 and 20 represent milliliters. Mixing 30 mL of the 60% solution with 20 mL of the 10% solution will produce a hypothetical 50 mL (30 mL + 20 mL) of the final 40% solution.

The basic definition of a fraction is a comparison of a part to the whole. The contribution of the 60% solution to the final mixture is represented this way.

$$\frac{\text{30 mL of 60\% solution}}{\text{50 mL of 40\% final solution}}$$

Once this relationship has been fixed, calculate the specific amount of 60% solution that is to be mixed with 10% solution to yield the desired amount of 40% final solution by using a proportion.

$$\frac{\text{30 mL of the 60\% solution}}{\text{50 mL of the 40 \% solution}} = \frac{x \text{ mL of the 60\% solution}}{\text{1000 mL of the 40\% final solution}}$$

Cross-multiply.

$$50x = 30 \times 1000$$

$$50x = 30{,}000$$

Divide both sides of the equation by 50.

$$\frac{50x}{50} = \frac{30{,}000}{50}$$

$$x = 600$$

Looking at the units in the proportion at the start of the problem shows that x equals 600 mL of 60% dextrose solution.

To complete the calculation, determine how much 10% dextrose solution needs to be mixed. Take the final amount of 1000 mL and subtract the amount that the 60% solution contributed to it.

$$\text{final volume} - \text{initial volume} = \text{diluent volume}$$

$$1000 \text{ mL total} - 600 \text{ mL of } 60\% \text{ solution} = 400 \text{ mL of } 10\% \text{ solution}$$

On the exam, eliminate any impossible answer choices. In this case, any answer in which the amount of 10% solution is equal to or greater than the amount of 60% solution used. Eliminating distractor answers is a helpful way to narrow the choices and improve the likelihood of correctly answering the question.

One additional warning about alligation questions on the exam: It is common to see an incorrect answer choice that switches the concentrations. For the example above, consider the following distractor choices:

a. 500 mL of 10% and 500 mL of 60%
b. 600 mL of 10% and 400 mL of 60%
c. 400 mL of 10% and 600 mL of 60%
d. 400 mL of 40% and 600 mL of 60%

By process of elimination, it is clear that answer *a* is incorrect because it does not use more of the 60% than the 10%. Answer *b* has the correct numbers applied to the wrong solutions. This is an attractive incorrect answer. Answer *d* uses 40% as part of the answer. The final concentration cannot be part of a correct answer choice because it does not even exist until it is mixed. Any answer choice that contains the final-strength solution or mixture is incorrect.

If this were an actual test question, you could have arrived at the correct answer merely by inspecting your answer choices after setting up the alligation box. Alligation problems take practice. Use the sample questions to sharpen your skills.

Oral and IV Dosages

Oral dosage calculations were discussed earlier in this chapter using liquid medication. Many oral medications are in solid dosage forms, such as pills, tablets, and capsules. The approach to solving these problems is the same.

A good way to approach dosage calculation problems is to develop a method that can be used in any circumstance. Earlier in this chapter, medications were discussed in terms of concentrations, typically expressed in milligrams per milliliters. But other expressions of concentration exist as well. The following examples calculate oral dosage using medication in solid dosage form. In the first example, calculate the dosage of lamotrigine, an anticonvulsant medication used in hospital and outpatient settings.

Example 11

Ordered: Lamotrigine 87.5 mg PO q12h
On hand: Lamotrigine 25 mg scored tablets

Think of the 25 mg lamotrigine tablets in terms of a concentration and state the solid dosage of the drug as a concentration (25 mg lamotrigine/1 tablet). Then use a proportion to solve the problem.

$$\frac{25 \text{ mg lamotrigine}}{1 \text{ tablet}} = \frac{87.5 \text{ mg lamotrigine}}{x \text{ tablets}}$$

Cross-multiply.

$$25x = 87.5 \times 1$$

$$25x = 87.5$$

Divide both sides of the equation by 25.

$$\frac{25x}{25} = \frac{87.5}{25}$$

$$x = 3.5$$

Express the numerical answer as a unit: 3.5 tablets equal an 87.5 mg dose.

Keep in mind that not all tablets are scored. Do not assume that a solid dosage form is scored. Scored tablets usually have a line down the middle with an equivalent amount of drug distributed on each side of the line.

Example 12 uses an oral liquid dosage of haloperidol liquid concentrate. Haloperidol is a potent antipsychotic medication used in acute care and psychiatric hospitals, nursing homes, and outpatient settings.

Example 12

Ordered: Haloperidol 10 mg PO t.i.d.
On hand: Haloperidol 2 mg/mL oral concentrate

Use a proportion to solve the problem. On the left side of the proportion enter the strength or concentration and the right side enter the amount to be dispensed.

$$\frac{\text{haloperidol 2 mg}}{1 \text{ mL}} = \frac{\text{haloperidol 10 mg}}{x \text{ mL}}$$

Cross-multiply.

$$2x = 10 \times 1$$

$$2x = 10$$

Divide both sides by 2.

$$\frac{2x}{2} = \frac{10}{2}$$

$$x = 5$$

Looking back at the proportion, 5 mL of the 2 mg/mL haloperidol oral concentrate is needed to provide the requested dose of 10 mg haloperidol.

The procedure for determining parenteral dosing is the same as for other dosage forms. Example 13 uses the drug Neulasta, a medication used to boost the white blood cell count of a patient who has become neutropenic (low white blood cell count) due to chemotherapy treatment for cancer.

Example 13

Ordered: Neulasta 6 mg SQ
On hand: Neulasta 10 mg/mL

As in previous examples, use a proportion to calculate the desired dosage to draw into the syringe. On the left side of the proportion, enter the strength or concentration of the drug, and on the right side, set up the desired amount to dispense.

$$\frac{10 \text{ mg}}{1 \text{ mL}} = \frac{6 \text{ mg}}{x \text{ mL}}$$

Cross-multiply.

$$10x = 6 \times 1$$

$$10x = 6$$

Divide both sides of the equation by 10.

$$\frac{10x}{10} = \frac{6}{10}$$

$$x = 0.6$$

According to the original proportion, it will take 0.6 mL of the 10 mg/mL solution to equal the requested dose of 6 mg.

IV Flow Rates

Many students find calculating intravenous flow rates daunting. That should not be the case if the problem is approached in a consistent, methodical fashion.

In simple terms, flow rate represents the amount of fluid that infuses into a patient over a given period of time. By knowing the flow rate and the amount of time that an infusion has to run, it is possible to calculate the exact amount of fluid that will be delivered. Example 14 illustrates the same concept in terms of everyday life.

Example 14

A car traveled at 50 miles per hour for 2½ hours. How far did the car travel?

To calculate the answer, use the method for calculating IV flow rates. Begin by writing 50 mph as a fraction.

$$\frac{50 \text{ miles}}{1 \text{ hr}}$$

Use the fraction to set up a proportion.

$$\frac{50 \text{ miles}}{1 \text{ hr}} = \frac{x \text{ miles}}{2.5 \text{ hr}}$$

Cross-multiply.

$$1x = 50 \times 2.5$$

$$x = 125$$

Based on the original proportion, translate the answer to the units, in this case, miles. The car traveled 125 miles in 2.5 hours.

Example 15 applies the same calculation method to a simple IV flow rate problem.

Example 15

A patient has an intravenous normal saline infusion running in at a rate of 125 mL/hr. How much fluid will the patient receive during an infusion that lasts 8 hours?

Use the same procedure as in Example 14.

$$\frac{125 \text{ mL}}{1 \text{ hr}} = \frac{x \text{ mL}}{8 \text{ hr}}$$

Cross-multiply.

$$1x = 125 \times 8$$

$$x = 1000$$

Based on the original proportion, the units are milliliters. The patient will receive 1000 mL or 1 L of fluid. On the exam, the answer may be written in milliliters or liters, requiring you to think about the conversion between units.

Now look at a method for actually determining the IV flow rate.

The rate of flow is defined as the volume of fluid over a period of time. The volume may be expressed in milliliters, liters, or drops. (Drops will be discussed later.) The time component of an IV flow rate may be expressed in terms of hours or minutes. When answering questions on the exam, pay close attention to the units of measure in the question.

Example 16

A patient receives 1.5 L of IV total parenteral nutrition over the course of 12 hours. What is the rate of flow in milliliters per hour?

To solve this problem, use a proportion. On the left side, enter the amount of fluid infused and the amount of time it took. On the right side, determine the rate of flow based on the number of milliliters delivered in 1 hour. The infusion rate is consistent throughout the 12 hours. However, instead of calculating the infusion for 12 hours, calculate the flow for 1 hour.

Make the units equivalent on both sides of the equation.

$$\frac{1.5\text{L}}{12\text{ hr}} = \frac{x\text{ mL}}{1\text{ hr}}$$

Convert 1.5 L to milliliters. (You should be able to do this step in your head.)

$$\frac{1500\text{ mL}}{12\text{ hrs}} = \frac{x\text{ mL}}{1\text{ hr}}$$

$$\frac{x\text{ mL}}{1.5\text{L}} = \frac{1000\text{ mL}}{1\text{L}}$$

$$x = 1500\text{ mL}$$

Cross-multiply.

$$12x = 1500 \times 1$$

$$12x = 1500$$

Divide both sides by 12.

$$\frac{12x}{12} = \frac{1500}{12}$$

$$x = 125$$

Translate the numeric answer into units, in this case, milliliters per hour. The rate of flow is 125 mL/hr.

As previously stated, flow rates may be expressed in terms of minutes instead of hours, as in Example 17.

Example 17

A patient receives 2640 mL of IV lactated Ringer's solution over 24 hours. What is the flow rate in milliliters per minute?

Many techniques and shortcuts are available to solve this problem. However, it is best to work step-by-step and use a consistent approach to avoid mistakes.

Calculate the flow rate in milliliters per hour. (Note that this is an intermediate step, and not the form of measure for the final answer.)

$$\frac{2640 \text{ mL}}{24 \text{ hr}} = \frac{x \text{ mL}}{1 \text{ hr}}$$

Cross-multiply.

$$24x = 2640 \times 1$$

$$24x = 2640$$

Divide both sides by 24.

$$\frac{24x}{24} = \frac{2640}{24}$$

$$x = 110$$

Identify the unit of measure from the right side of the proportion. The proportion indicates that the intermediate answer is 110 mL/hr. However, this is not the final answer. The problem asked for the flow rate in milliliters per minute. Calculate the final answer by converting 110 mL/hr to milliliters per minute.

Because there are 60 minutes in 1 hour, 110 mL/hr equals 110 mL/60 min. Use this information to do a simple conversion using a proportion to get the flow rate in milliliters per minute.

$$\frac{110 \text{ mL}}{60 \text{ min}} = \frac{x \text{ mL}}{1 \text{ min}}$$

Cross-multiply.

$$60x = 110 \times 1$$

$$60x = 110$$

Divide both sides by 60.

$$\frac{60x}{60} = \frac{110}{60}$$

$$x = 1.83333 \text{ (round to 1.83)}$$

Identify the unit of measure from right side of the proportion where x was first introduced. The final answer is 1.83 mL/min.

The next example calculates infusion time. The concepts are the same but the application used for these problems is slightly different.

Example 18

A 100-mL minibag of solution containing 20 mEq of KCl is piggybacked into a continuous D_5W solution and is infusing into a patient at a rate of 4 mL/min. How long will it take to complete the infusion?

Begin by setting up a proportion.

$$\frac{4 \text{ mL}}{1 \text{ min}} = \frac{100 \text{ mL}}{x \text{ min}}$$

Note that the proportion must be set up in minutes so the units of measure are the same on both sides.

Cross-multiply.

$$4x = 100 \times 1$$

$$4x = 100$$

Divide both sides by 4.

$$\frac{4x}{4} = \frac{100}{4}$$

$$x = 25$$

Identify the units from the right side of the proportion. It will take 25 min to run 100 mL of IV fluid. To calculate how many hours it would take to complete the infusion, convert 25 minutes into the equivalent time in hours.

$$\frac{60 \text{ min}}{1 \text{ hr}} = \frac{25 \text{ min}}{x \text{ hr}}$$

Cross-multiply.

$$60x = 25 \times 1$$

$$60x = 25$$

Divide both sides by 60.

$$\frac{60x}{60} = \frac{25}{60}$$

$$x = 0.4 \text{ hr}$$

The original proportion is based on hours, so the answer is 0.4 hours, which is equivalent to 25 minutes. Either 25 min or 0.4 hr would be correct. On the certification exam, be sure to provide your answer in the correct unit of measure.

A pharmacy technician may also be asked to calculate IV flow rates in drops. Each IV infusion set has a particular drop factor—a certain number of drops will equal 1 mL of volume. The most common drop factors are listed in Table 2.3. (The abbreviation gtt stands for *guttae*, which is *drops* in Latin.)

The larger the drop factor, the smaller the individual drops. A 10-drop set requires 10 gtt to add up to 1 mL of volume. A 60-drop set requires 60 gtt. The drops in a 60-drop set are frequently called *microdrops* because they are so small. Example 19 calculates an IV infusion rate in drops.

TABLE 2.3 Common Drop Factors

10 gtt = 1 mL
15 gtt = 1 mL
20 gtt = 1 mL
60 gtt = 1 mL

Example 19

A patient is to receive 200 mL of IV 20% fat emulsion over 10 hours, using a 15-drop infusion set. What should the flow rate be set to in drops per minute?

The approach to this problem is the same as in earlier problems. Once we get the flow rate in milliliters per minute, we do one more conversion to get the final answer. Begin by setting up the proportion.

$$\frac{200 \text{ mL}}{10 \text{ hr}} = \frac{x \text{ mL}}{1 \text{ hr}}$$

Cross-multiply.

$$10x = 200 \times 1$$

$$10x \times 200$$

Divide both sides by 10.

$$\frac{10x}{10} = \frac{200}{10}$$

$$x = 20$$

Based on the original proportion, the units are milliliters. The intermediate answer is 20 mL/hr.

Next, convert the flow rate from milliliters per hour to milliliters per minute by substituting 60 minutes for 1 hour, and setting up a new proportion.

$$\frac{20 \text{ mL}}{60 \text{ min}} = \frac{x \text{ mL}}{1 \text{ min}}$$

Cross-multiply.

$$60x = 20 \times 1$$

$$60x = 20$$

Divide both sides by 60.

$$\frac{60x}{60} = \frac{20}{60}$$

$$x = 0.33333 \text{ (round to 0.33)}$$

Based on the original proportion, the units are milliliters, and the converted intermediate answer is 0.33 mL/min. In the final step, apply the drop factor to convert the volume from milliliters to drops. Remember, the drop factor varies, depending on the infusion set in use. For this problem it is a 15-drop set. In a 15-drop set, the following relationship exists between drops and milliliters.

$$15 \text{ gtt} = 1 \text{ mL}$$

Take each side of this equation and divide by 1 mL.

$$\frac{15 \text{ gtt}}{1 \text{ mL}} = \frac{1 \text{ mL}}{1 \text{ mL}}$$

Keep in mind that any number (except zero) divided by itself equals 1. The equation now reads

$$\frac{15 \text{ gtt}}{1 \text{ mL}} = 1$$

The importance of this is that any number can be multiplied by 1, and the value does not change. In this instance, the expression for the number 1 will be 15 gtt/1 mL.

Take the flow rate in milliliters per minute and multiply it by the conversion factor.

$$\frac{15 \text{ gtt}}{1 \text{ mL}} \times \frac{0.33 \text{ mL}}{1 \text{ min}} = \frac{x \text{ gtt}}{\text{min}}$$

Canceling out the units of measure further simplifies the calculation.

$$\frac{0.33}{1 \text{ min}} \times \frac{15 \text{ gtt}}{1} = \frac{x \text{ gtt}}{\text{min}}$$

$$\frac{4.95 \text{ gtt}}{\text{min}} \text{ (round down to } \frac{4 \text{ gtt}}{\text{min}}\text{)}$$

When rounding a fractional portion of a drop, always round *down* to the last full drop, even if the fractional drop is more than one-half of a drop.

The conversion process is the same for all drop factors. Keep in mind that for the final conversion from milliliters per minute to drops per minute, the conversion factor will be the drop factor divided by 1 mL.

Because all of these expressions have a value of 1, any flow rate in milliliters per minute may be multiplied by the appropriate conversion factor and it will not change the value. It will, however, convert the units.

Business Math in the Pharmacy

The pharmacy not only serves healthcare needs but also functions as a business. The certification exam is likely to include some business-related math problems.

Markup

If a pharmacy or any business sold goods for the same price it paid suppliers, there would be no profit. In fact, after accounting for overhead, the business would be operating at a loss. That is why pharmacies mark up products above the purchase price. The markup is the difference between the selling price and the purchase price and is expressed in dollars and cents.

$$\text{selling price} - \text{purchase price} = \text{markup}$$

The following example calculates the markup for crutches.

Example 20

If a pharmacy purchased a set of crutches for $15.50 and sells them to the public for $25.00, what is the markup?

Translate the problem into an equation.

$$\text{selling price} - \text{purchase price} = \text{markup}$$

$$\$25.00 - \$15.50 = \$9.50$$

The markup is $9.50.

Markup Rate

Any retail operation, including a pharmacy, needs to know how much to mark up items to operate at a profit. This concept is called the markup rate and is expressed as a percentage.

$$\frac{\text{markup}}{\text{purchase price}} \times 100 = \text{markup rate}$$

When calculating markup, think like a business, not like a consumer. The purchase price reflects what the *pharmacy* paid, not the consumer price. Building on the previous example, Example 21 calculates the markup rate for crutches.

Example 21

If a pharmacy purchases a set of crutches for $15.50 and sells them to the public for $25.00, what is the markup rate?

Put the correct values into the appropriate formula.

$$\frac{\text{markup}}{\text{purchase price}} \times 100 = \text{markup rate}$$

$$\frac{\$9.50}{15.50} \times 100 = \text{markup rate}$$

$$0.61 \times 100 = 61\%$$

The markup rate is 61%.

Example 22

The pharmacy purchases melatonin 3 mg for $1.20 per bottle of 120 tablets and marks up the price by 30%. What is the selling price?

Take the pharmacy's purchase and calculate an additional 30%.

$$\frac{\text{purchase price} \times \text{markup rate}}{100} = \text{markup}$$

$$\frac{\$1.20 \times 30\%}{100} = \text{markup}$$

$$\$1.20 \times 0.3 = \$0.36$$

The markup is $0.36 per bottle. To calculate the selling price, add the markup to the purchase price.

$$\text{purchase price} + \text{markup} = \text{selling price}$$

$$\$1.20 + \$0.36 = \$1.56$$

The purchase price plus a 30% markup equals $1.56.

Discount

Like many other retail establishments, pharmacies offer discounts on certain items from time to time. Use the following equation to calculate a discount.

$$\begin{matrix}\text{usual} \\ \text{sales price}\end{matrix} - \begin{matrix}\text{discounted} \\ \text{sales price}\end{matrix} = \text{discount}$$

Much like markup, a discount is expressed in dollars and cents.

Example 23

A pharmacy usually sells loratidine 10 mg tablets #20 for $4.25. However, the sale price is $3.50. What is the discount?

$$\text{usual sales price} - \text{discounted sales price} = \text{discount}$$

$$\$4.25 - \$3.50 = \$0.75$$

The discount is $0.75.

Discount Rate

The discount rate is similar to a markup rate and refers to selling certain goods for less than the usual sales price. A discount rate also applies when a wholesaler sells products to a pharmacy below the usual price. The formula for calculating a discount price uses the discount rate, which is expressed as a percentage of the purchase price to be subtracted from the purchase price.

$$\begin{matrix}\text{usual}\\\text{purchase}\\\text{price}\end{matrix} - \left(\begin{matrix}\text{usual}\\\text{purchase}\\\text{price}\end{matrix} \times \begin{matrix}\text{discount}\\\text{rate}\end{matrix}\right) = \begin{matrix}\text{discount}\\\text{price}\end{matrix}$$

Example 24

A carton of hydrogen peroxide usually costs the pharmacy $30.00. However, if the invoice is paid within two weeks, the pharmacy receives a 15% discount. Calculate the discount price for a carton of hydrogen peroxide.

Insert the numbers from the problem statement to the formula.

$$\$30.00 - (\$30.00 \times 15\%) = \text{discount price}$$

$$\$30.00 - (\$30.00 \times 0.15) = \text{discount price}$$

$$\$30.00 - (\$4.50) = \text{discount price}$$

$$\$25.50 = \text{discount price}$$

Another way to look at this calculation is that the pharmacy is paying only 85% of the usual price. Multiply $30.00 by 85% to get the discount price.

Days' Supply

Pharmacy technicians may also be asked to calculate the days' supply of a medication for insurance and refills on a daily basis. Days' supply problems are likely to appear on the exam. To calculate days' supply, determine the amount of medication required per day and then multiply it by the number of days prescribed.

Example 25

The prescription is for baclofen, 10 mg Sig: 1 tab PO t.i.d. #90, 1 refill. Calculate the days' supply for the patient profile.

To solve this problem, collect certain information from the problem statement (the prescription): the number of tablets per dose; the number of doses prescribed per day; the number of tablets to be dispensed. Set up the calculation to determine the maximum number of tablets taken in a day.

$$\frac{1 \text{ tablet}}{1 \text{ dose}} \times \frac{3 \text{ doses}}{1 \text{ day}}$$

Cancel the units and multiply the numerator and then the denominator values.

$$\frac{1 \text{ tablet}}{1} \times \frac{3}{1 \text{ day}} = \frac{x \text{ tablet}}{\text{day}}$$

$$x = \frac{3 \text{ tablets}}{\text{day}}$$

Use this number to set up a proportion to calculate the days' supply.

$$\frac{3 \text{ tablets}}{1 \text{ day}} = \frac{90 \text{ tablets}}{x \text{ days}}$$

$$3x = 90 \times 1$$

$$3x = 90$$

$$x = \frac{90}{3}$$

$$x = 30$$

Based on the original proportion, the units are days. If the patient takes the maximum dose of three tablets per day, the days' supply would be 30 days.

The same process can be used for oral medication in liquid form. This is important in terms of choosing the most appropriate container and the amount to dispense, and for insurance information.

Example 26

The prescription is for azithromycin oral suspension, a macrolide antibiotic. The prescription reads: Azithromycin Oral Suspension 200 mg/5 mL, Sig 1 tsp po on day 1 then ½ tsp qam x 4 days. How much medication should be dispensed?

The medication is dispensed as 1 teaspoon per dose on the first day. This is equivalent to 5 mL. On days 2 to 5 the patient receives ½ teaspoon, or 2.5 mL. The duration of the therapy is 5 days.

Calculate the problems as follows:

$$\frac{5\ \text{mL}}{1\ \text{dose}} \times \frac{1\ \text{dose}}{1\ \text{day}} \times 1\ \text{day} = x$$

After canceling the units, solve for x in mL.

$$x = \frac{5\ \text{mL}}{1\ \text{day of therapy}}$$

Do not stop here though. Calculate the quantity for the 4 remaining days.

$$\frac{2.5\ \text{mL}}{1\ \text{dose}} \times \frac{1\ \text{dose}}{\text{day}} \times 4\ \text{days} = x$$

Again, cancel the units and solve for x in mL.

$$x = \frac{10\ \text{mL}}{4\ \text{days of therapy}}$$

According to the calculation, the prescription calls for 5 mL of azithromycin oral suspension 200 mg/5ml for the first day's dose and 10 mL for the following 4 days of therapy for a total of 15 mL of azithromycin oral suspension 200 mg/5 mL. This volume is equivalent to 0.5 fluid ounces.

The same concepts are used in Example 27 to determine how long a liquid medication will last.

Example 27

A patient presents the following prescription: cefaclor 250 mg/5 mL, Sig: ¾ tsp PO t.i.d. Disp: 80 mL. How long will this medication last?

First, determine how much medication (in milliliters) is to be taken each day. Calculate the amount in a single dose. Keep in mind that 1 tsp equals 5 mL.

$$\frac{3/4\ \text{tsp}}{1\ \text{dose}} \times \frac{5\ \text{mL}}{1\ \text{tsp}} =$$

$$\frac{3/4}{1\ \text{dose}} \times 5\ \text{mL} = \frac{3.75\ \text{mL}}{\text{dose}}$$

Calculate the volume needed for the prescribed number of doses per day.

$$\frac{3.75\ \text{mL}}{1\ \text{dose}} \times \frac{3\ \text{doses}}{1\ \text{day}} =$$

$$\frac{3.75\ \text{mL}}{1\ \text{dose}} \times \frac{3\ \text{doses}}{1\ \text{day}} = \frac{11.25\ \text{mL}}{\text{day}}$$

The patient will need 11.25 mL of the medication for each day.

Determine how long the dispensed volume (80 mL) of cefaclor will last using the daily amount to be taken.

$$80 \text{ mL} \times \frac{1 \text{ day}}{11.25 \text{ mL}} =$$

$$80 \text{ mL} \times \frac{1 \text{ day}}{11.25 \text{ mL}} = 7.11 \text{ days (rounded down to 7 days)}$$

Remember that multiplying by a fraction is equivalent to dividing by the inverse of the fraction.

Body Weight and Surface Area Dose Calculations

Particularly when dosing chemotherapy and pediatric patients, the dose for a specific patient may be calculated based on the patient's body weight or a combination of body weight and height.

Example 28

Sally S., a 5-year-old patient, has developed a seizure disorder. She is hospitalized and the doctor wants to start divalproex sodium delayed release tablets. Sally weighs 40 pounds. The doctor orders her first dose as "Depakote 15 mg/kg." Calculate the dose Sally should take.

In this example, Sally's weight is given in pounds, but the drug is dosed in milligrams per kilogram.

Calculate Sally's weight in kilograms.

$$\frac{x \text{ kg}}{40 \text{ lbs}} = \frac{1 \text{ kg}}{2.2 \text{ lbs}}$$

$$x \text{ kg} \times 2.2 \text{ lbs} = 1 \text{ kg} \times 40 \text{ lbs}$$

$$x = 18.18 \text{ kg}$$

Calculate the dose.

$$\frac{x \text{ mg}}{18.18 \text{ kg}} = \frac{15 \text{ mg}}{1 \text{ kg}}$$

$$1x = 15 \times 18.18$$

$$x = 272.7 \text{ mg}$$

Based on the physician's order, the correct dose is 272.7 mg. Depakote is available as 125 mg, 250 mg, and 500 mg tablets. The tablets cannot be crushed or broken. What dose is the closest to the physician-recommended dose? The pharmacist will discuss the options available with the doctor.

Body Surface Area

Body surface area (BSA) is a measurement based on a patient's height and weight. It is expressed as "m^2." A nomogram is used to calculate a patient's BSA. Many chemotherapy drugs used to treat cancers are dosed using BSA. On the exam, the patient's body surface area will be given in questions requiring BSA dose calculations.

Example 29

A chemotherapy admixture pharmacy technician in a busy oncology unit is asked to calculate the dose for a patient receiving chemotherapy. The patient is prescribed cyclophosphamide 400mg/m^2 on day 1 of chemotherapy. The patient's BSA is 1.85 m^2. What is the correct dose in milligrams?

Although the terminology may be different than for other calculations, by setting up the ratio equivalence and making sure the units are in the right location, the actual problem is easy to solve.

$$\frac{x \text{ mg}}{1.85 \text{ m}^2} = \frac{400 \text{ mg}}{1 \text{ m}^2}$$

$$x \text{ mg} \times 1 \text{ m}^2 = 400 \text{ mg } x \text{ } 1.85 \text{ m}^2$$

$$x = 740 \text{ mg}$$

Temperature Calculations

A pharmacy technician may be asked to monitor the refrigerator and freezer temperatures daily to ensure the pharmaceuticals are properly stored. Two different systems of measurement may be used: Fahrenheit or Celsius. The technician should be able to calculate the equivalent temperature using the following conversion formulas.

Celsius to Fahrenheit $°F = (9/5 \text{ x } °C) + 32$

Fahrenheit to Celsius $°C = 5/9\ (°F - 32)$

Example 30

NuvaRings must be kept refrigerated at a temperature between 36°F and 45°F before dispensing. Calculate the equivalent temperatures in degrees Celsius.

Calculate the Celsius equivalent of 36°F.

$$°C = 5/9\ (36 - 32)$$

$$°C = 2.2$$

Calculate the Celsius equivalent of 45°F

$$°C = 5/9\,(45 - 32)$$

$$°C = 7.2$$

The equivalent range in Celsius is 2.2° to 7.2°

DEA Number Checksum Formula

Although most pharmacies today have a computer system that verifies a physician's DEA number, it is possible to verify the number by hand using the following formula.

Step 1: Add the first, third, and fifth digits of the DEA number.

Step 2: Add the second, fourth, and sixth digits of the DEA number.

Step 3: Double the sum obtained in Step 2.

Step 4: Add the results of Steps 1 and 3. The last digit of the sum should match the last digit of the DEA number.

Example 31

Check the validity of Dr. Jones' DEA number: BJ2243551.

Step 1: $2 + 4 + 5 = 11$

Step 2: $2 + 3 + 5 = 10$

Step 3: $10 \times 2 = 20$

Step 4: $11 + 20 = 31$

The last digit of the sum in Step 4 matches the last digit of the DEA number. The number is valid.

Calculations only become easier with practice. Use the Skills Quiz, Thinking Beyond the Exam, and the Calculation Practice Exam to hone your skills.

Skills Quiz

Select the best answer from the choices provided.

1. A 3-year-old patient has otitis media. The doctor gives his mother a prescription for Augmentin oral suspension 200 mg/5 mL, Sig: ¾ tsp PO t.i.d. for 7 days. How many milligrams will the patient get per dose?
   a. 150 mg
   b. 200 mg
   c. 267 mg
   d. 450 mg

2. A patient is in the ICU with hyponatremia. The doctor orders 500 mL of 3% NaCl solution to be given over the next 8 hours. How many milligrams of NaCl will the patient receive at the end of the 8 hours?
   a. 15 mg
   b. 500 mg
   c. 1500 mg
   d. 15,000 mg

3. Epinephrine 1:10,000 is used during a pediatric code. How many milligrams of epinephrine are given in 10 mL?
   a. 0.001 mg
   b. 0.01 mg
   c. 0.1 mg
   d. 1 mg

4. You are asked to make a 5% zinc oxide ointment using 10% zinc oxide ointment and petrolatum. How many grams of each ingredient will you need to make 4 oz of 5% zinc oxide ointment?
   a. 50 g of 10% zinc oxide, 50 g of petrolatum
   b. 60 g of 10% zinc oxide, 60 g of petrolatum
   c. 120 g of 5% zinc oxide, 60 g of petrolatum
   d. 30 g of 10% zinc oxide, 90 g of petrolatum

5. A patient has a prescription for risperidone 0.75 mg PO b.i.d. How many risperidone 0.5 mg tablets are needed for a 30-day supply?
   a. 3 tablets
   b. 60 tablets
   c. 90 tablets
   d. 120 tablets

6. Dexamethasone oral solution is available as 0.5 mg/5 mL. A patient has to take 4 mg before chemotherapy. How many teaspoons of the medication will the patient ingest?
   a. 20 tsp
   b. 8 tsp
   c. 4 tsp
   d. 0.8 tsp

7. Cefazolin 1 g in 50 mL of D_5W is to be given over 20 minutes. What is the IV rate per hour?
   a. 2.5 mL/hr
   b. 50 mL/hr
   c. 125 mL/hr
   d. 150 mL/hr

8. Using a 60 gtt/mL microdrop set with a rate of 20 gtt/min, how many hours will it take to empty a 250 mL bag of D_50?
   a. 1.25 hr
   b. 12.5 hr
   c. 4.5 hr
   d. 250 hr

9. Your pharmacy buys bottles of Tylenol 325 mg for $3.66 per bottle of 100 tablets. What price would the pharmacy sell them for at a markup rate of 40%?
   a. $1.46
   b. $2.20
   c. $5.12
   d. $5.75

10. A Pro Air HFA Inhaler is ordered with Sig: 2 puffs q4h p.r.n. for shortness of breath. What is the minimum number of days a 200-dose inhaler will last?
    a. 17 days
    b. 25 days
    c. 33 days
    d. 50 days

Thinking Beyond the Exam

While working in the IV lab at a hospital, you notice that another staff member has made a serious error in calculating the dose of a chemotherapy IV drug. The concentration will be nearly 10 times weaker than prescribed. You see this staff member walking into the compounding lab with all the compounding supplies in hand. What steps would you take to prevent this error from occurring? What if this staff member is a pharmacy technician? A pharmacist?

Calculation Practice Exam

Complete the following practice exam to assess your understanding of concepts and skills critical to practicing as a safe and effective pharmacy technician. The answer key at the back of this textbook includes the answers and the calculations required to answer each question.

1. Patient A.J. was given 1 mL of fluphenazine decanoate 25 mg/mL two weeks ago. He is not due for his next dose for another two weeks. The physician wants to give an extra dose of 6.25 mg today and increase the monthly dose to 37.5 mg. How many milliliters should be administered today?
   a. 0.25 mL
   b. 1.5 mL
   c. 1 mL
   d. 0.5 mL

2. A patient is extremely agitated and the physician prescribes haloperidol 5 mg IM, lorazepam 2 mg IM, and diphenhydramine 50 mg IM. The haloperidol is available as 5 mg/mL, the lorazepam as 2 mg/mL, and the diphenhydramine as 25 mg/mL. The haloperidol and lorazepam may be mixed in the same syringe as long as the total volume is less than 3 mL. What is the volume for injection of the diphenhydramine?
   a. 1 mL
   b. 2 mL
   c. 3 mL
   d. 4 mL

3. A patient in the Emergency Department needs to be treated with a one-time dose of ceftriaxone 125 mg IM and azithromycin 2 g orally. The pharmacy stocks ceftriaxone 1 g vials that are to be diluted with lidocaine 1% 2.8 mL to a final concentration of 250 mg/mL. Azithromycin is stocked as 250 mg tablets. How many milliliters of the diluted solution of ceftriaxone should be administered, and how many tablets of azithromycin should be taken orally?
   a. 0.5 mL, 4 tablets
   b. 0.25 mL, 8 tablets
   c. 0.5 mL, 8 tablets
   d. 2 mL, 8 tablets

4. The pharmacy receives a prescription for guanfacine 0.5 mg po t.i.d. A month's supply is to be dispensed. Guanfacine is available only as 1 mg tablets. How many tablets should be dispensed?
   a. 90 tablets
   b. 60 tablets
   c. 45 tablets
   d. 30 tablets

5. A patient takes Vicodin 5/500 (hydrocodone/acetaminophen) 2 tablets at bedtime, Advil (ibuprofen) 200 mg b.i.d., and Tylenol (acetaminophen) 325 mg, 2 tablets at noon, for chronic pain. How many milligrams of acetaminophen will the patient take daily?
   a. 650 mg
   b. 1050 mg
   c. 1000 mg
   d. 1650 mg

6. An alcohol detox protocol commonly calls for the patient to receive thiamine 100 mg IM upon admission. The vial of thiamine is 200 mg/mL. How many doses are in one vial?
   a. 1
   b. 2
   c. 3
   d. 4

7. Levothyroxine tablets are available in 25 mcg, 50 mcg, 75 mcg, 88 mcg, 100 mcg, 125 mcg, 137 mcg, 150 mcg, 200 mcg, and 300 mcg. The physician wants the patient to take 62.5 mcg orally daily. Which strength should be used to fill the prescription, and how many should be dispensed for a 90-day supply?
   a. 25 mcg, 75 tablets
   b. 50 mcg, 135 tablets
   c. 125 mcg, 45 tablets
   d. 137 mcg, 45 tablets

8. Calculate the quantity of ingredients needed to make 24 jars of a compounded ointment. Each jar is 4 ounces. The recipe is
   Hydrocortisone 10%
   Menthol 0.5%
   Aquaphor qs ad

   How many grams of hydrocortisone powder will be needed to compound the 24 jars?
   a. 288 g
   b. 2880 g
   c. 9.6 g
   d. 12 g

9. How many grams of menthol crystals will be needed to make 24 jars of 4 ounces each if the strength of menthol is 0.5%?
   a. 0.144 g
   b. 0.014 g
   c. 0.6 g
   d. 14.4 g

10. A child is prescribed fluoxetine 20 mg/5 mL oral solution. The dose is 1.25 mL per day. How many milligrams of fluoxetine will the child receive daily?
    a. 1.25 mg
    b. 4 mg
    c. 5 mg
    d. 25 mg

11. Before a colonoscopy, the patient must drink 17 grams of Miralax (polyethylene glycol powder) in 8 ounces of water every 15 minutes for 4 hours as a bowel prep. What size bottle of Miralax should the patient purchase to complete the entire prep?
    a. 170 g
    b. 255 g
    c. 357 g
    d. 510 g

12. Lamotrigine (Lamictal) must be slowly titrated when starting therapy. The physician wants the patient to take 25 mg po qam × 14 days, 50 mg po qam × 14 days, then 25 mg po qam and 50 mg po qhs × 14 days. How many 25 mg tablets need to be dispensed to complete the first six weeks of therapy?
    a. 42 tablets
    b. 56 tablets
    c. 84 tablets
    d. 98 tablets

13. When repackaging bulk medications into unit dose packages, the beyond-use date must be calculated as one year from the date of repackaging if the manufacturer's expiration date is greater than 1 year for the date of packaging. If the manufacturer's expiration date is less that 1 year, then the new beyond-use date is only 50% of the time remaining. If the date you repackage is 7/15/2016 and the levofloxacin 500 mg tablets have a manufacturer's expiration date of 5/2020, what beyond-use date will be on the unit dose packaging?
    a. 1/1/2017
    b. 7/15/2017
    c. 5/31/2017
    d. 5/31/2020

14. State Medicaid law requires certain medications to be dispensed as a 90-day supply. A patient has a prescription for Xopenex (levalbuterol) Inhaler 2 puffs po QID. How may inhalers, each with 120 puffs, will be dispensed for a 3-month supply?
    a. 1
    b. 3
    c. 5
    d. 6

15. The dose of amoxicillin for a child is 50 mg/kg/day. How many milligrams should a 20-kg child receive per dose if the daily dose is divided into 8-hour intervals?
    a. 1000 mg
    b. 500 mg
    c. 333 mg
    d. 100 mg

16. The prescription is for cephalexin 250 mg/5 mL Take 1 tsp po QID × 14 days. How much should be dispensed to complete the 14-day therapy?
    a. 100 mL
    b. 150 mL
    c. 210 mL
    d. 300 mL

17. A diabetic is prescribed to check their blood sugar "AC breakfast, 2 hr PC lunch, AC dinner and at bedtime." Calculate the minimum number of 100-count containers of glucometer strips needed for a 3-month supply.
    a. 1 container
    b. 2 containers
    c. 3 containers
    d. 4 containers

18. Insulin is usually in a concentration of 100 units/mL. Mrs. Jones has a Lantus (insulin glargine) Solostar prescription, and she is going to inject 70 units Q HS. How many Lantus Solostar, pens will be needed for a 30-day supply? Each pen contains 3 mL of Lantus insulin.
    a. 1
    b. 5
    c. 7
    d. 10

19. Mr. Jones has insulin resistance and requires 125 units of U-100 regular insulin t.i.d. AC. The doctor decides to change to U-500 regular insulin. How many milliliters of U-500 insulin will be given per dose?
    a. 1.25 mL
    b. 1 mL
    c. 0.75 mL
    d. 0.25 mL

20. Calculate the number of warfarin 2.5 mg tablets to be dispensed for a 30-day supply if a patient takes warfarin 2.5 mg po daily × 2 days, then warfarin 3.75 mg po daily × 1 day, then repeats the cycle for a total of 30 days.
    a. 30 tablets
    b. 35 tablets
    c. 45 tablets
    d. 70 tablets

21. A 15 gtt/mL drop set will be used to administer 1 g of vancomycin in 250 mL of normal saline over 1 hour. How many drops per minute will the vancomycin administration rate?
    a. 37.5 gtt/min
    b. 62.5 gtt/min
    c. 375 gtt/min
    d. 625 gtt/min

22. A prescription arrives at the pharmacy for OxyContin 10 mg. The prescriber is not in the pharmacy computer and is unknown to you. A DEA number is on the prescription. Which number is the legal DEA number for a Dr. Janine Crosby?
    a. JC5497217
    b. AJ5497211
    c. BC5497210
    d. MC5497218

23. A prescription for a compounded topical acne treatment must be made using clindamycin capsules and alcohol. The final solution is to be 0.5% and the total volume is 30 mL. How many capsules of clindamycin 150 mg will be needed?
    a. 1
    b. 2
    c. 3
    d. 4

24. A patient has a $500 deductible on her prescription insurance plan; the plan then pays all but $10 of each prescription. The patient has already paid $493 of the deductible and has a new prescription to fill. The cost of the prescription is $29.65. How much is the patient required to pay?
    a. $7
    b. $10
    c. $12.65
    d. $17

25. A patient is on TPN and must receive a total of 3 L in a day. What is the infusion rate?
    a. 42 mL/hr
    b. 75 mL/hr
    c. 100 mL/hr
    d. 125 mL/hr

26. Azithromycin powder for oral solution contains 1200 mg. You will add 12.5 mL to the bottle for a final volume of 15 mL. What is the final concentration of the oral solution?
    a. 80 mg/mL
    b. 96 mg/mL
    c. 100 mg/mL
    d. 120 mg/mL

27. You are in charge of reordering for the pharmacy. The minimum level for amoxicillin is set at 300 capsules and the maximum level at 750 capsules. Today, five prescriptions are filled for amoxicillin in the following quantities: 30, 30, 60, 8, and 45. You started the day with 420 capsules. How many bottles of 100 capsules will you order?
    a. 0
    b. 1
    c. 3
    d. 5

28. The pharmacy filled 120 prescriptions today. Third-party payment was received on 97 of them and the rest were paid for in cash. What percentage of the filled prescriptions was covered by third-party payment?
    a. 97%
    b. 81%
    c. 67%
    d. 19%

29. An insurance plan calculates the pharmacy payment for a prescription as AWP – 5% plus a dispensing fee. A prescription for 30 tablets of lisinopril 10 mg is paid at $13.16. If the AWP for lisinopril 10 mg is $26.59 for 100 tablets, what is the dispensing fee paid to the pharmacy?
    a. $5.58
    b. $7.58
    c. $7.98
    d. $8.38

30. When a patient is on clozapine, regular WBC and ANC levels must be measured; if the lab test shows that the WBC dropped more than 2 points, the test should be repeated to double-check the value. At the last test, the patient had a WBC of 7.6 and ANC of 3.6. The patient's WBC level would need to be above_______ to avoid retesting.
    a. 1.6
    b. 3.6
    c. 5.6
    d. 7.6

31. To prevent cardiac toxicity, doxorubicin has a lifetime limit of 550 mg/m^2. A patient with a body surface area of 2.1 m^2 has already received 400 mg of doxorubicin. How many more milligrams may the patient receive before reaching the lifetime limit?
    a. 150 mg
    b. 550 mg
    c. 755 mg
    d. 1155 mg

32. Over the course of the last month, the pharmacy has sold 2700 doses of Suboxone 2 mg/0.5 mg films, the least amount of any month in the last year. Over the last 12 months, the largest quantity sold in any one month was 3500 doses. Calculate the minimum number needed to have on hand so that the pharmacy does not run out and it is the maximum to stock. (Suboxone is sold in boxes of 30 films.)
    a. 30 films minimum, 120 films maximum
    b. 120 films minimum, 150 films maximum
    c. 90 films minimum, 120 films maximum
    d. 30 films minimum, 90 films maximum

33. The pharmacy needs to make a very weak solution of sodium chloride for a patient. The concentration ordered is 0.225%. On hand, the pharmacy has NaCl 0.9%, NaCl 0.45%, and sterile water for injection. How much of the appropriate solutions will be needed to make a liter of the 0.225% NaCl solution?
    a. 500 mL of 0.9% NaCl and 500 mL of 0.45% NaCl
    b. 250 mL of 0.9% NaCl and 750 mL of 0.45% NaCl
    c. 500 mL of 0.45% NaCl and 500 mL of sterile water
    d. 225 mL of 0.9% NaCl and 775 mL of sterile water

34. The physician has a patient who needs a Magic Mouthwash combination of diphenhydramine elixir, lidocaine 2% viscous, and Mylanta in a ratio of 1:1:1. How much of each ingredient will be needed to make an 8-ounce bottle?
    a. 30 mL
    b. 40 mL
    c. 60 mL
    d. 80 mL

35. Dopamine for infusion is available in a concentration of 400 mg/500 mL. A patient weighing 50 k is started on an infusion at the rate of 5 mcg/kg/min and over time titrating by 5 mcg/kg/min the patient is receiving 20 mcg/kg/min. Calculate the infusion rate in mL/hr at the 20 mcg/kg/min dose.
    a. 60 mL/hr
    b. 75 mL/hr
    c. 100 mL/hr
    d. 750 mL/hr

36. A pediatric patient needs 1 mg of propranolol orally b.i.d. Because this is not available commercially, it will need to be compounded from propranolol tablets. The final concentration should be 1 mg/5 mL of simple syrup. The patient will need a 2-week supply before seeing the doctor again. How many 10-mg propranolol tablets will be needed to make the 150-mL of a 1 mg/5 mL solution?
    a. 2
    b. 3
    c. 4
    d. 5

37. A patient takes a total of 200 mL of fluoxetine oral solution in an overdose attempt. The physician wants to know how many total milligrams of fluoxetine the patient took. (Fluoxetine is manufactured in 20 mg/5 mL strengths.)
    a. 4000 mg
    b. 1000 mg
    c. 800 mg
    d. 50 mg

38. If you compound a lidocaine solution with 10 g of lidocaine powder, USP in 200 mL of sterile water, what is the final concentration of the solution?
    a. 1%
    b. 5%
    c. 10%
    d. 20%

39. You compound a 4-ounce jar of 10% hydrocortisone in Eucerin cream for a prescription. When you check the original prescription, it was written for 5% hydrocortisone in Eucerin cream. How much more Eucerin will need to be added to the original ointment to make it 5%?
    a. 50 g
    b. 60 g
    c. 120 g
    d. 240 g

40. To make a profit on over-the-counter analgesic products, the pharmacy owner wants them marked up 30% over the acquisition cost. If a case of 12 bottles of Ecotrin costs $71.52, how much should each bottle cost?
    a. $7.75
    b. $5.96
    c. $1.80
    d. $9.30

41. A pediatric heparin drip set (60 gtt/mL) is infusing at 15 gtt/min. What is the rate in mL/hr?
    a. 0.25 mL/hr
    b. 15 mL/hr
    c. 60 mL/hr
    d. 120 mL/hr

42. Each year patients are advised to receive an influenza vaccination. A vial of influenza vaccine has 5 mL and a dose is 0.5 mL. How many doses are available in 10 vials of flu vaccine?
    a. 5
    b. 10
    c. 50
    d. 100

43. A pharmacy charges $25 for a flu vaccination and pays $125 per 5 mL vial of vaccine. What is the monetary profit if the entire vial is used? (1 dose = 0.5 mL)
    a. $125
    b. $95
    c. $47.50
    d. $9.50

44. An infusion of 1 L of D_5W is started at 8 a.m. and a new liter bag needs to be started at noon when the first liter runs out. What is the rate of the D_5W infusion?
    a. 75 mL/hr
    b. 125 mL/hr
    c. 187.5 mL/hr
    d. 250 mL/hr

45. The pharmacy medication refrigerator is to be kept between 36°F and 45°F. Your thermometer is calibrated in Celsius and reads 5°C. What is the temperature in Fahrenheit?
    a. 34.8
    b. 39
    c. 41
    d. 56
46. If the maximum recommended dose of valproic acid and its derivatives (divalproex sodium) is 60 mg/kg/day, what would be the maximum daily dose for a 120-pound patient?
    a. 3250 mg
    b. 7250 mg
    c. 3500 mg
    d. 1000 mg
47. What is the ratio strength of a solution of atropine Sulfate 10 mg in 10 mL?
    a. 1:100
    b. 1:1000
    c. 2:1000
    d. 1:10,000
48. What is the final concentration of an erythromycin topical solution if 1 g of erythromycin powder is dissolved in 50 mL of solvent?
    a. 0.2%
    b. 0.5%
    c. 1%
    d. 2%
49. Predental work treatment with amoxicillin 2 g is ordered. The dentist wants the patient to have enough for three different dental appointments. If the prescription is filled with 250 mg capsules, how many capsules will be dispensed?
    a. 8 capsules
    b. 16 capsules
    c. 24 capsules
    d. 32 capsules
50. A Combivent inhaler has 200 metered doses per inhaler. The patient is to take two puffs po QID. How many days will one inhaler last?
    a. 50
    b. 30
    c. 25
    d. 20

Pharmacology for Technicians

3

Learning Objectives

- Identify the generic name, brand name, and indication for the most frequently prescribed drugs in community and hospital pharmacy practice.
- Know the side effects and adverse reactions for central nervous system, cardiovascular, anti-infective, endocrine, respiratory, gastrointestinal, and renal drugs.
- Identify common medications that require auxiliary labels and administration instructions.
- Recognize common medications that can cause severe allergic or withdrawal reactions.
- Name drugs that can interact with cholesterol-lowering drugs to cause muscle fatigue.
- Discuss unique patient counseling recommendations for bisphosphonates.
- Identify a serious, life-threatening drug interaction caused by erectile dysfunction drugs.
- Contrast the labeling requirements of over-the-counter drugs and dietary supplements.
- Define the pharmacy technician's role with regard to OTC drugs and dietary supplements.

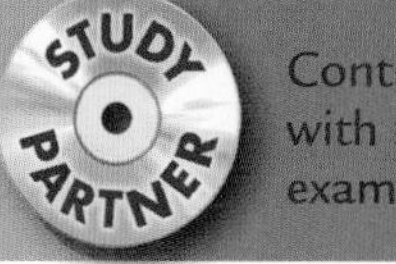

Continue your review with more than 1,000 exam-style questions.

There are many drugs on the market for many indications, but it is important to remember that lifestyle changes remain the cornerstone of good health. Lifestyle changes include maintaining a good weight with a healthy diet, getting sufficient daily exercise, refraining from smoking, using alcohol in moderation, following safe sexual practices, and always wearing a seat belt.

This chapter reviews and discusses the basic pharmacology of the most commonly dispensed drugs in the community and hospital pharmacy. The pharmacy technician should have a clear understanding of the generic and trade names of the most common medications, their primary indications, and common side effects. This knowledge is important to function effectively in the pharmacy. This information is also covered on the certification exam. Essential pharmacology information is necessary to better understand the use of auxiliary labels to enhance patient education and compliance with the prescribed medication.

Classification of Drugs

Pharmacology is defined as the scientific study of drugs and how they work (the mechanism of action) along with side effects, adverse reactions, and drug interactions. Pharmacists spend several years studying basic and applied pharmacology for thousands of drugs. Questions about how drugs work, dosages, side effects, adverse reactions, drug interactions, and drug use in pediatrics, geriatrics, during pregnancy, or with lactating women must always be directed to the pharmacist who has the necessary expertise and experience in these areas.

There are several ways to classify drugs. Facts and Comparisons® is a primary reference for drug classifications. It categorizes drugs based on an organ system and mechanism of action or chemical name. For example, metoprolol ER (Toprol XL) and lisinopril (Prinivil, Zestril) are both used to treat high blood pressure, but each drug lowers the blood pressure in different ways. That is, the mechanism of pharmacological action is different. Metoprolol is a beta adrenergic blocker that slows heart rate, whereas lisinopril is an angiotensin-converting enzyme inhibitor (ACE inhibitor), which causes a dilation of the blood vessels.

In the hospital setting, the American Hospital Formulary Service (AHFS) serves as a primary reference for drug information. Although there is some overlap with community pharmacies in terms of drugs dispensed, drugs used in hospital settings include injectable antibiotic and biotechnology drugs outlined later in the chapter.

Central Nervous System Agents

The central nervous system (CNS) consists of specialized nerve cells called neurons, which are located in the brain and spinal cord. Neurons within the CNS communicate with other neurons primarily through chemicals known as neurotransmitters. Prescribed drugs alter neurotransmitter activity at the neuron, producing both therapeutic effects and side effects.

Analgesic and Anti-inflammatory Agents

As seen in Table 3.1, there are multiple medications in the subcategory of analgesic and anti-inflammatory agents. Because narcotic analgesics are considered CNS depressants that can cause drowsiness, it is best to avoid using them with other CNS depressants, such as psychiatric medications, sleeping medications, or alcohol. Narcotic analgesics can cause stomach upset and constipation. It is recommended that these medications be taken with a snack, and if constipation occurs, a stool softener or short-term laxative may be recommended. Many oxycodone, hydrocodone, and codeine preparations also contain acetaminophen (or APAP), which is found in many prescription and over-the-counter (OTC) products. Large doses of acetaminophen (more than 3 grams per day) damage the liver, especially if combined with alcohol.

Forged prescriptions and addiction are more common with narcotic analgesics, especially OxyContin. No refills are permitted for Schedule II narcotics such as oxycodone or morphine. Prescription drug abuse is the number one drug problem in the United States, and hydrocodone combination drugs are far and away the number one prescribed drug. Suboxone is a combination drug that is primarily used to treat narcotic addiction. In the hospital setting, injections of morphine, meperidine (Demerol), and hydromorphone (Dilaudid) are commonly used for temporary relief of severe pain. For terminally ill hospice or cancer patients, around-the-clock narcotics, administered via subcutaneous infusion pumps, controlled-released solid dosage forms, or patches are commonly and appropriately used to provide comfort and pain relief.

Non-narcotic pain relief medications include acetaminophen (Tylenol) and lidocaine (Lidoderm). Acetaminophen is used in children and adults as a fever reducer and pain reliever that will not upset the stomach. It is contained in many OTC and prescription medications. Acetaminophen *must not* be used with alcohol. Lidocaine is available as a patch that is worn 12 hours on and then removed for 12 hours to relieve chronic pain. These non-narcotic pain relief medications may reduce the dose or frequency of the more addicting narcotic medications. Tramadol is another non-narcotic analgesic that is centrally acting. While not identified by the DEA as a controlled medication, it may cause some physical or psychological dependence.

The anti-inflammatory drugs listed in Table 3.1 are commonly called NSAIDs, or nonsteroidal anti-inflammatory drugs. If a patient is allergic to aspirin, an NSAID cannot be used. The anti-inflammatory agents can cause serious gastrointestinal (GI) bleeding if taken in large doses for an extended period of time, especially in the elderly. It is recommended that NSAIDs always be taken with food, milk, or a snack. Ibuprofen, naproxen, and aspirin are also available as OTC drugs. These drugs may negate the beneficial blood-thinning effects of aspirin when taken at the same time. Celebrex (celecoxib), a COX-2 selective inhibitor, is less likely to cause GI side effects and bleeding, but it is much more costly. If a patient is allergic to sulfa drugs, Celebrex is contraindicated.

TABLE 3.1 Analgesic and Anti-inflammatory Central Nervous System Agents

Generic Name	Trade Name	Classification
Pain Relief		
buprenorphine/naloxone	Suboxone	narcotic analgesic/antagonist
codeine	various generics	narcotic analgesic
fentanyl	Duragesic, Actiq	narcotic analgesic patch
hydrocodone/APAP	Lortab, Norco, Vicodin	narcotic analgesic
hydromorphone	Dilaudid	narcotic analgesic
lidocaine	Lidoderm	anesthetic analgesic
morphine	MS Contin, MSIR	narcotic analgesic
oxycodone	OxyContin	narcotic analgesic
oxycodone/APAP	Percocet, Endocet	narcotic analgesic
tramadol	Ultracet, Ultram	central analgesic
Anti-Inflammatory		
celecoxib	Celebrex	COX-2 inhibitor
ibuprofen	Motrin	NSAID
meloxicam	Mobic	NSAID
naproxen	Naprosyn	NSAID

Antianxiety and Hypnotic Agents

As seen in Table 3.2, many antianxiety and sleep medications are commonly dispensed in the community pharmacy. These drugs are also CNS depressants with the same limitations as the narcotic analgesics. The benzodiazepines, as well as zolpidem, are controlled drugs that generate some degree of physical or psychological dependence if used long term. Refills of Schedule III and IV drugs are limited to five times or six months, and prescriptions must also be monitored for forgeries, early refills, and abuse. Most of these medications are recommended for short-term or p.r.n. use. In practice, many are used on a long-term, routine basis for anxiety or insomnia. Benzodiazepines are also used to stop tonic-clonic seizures. They are administered by injection in the hospital or rectally at home.

TABLE 3.2 Antianxiety and Hypnotic Central Nervous System Agents

Generic Name	Trade Name	Classification
Anxiety		
alprazolam	Xanax	benzodiazepine
clonazepam	Klonopin	benzodiazepine
diazepam	Valium, Diastat	benzodiazepine
lorazepam	Ativan	benzodiazepine
Insomnia		
zolpidem	Ambien	hypnotic

Antidepressant Agents

It is interesting to note that among the most common CNS agents in use in the United States, 12 are used primarily for the treatment of depression. As shown in Table 3.3, these drugs work through different mechanisms (listed under classification). Antidepressants primarily act on neurotransmitters (brain chemicals) like serotonin, norepinephrine, and dopamine to achieve a therapeutic effect. Although all are used to treat depression, medication and dose must be individually tailored to each patient to achieve the correct therapeutic response. Antidepressants carry black box warnings because of the increased risk of suicidal thoughts and behavior in children, adolescents, and young adults. Amitriptyline is an older drug used for both depression and to enhance the effect of pain medications or to prevent migraine headaches. Amitriptyline can cause a dry "cotton" mouth and blurry vision. This drug, along with trazodone, can cause drowsiness and is sometimes prescribed as a sleep medication. Male patients taking trazodone should be warned about the risk of priapism, or a prolonged painful erection. Other drugs, such as fluoxetine, venlafaxine, and duloxetine, may cause insomnia if given at bedtime. Venlafaxine and duloxetine should be used cautiously in patients with high blood pressure.

First-generation antipsychotics, including chlorpromazine (Thorazine) and thioridazine (Mellaril), are rarely prescribed today because of a higher incidence of side effects. Aripiprazole, olanzapine, quetiapine, and risperidone are considered atypical antipsychotics but are often used to augment the antidepressant effect of traditional antidepressants. In addition to bipolar depression, these drugs are used in adults to treat schizophrenia and severe agitation. These drugs may cause or aggravate diabetes and high cholesterol and should be used cautiously in elderly patients due to potential

TABLE 3.3 Antidepressant Central Nervous System Agents

Generic Name	Trade Name	Classification
Depression		
aripiprazole	Abilify	serotonin, dopamine
citalopram	Celexa	SSRI
duloxetine	Cymbalta	SSRI/NE/DA
escitalopram	Lexapro	SSRI
fluoxetine	Prozac	SSRI
olanzapine	Zyprexa	serotonindopamine
paroxetine	Paxil, Paxil CR	SSRI
quetiapine	Seroquel	serotonin, dopamine
risperidone	Risperdal	serotonin, dopamine
sertraline	Zoloft	SSRI
trazodone	Desyrel	triazolopyridine
venlafaxine	Effexor, Effexor ER	SSRI/NE
Depression, Pain Relief		
amitriptyline	Elavil	tricyclic

SSRI = selective serotonin reuptake inhibitor NE=norepinephrine DA=dopamine

cardiovascular adverse reactions. If the patient experiences any rigidity, tremor, or involuntary muscle twitching, the physician should be notified immediately.

Several prescription (and some OTC) drugs, such as tramadol and cyclobenzaprine, can cause an unsafe level of serotonin when used with SSRI (selective serotonin reuptake inhibitor) antidepressants. Alcohol should not be used when any of these drugs are prescribed. Patient education and compliance are important while taking antidepressants. A patient may experience a withdrawal reaction if the drug is stopped abruptly.

Miscellaneous CNS Agents

Drugs that stimulate the CNS are listed in Table 3.4. Drugs for attention deficit hyperactivity disorder (ADHD) are frequently used in pediatric patients, sometimes in combination with other drugs. These drugs commonly cause insomnia and loss of appetite and should be administered in the morning or early afternoon. New uses for older drugs include the use of guanfacine (Tenex and Intuniv) and clonidine (Kapvay and Catapres) for ADHD in children to augment or even replace traditional stimulants.

Other CNS agents, such as memantine, are used to slow the progression of mild to moderate Alzheimer's disease. These are potent medications that alter brain chemistry to achieve the desired therapeutic response. Memantine is sometimes used in combination with donepezil (Aricept). Drowsiness is a common side effect. Donepezil is metabolized through the CYP 3A4 isoenzyme system in the liver and is susceptible to more interactions than memantine. The main side effects are GI-related diarrhea, nausea, and vomiting.

TABLE 3.4 Miscellaneous Central Nervous System Agents

Generic Name	Trade Name	Classification	Indication
amphetamine salts	Adderall	CNS stimulant	ADHD
carisoprodol	Soma	skeletal	muscle spasms
cyclobenzaprine	Flexeril	skeletal	muscle spasms
gabapentin	Neurontin	anticonvulsant, analgesic	pain, seizures
lisamfetamine	Vyvanse	CNS stimulant	ADHD
memantine	Namenda	brain receptor antagonist	Alzheimer's disease
methylphenidate	Concerta, Ritalin	CNS stimulant	ADHD
metoclopramide	Reglan	prokinetic agent	nausea, heartburn, gastroparesis
ondansetron	Zofran	brain receptor antagonist	nausea, vomiting
pregabalin	Lyrica	anticonvulsant, analgesic	pain, seizures
promethazine	Phenergan	antidopaminergic	nausea

Gabapentin and Lyrica were initially used as anticonvulsant drugs to control epileptic seizures. Today, these drugs are primarily used to reduce nerve pain associated with diabetes, shingles, and spinal cord injury. Gabapentin is also used as a mood stabilizer and for anxiety in psychiatric medicine, and in the treatment of restless leg syndrome. Lyrica is sometimes prescribed for muscle fatigue (fibromyalgia). The most common side effects are drowsiness, dizziness, and swelling of the ankles. OTC antacids, such as Mylanta or Maalox, interfere with the absorption of gabapentin. It is recommended that the drug be administered at least one hour before or two hours after the patient takes an antacid.

The muscle relaxants cyclobenzaprine and carisoprodol are commonly prescribed with narcotic analgesics and anxiolytics. They are indicated for short-term treatment of muscle spasm; however, they are often used long term. Promethazine (Phenergan) is commonly used in tablet, liquid, injection, or suppository form for the treatment of nausea and vomiting from a viral illness. Metoclopramide is used to treat heartburn and gastroparesis (or slow stomach emptying) in diabetics. It is commonly given 30 minutes before each meal and at bedtime. Metoclopramide can cause severe abnormal muscle movements called tardive dyskinesias with long-term use. Metoclopramide and ondansetron are often used to treat severe nausea and vomiting resulting from chemotherapy. Ondansetron is available as an oral disintegrating tablet (ODT), syrup, and as an injection for pediatric patients or those too sick to swallow tablets. Common side effects with all these drugs are drowsiness and dizziness. As with most CNS drugs, alcohol must be avoided.

Cardiovascular Agents

Heart disease is a major disease threat in the United States and includes such conditions as high blood pressure (hypertension). The complications of untreated or undertreated hypertension are renal and congestive heart failure, angina pectoris (severe chest pain), stroke, and heart attack. The presence of heart disease may be genetic, but it is often the result of poor lifestyle choices as well. Examples of poor lifestyle choices include smoking, obesity, and lack of exercise. Elevated cholesterol is an important and independent risk factor for heart disease.

Antihypertensive Agents

There are many antihypertensive agents (see Table 3.5) that work to lower blood pressure by dilating blood vessels, decreasing heart rate, and increasing the elimination of salt from the body. Often, more than one drug is needed to reach the desired blood pressure range, usually below 140 mm Hg for the systolic reading. In fact, many antihypertensives are combined with a diuretic such as hydrochlorothiazide (HCTZ). The most frequently prescribed calcium channel blocker (CCB) today is amlodipine. Other less frequently prescribed CCBs include verapamil, diltiazem, nicardpine, and nifedipine. Verapamil can frequently cause constipation, whereas amlodipine and nifedipine can cause headache, fast heart rate, and, in some cases, ankle swelling. Nicardipine is used orally and intravenously to control blood pressure and chest pain. Diltiazem and verapamil, along with most statins used to treat high cholesterol, should not be taken with grapefruit juice, as this may decrease metabolism and increase the risk of side effects.

Beta-adrenergic blockers include atenolol, metoprolol, and the newest agent nebivolol. Metoprolol succinate is available in an extended-release dosage form; metoprolol tartrate is an immediate-release dosage form. These different salts cannot be

TABLE 3.5 Antihypertensive Cardiovascular Agents

Generic Name	Trade Name	Classification
Hypertension		
amlodipine	Norvasc	calcium channel blocker
atenolol	Tenormin	beta-adrenergic blocker
metoprolol	Lopressor, Toprol	beta-adrenergic blocker
nebivolol	Bystolic	beta-adrenergic blocker
nicardipine	Cardene	calcium channel blocker
Hypertension, Heart Failure		
benazepril	Lotensin	ACE inhibitor
enalapril	Vasotec	ACE inhibitor
lisinopril	Prinivil, Zestril	ACE inhibitor
losartan	Cozaar	ARB
olmesatran	Benicar	ARB
ramipril	Altace	ACE inhibitor
valsartan	Diovan	ARB

interchanged. They are generally well tolerated, but a patient must not run out of these medications. If the drug is withdrawn for 48 to 72 hours, blood pressure can rebound to unsafe levels, leading to severe chest pain or even a heart attack (myocardial infarction). Diabetics who are prone to low blood sugar must use these drugs with caution because they can mask the symptoms of hypoglycemia.

Angiotensin-converting enzyme (ACE) inhibitors and their first cousins, angiotensin receptor blockers (ARBs), are frequently used to treat hypertension and heart failure. These drugs also protect the kidneys from the damage caused by diabetes and hypertension. ACE inhibitors (and ARBs) can retain potassium and must be used with caution in patients on potassium supplements, potassium-sparing diuretics (covered later in this chapter and in Table 3.14), or patients with declining kidney function.

The most common side effect of the ACE inhibitors is a drug-induced dry cough caused by the buildup of bradykinin in the lungs. If the cough continues, an ARB is usually prescribed. The most serious adverse effect of ACE inhibitors is angioedema, which can be a life-threatening allergic reaction manifested by a swelling of the tongue, lips, or eyes. If these symptoms present, the drug must be discontinued immediately and the patient should receive emergency care.

Antihyperlipidemic Agents

Antihyperlipidemic cardiovascular agents include medications that can lower cholesterol as well as triglyceride levels. A patient's total cholesterol consists of two main types: LDL, or bad cholesterol, and HDL, or good cholesterol. Medical history and risk factors determine an individual's target LDL cholesterol level. Antihyperlipidemic agents (see Table 3.6), commonly referred to as statins, prevent the production of cholesterol by blocking a key enzyme in the liver. These drugs vary in dose and potency but can lower LDL cholesterol up to 50 percent or more. Muscle fatigue is a common side effect, especially when these drugs are combined with other agents, such as gemfibrozil, verapamil, diltiazem, macrolide antibiotics, and amiodarone.

TABLE 3.6 Antihyperlipidemic Cardiovascular Agents

Generic Name	Trade Name	Classification
Cholesterol		
atorvastatin	Lipitor	HMG CoA reductase inhibitor
ezetimibe	Zetia	Absorption blocker
lovastatin	Mevacor	HMG CoA reductase inhibitor
nicotinic acid	Niaspan	Inhibits FFA, increases LPL
pravastatin	Pravachol	HMG CoA reductase inhibitor
rosuvastatin	Crestor	HMG CoA reductase inhibitor
simvastatin	Zocor	HMG CoA reductase inhibitor
simvastatin-ezetimibe	Vytorin	HMG CoA reductase inhibitor, absorption blocker
Triglycerides		
fenofibrate	TriCor	antihyperlipidemic
omega-3 fatty acid	Lovaza	antihyperlipidemic

Nicotinic acid (Niaspan) is a B-3 vitamin with a broad spectrum of activity. In large doses, it lowers LDL and triglycerides and improves HDL. It is thought to work by inhibiting the breakdown of free fatty acids in the liver and/or increasing lipoprotein lipase (LPL) activity. It is available as a prescription and OTC drug, but liver function should be tested periodically in patients using this drug. The dose must be slowly titrated over several weeks to avoid flushing and headache. Flushing can be avoided by pre-dosing with aspirin 30 minutes before taking the Niaspan. Niaspan is usually taken at bedtime with a small snack.

Fenofibrate primarily lowers triglycerides rather than cholesterol and is generally well tolerated; however, it must be used with caution with statins as well as warfarin and other blood thinners. Omega-3 fatty acids are the prescription equivalent of fish oil; they are effective in lowering the triglycerides in patients who are allergic or intolerant to seafood. Salmon is high in omega-3 fatty acids and can help naturally lower triglycerides. Lovaza is a "prescription only" omega-3 fatty acid.

Miscellaneous Cardiovascular Agents

In addition to hypertension and cholesterol, other agents (see Table 3.7) are used to treat abnormal heart beats, heart failure, and severe chest pain.

The agents for heart failure all work differently and are sometimes used in combination or with the ACE inhibitors previously discussed. Digoxin is an older drug, and its serum blood levels should be measured to prevent toxic levels and side effects, including arrhythmias and death. The drug can slow down the heart rate and cause nausea and vomiting when toxic levels are reached, especially if blood potassium levels are low (less than 3.5 mEq/L).

Isosorbide belongs to the nitrate family; nitroglycerin is the most commonly known drug of this group. The nitrates all work similarly; they dilate the blood vessels, particularly those of the heart, to relieve chest pain or reduce the workload on the heart. Isosorbide is available as both a mononitrate (Ismo, Imdur) and a dinitrate (Isordil). The mononitrate is preferred because it has a longer duration action. Nitrates can cause a headache and a dangerous drop in blood pressure when combined with erectile dysfunction drugs, including Viagra, Levitra, and Cialis. Nitroglycerin sublingual (under the tongue) tablets are sensitive to air and light and should be replaced every three to six months to assure potency. Nitroglycerin is often taken at the first sign of chest pain with repeated doses every five minutes for three doses. If chest pain continues, the patient is advised to take a crushed aspirin tablet and get to the emergency room as quickly as possible.

Carvedilol is commonly used as a core drug in the treatment of heart failure. It has both beta-adrenergic and alpha-adrenergic blocking action to lower demands on a compromised heart. It is also available in a Coreg CR (controlled release) dosage formulation. All beta blockers must be used with caution in patients with asthma and chronic obstructive pulmonary disease (COPD), or with drugs that lower heart rate, such as digoxin and verapamil.

TABLE 3.7 Miscellaneous Cardiovascular Agents

Generic Name	Trade Name	Classification	Indication
carvedilol	Coreg	alpha/beta blocker	heart failure
digoxin	Lanoxin	inotropic agent	heart failure
isosorbide	Imdur, Ismo, Isordil	vasodilator	angina pectoris, heart failure

Systemic Anti-infective Agents

Most systemic anti-infective agents (see Table 3.8) are antibiotics with different mechanisms of action. They include penicillin derivatives as well as sulfa drugs, tetracyclines, macrolides, lincosamides, antifungals, and antivirals. Penicillin and its derivatives, amoxicillin and amoxicillin/clavulanate, are commonly used to treat upper respiratory and ear infections in adult and pediatric patients. These drugs are generally well tolerated, but these derivatives of penicillin may cause diarrhea and yeast infections. Yogurt or probiotics often offset diarrhea, but yeast infections may require treatment with OTC or prescription drugs. It is important for the technician to double-check the allergy history in the patient profile before dispensing any antibiotic prescription. Ampicillin/sulbactum and nafcillin are used in the hospital to treat infections resistant to traditional penicillins.

TABLE 3.8 Systemic Anti-infective Agents

Generic Name	Trade Name	Classification
Infection		
amoxicillin	Amoxil	aminopenicillin
amoxicillin-clavulanate	Augmentin	aminopenicillin
ampicillin-sulbactum	Unasyn	aminopenicillin
azithromycin	Z-Pak	macrolide
ceftazolin	Ancef	cephalosporin
ceftazidime	Fortaz, Tazicef	cephalosporin
ceftriaxone	Rocephin	cephalosporin
cephalexin	Keflex	cephalosporin
ciprofloxacin	Cipro	fluoroquinolone
gentamicin	generic only	aminoglycoside
levofloxacin	Levaquin	fluoroquinolone
nafcillin	generic only	penicillinase resistant penicillin
penicillin	Veetids, Pen VK	natural penicillin
sulfamethoxazole-trimethoprim	Bactrim, Septra	sulfonamide
vancomycin	Vancocin	glycopeptide
Infection, Acne		
clindamycin	Cleocin	lincosamide
doxycycline	Doryx, Vibramycin	tetracycline
metronidazole	Flagyl	antiprotozoan
Fungal Infection		
fluconazole	Diflucan	antifungal
Viral Infection		
acyclovir	Zovirax	herpes infections

The cephalosporins are a frequently prescribed class of antibiotics in the hospital and community and are generally well-tolerated. Fewer than 5 percent of those allergic to penicillin may develop a rash with cephalosporins, so the patient (or parent) should be so advised. If the patient has an anaphylactic reaction (severe allergy) to penicillin, cephalosporins should be avoided. Each generation of the parenteral cephalosporins has activities against different microorganisms. The fluoroquinolones are a class of potent antibiotics that include ciprofloxacin and levofloxacin; they should not be taken with milk, dairy products, or antacids. They can cause rare but serious ruptured tendons or severe tendonitis with strenuous exercise. The FDA-mandated MedGuide describes this reaction to consumers. Ciprofloxacin and levofloxacin may also interact with diabetic medications to further lower blood sugar.

Doxycycline is an all-purpose antibiotic commonly used to treat acne and Lyme disease. It cannot be used in pregnant women or children younger than 8, and must not be taken at the same time as dairy, antacids, iron, or calcium. As with many antibiotics (and sulfa), the patient should take precaution in the sun because these agents enhance sunburn. Azithromycin, a macrolide, is commonly prescribed in tablet (Z-Pak) or suspension form for the treatment of upper respiratory infections in adults and children. Azithromycin has the advantage of a five-day course of therapy, which may improve patient compliance. The drug should be taken with a meal or snack to lessen GI side effects. Unlike most antibiotic suspensions, this one can be kept at room temperature. Azithromycin may interact with other drugs, including the blood thinner warfarin, and use must be assessed by the pharmacist.

The most commonly prescribed sulfa drug is a combination of sulfamethoxazole and trimethoprim, which have a mutually beneficial effect on bacteria. This drug is commonly used to treat urinary tract infections and ear infections. Sulfa drugs should be taken with large quantities of water and must be used cautiously with blood thinners and other drugs.

Clindamycin is an alternative antibiotic for use in patients who are allergic to penicillin; it can cause severe diarrhea. Clindamycin is commonly prescribed for a dental infection as it has anaerobic coverage, which is common in the oral cavity. If patients develop serious bloody diarrhea, they should contact their physicians immediately as they may have developed colitis from the antibiotic or a Clostridium difficile infection.

Clindamycin and metronidazole are used in the hospital to treat or prevent severe anaerobic infections post-surgery. They are also used topically to treat acne in adolescents and adults. Metronidazole is also frequently prescribed for five to seven days to treat vaginal infections. The use of alcohol with this drug could cause severe nausea.

Several antibiotics listed in Table 3.8 are commonly used in the hospital and administered intravenously. Vancomycin is commonly the drug of choice to treat methicillin-resistant staph aureus (MRSA). Kidney function must be carefully monitored and drug blood levels are frequently measured to assure correct dosing. If the MRSA infection is vancomycin resistant, ertapenum (Invanz) and other antibiotics serve as alternatives. Oral vancomycin is used to treat *Clostridium difficile* infection of the intestinal tract. Gentamicin is a parenteral antibiotic that is frequently used to treat serious infections; it is sometimes combined with another antibiotic to overcome resistance. Kidney function must be carefully monitored with the aminoglycoside antibiotics, and blood levels are frequently monitored to adjust dosing. Excessively high levels of aminoglycosides and long-term use will cause hearing loss and kidney damage. Most antibiotics can cause gastrointestinal side effects.

The antifungal drug fluconazole is commonly prescribed as a one-time or short-term oral treatment for yeast infections. Acylovir is used orally, topically (Zovirax), and parentally to treat viral herpes infections.

Endocrine and Metabolic Agents

The various endocrine and metabolic agents that are frequently prescribed in the community pharmacy setting are covered in the next sections. These drugs vary from hormones and birth control pills to drugs that treat bone loss, diabetes, thyroid conditions, inflammatory diseases, and gout.

Estrogens and Birth Control Agents

In postmenopausal women, or those who have had a hysterectomy, hormone replacement therapy with estrogen is often necessary to reduce symptoms such as hot flashes, insomnia, and emotional imbalance. Short-term use in low doses has been shown to be safe and effective. The major side effect of estrogens is nausea, and there is a concern about the increase in the risk of stroke and cancer with long-term (more than 5 years) use.

There are many prescription birth control pills available on the market. Most contain both an estrogen and a progestin to simulate pregnancy and thereby prevent ovulation. Some pill packets contain pills with varying amounts of hormone for each week of the month. Newer birth control pills, such as Seasonale and Seasonique, are available in 91-day supply packs that offer the convenience of menses once every three months. Most pills contain three weeks of active medication and one week of placebo or iron tablets. Birth control pills are quite effective if taken properly, and they are generally well accepted and tolerated. In women over age 35 who smoke, there is concern that birth control pills may increase the risk of stroke. The FDA mandates pharmacies dispense a MedGuide with birth control. NuvaRing is a once-a-month birth control device in which the hormones are slowly released intravaginally; this drug should be refrigerated before use.

TABLE 3.9 Estrogens and Contraceptives

Generic Name	Trade Name	Classification
Hormone Replacement Therapy		
conjugated estrogen	Premarin	sex hormone
Birth Control		
ethinyl estradiol/norethindrone	LoEstrin Fe-24	contraceptive
ethinyl estradiol/norgestimate	Tri-Nessa, Tri-Sprintec	contraceptive
ethinyl estradiol/drospirenone	Gianvi	contraceptive
etonogestrel-ethinyl	NuvaRing	contraceptive hormone estradiol
levonorgestrel/ethinylestradiol	Seasonale, Seasonique	contraceptive

Antidiabetic Agents

Diabetes drugs (see Table 3.10) all lower blood sugar but by different mechanisms of action. Often more than one drug is necessary to reduce blood sugar to target levels. Type I diabetics always require insulin injections. Type II diabetics may need oral medications and/or insulin injections.

The sulfonylureas, including glyburide and glipizide, are most likely to cause hypoglycemia (low blood sugar) and more likely to interact with other drugs (such as

TABLE 3.10 Diabetes Controlling Agents

Generic Name	Trade Name	Classification
glipizide	Glucotrol	sulfonylurea
glyburide	DiaBeta, Micronase	sulfonylurea
insulin glargine	Lantus	insulin
metformin	Glucophage	biguanide
pioglitazone	Actos	thiazolidinedione
sitagliptin	Januvia	DPP-4 inhibitor

Ciprofloxacin). These agents can cause photosensitivity to the sun, so sunscreen should be recommended as a precaution. Actos (pioglitazone) must be used with caution in patients with heart failure. Metformin is the most frequently prescribed diabetes drug; it is available in both an immediate-release and extended-release form. The drug should be taken with food, and the patient may need to take a vitamin B12 supplement while taking metformin long term.

Januvia is a relatively new treatment for Type II diabetes. It is most effective at controlling blood sugars after a meal. It is sometimes prescribed as Janumet, which is a combination of Januvia and metformin.

Many types of insulin are available, and they are the most common source of medication errors. Novolin and Humulin are different than NovoLog and Humalog. Many insulins come in mixtures of regular and slower release NPH insulin. For patient convenience, many are available as an insulin pen. Insulins can be sold without a prescription.

Needle and syringe prescription requirements vary by state, and insurers require a prescription for diabetic supplies. Medicare Part D plans cover diabetic supplies, but quantities vary and depend on whether the patient is insulin dependent. Medicare Part B may cover insulin supplies with a prescription and proper documentation and diagnostic codes from the prescriber.

Insulin glargine (Lantus) is the most commonly prescribed insulin; it is often taken at bedtime. It does not peak or trough but simply provides a level reduction of blood sugar over a 24-hour period. Insulins lose their potency if stored unrefrigerated for more than 28 days. The patient should be advised to date insulin and replace it every four weeks.

Miscellaneous Endocrine Agents

Bisphosphonates such as alendronate are indicated in the treatment of osteoporosis or bone loss (see Table 3.11). Bone loss often occurs in postmenopausal women or men over age 75 whose do not receive enough calcium. These drugs are taken daily, weekly, or monthly. To minimize the risk of esophageal erosions and decreased absorption, these drugs must be taken first thing in the morning, with water only, and not in a reclining position. This may present a problem in a bedridden or nursing home patient.

Hypothyroidism is a treatable disease and is especially common in women. Many physicians and some patients may request a brand name drug due to better tolerance or a more reliable therapeutic effect. Thyroid medication should be taken in the morning or on an empty stomach to increase absorption. It must not be taken at the same time as dairy, antacids, iron, or calcium or within two hours of ingestion of these substances.

TABLE 3.11 Miscellaneous Endocrine and Metabolic Agents

Generic Name	Trade Name	Classification
Osteoporosis, Hypercalcemia		
alendronate	Fosamax	bisphosphonate
Hypothyroidism		
levothyroxine	Levoxyl, Synthroid	thyroid hormone
Anti-Inflammatory		
dexamethasone	Decadron	corticosteroid
methylprednisolone	Medrol Dosepak	corticosteroid
prednisone	Deltasone	corticosteroid

Corticosteroids, including dexamethasone, prednisone, and methylprednisolone (Medrol dosepack) are used to treat a variety of inflammatory diseases, such as rheumatoid arthritis, asthma, allergic reactions, poison ivy/oak, ulcerative colitis, Crohn's disease, and gout. These drugs are usually prescribed for short-term use because of their side effects. They should be taken with food and may interfere with blood sugar or blood-thinning medications. Dexamethasone is sometimes used to reduce swelling in the brain in trauma victims.

Respiratory Agents

Asthma, chronic obstructive pulmonary disease (COPD), allergies, and coughing constrict the airways and cause inflammation, which results in shortness of breath and wheezing and decreases oxygen saturation in the blood. Table 3.12 contains a variety of common respiratory drugs used to treat these conditions.

Albuterol (and its chemical cousins levalbuterol, formeterol, and salmeterol) and Atrovent (ipratropium) or Spiriva (tiotropium) work in different ways to cause bronchodilation (relaxing of the airways) in the lungs in patients with asthma or COPD. Side effects include increases in heart rate and blood pressure with albuterol and derivatives. Atrovent and Spiriva cause dry mouth, eyes, and throat. These drugs are inhaled into the lungs and provide relief for shortness of breath. Albuterol is the fastest acting and should be used for acute attacks. Overuse may cause patients to develop a tolerance. Albuterol may be prescribed as a tablet, syrup, metered-dose inhaler (MDI), or sterile solution for nebulizer use.

Combivent combines ipratropium and albuterol. In essence, these drugs provide symptomatic relief only. Advair and Symbicort combine a bronchodilator with a corticosteroid. Corticosteroids work on the inflammatory component of asthma and COPD. Decreasing inflammation should reduce the number of acute attacks and the use of short-acting agents such as albuterol (Ventolin, ProAir). Keeping the metered dose inhaler (MDI) clean is important, and rinsing the mouth after using corticosteroids may prevent the development of a fungal infection in the mouth called thrush.

Montelukast (Singulair), available in tablet, chewable tablet, and granular form, is used to treat asthma and allergies. It neutralizes and prevents the release of chemicals called leukotrienes, which cause allergy symptoms. Intranasal steroids like Flonase

TABLE 3.12 Respiratory Agents

Generic Name	Trade Name	Classification
Asthma, COPD		
albuterol	ProAir, Ventolin	sympathomimetic
levalbuterol	Xopenex	sympathomimetic
COPD		
budesonide/formeterol	Symbicort	combination
fluticasone/salmeterol	Advair	combination
ipratropium	Atrovent	anticholinergic
ipratropium-albuterol	Combivent	combination
tiotropium	Spiriva	anticholinergic
Asthma, Allergy		
fluticasone	Flonase, Flovent	inhaled steroid
montelukast	Singulair	leukotriene receptor antagonist
Allergy		
fexofenadine (OTC)	Allegra	antihistamine
mometasone	Nasonex	inhaled steroid
Cough Suppressant		
guiafenesin/codeine	Cheracol, Robitussin AC	narcotic antitussive

and Nasonex are used routinely to prevent seasonal allergy symptoms from developing. Fexofenadine (Allegra) and loratidine (Claritin) are considered nonsedating antihistamines. Other common OTC antihistamines include cetirizine, chlorpheniramine, and diphenhydramine (Benadryl). Guaifenesin with codeine is a Schedule V drug and is commonly prescribed for short-term relief of moderate to severe cough. It may cause drowsiness. An OTC cough suppressant, dextromethorphan, may be as effective as codeine without the narcotic side effects, but remain vigilant for overuse as high doses cause hallucinations. Dextromethorphan is commonly shoplifted for abuse by minors.

Gastrointestinal Agents

The most frequently prescribed classes of gastrointestinal agents (see Table 3.13) are the proton pump inhibitors (PPIs) and the histamine-2 antagonists. These drugs work to either reduce or shut off the secretion of acid in the stomach, thus resolving the symptoms of heartburn, gastroesophageal reflux, and ulcer disease. Prilosec, Prevacid, Pepcid, and Zantac are available over the counter in a lower dose.

PPIs and ranitidine are well tolerated with only occasional reports of side effects, such as headache and dizziness. PPIs, such as omeprazole, can interfere with beneficial effects of the antiplatelet drug clopidogrel (Plavix); these drugs should not be taken together, and there is concern even if they are spaced 12 hours apart. Long-term use of

TABLE 3.13 Gastrointestinal Agents

Generic Name	Trade Name	Classification
esomeprazole	Nexium	proton pump inhibitor
famotidine	Pepcid (Rx, OTC)	histamine-2 antagonist
lansoprazole	Prevacid (Rx, OTC)	proton pump inhibitor
omeprazole	Prilosec (Rx, OTC)	proton pump inhibitor
pantoprazole	Protonix	proton pump inhibitor
ranitidine	Zantac	histamine-2 antagonist

PPIs has been reported to increase bone loss; the recommendation of an OTC calcium supplement, especially in older females, may be warranted. Some additional agents such as promethazine, ondansetron, and metoclopramide are listed in Table 3.4.

Renal and Genitourinary Agents

The most frequently prescribed renal and genitourinary agents are the phosphodiesterase (PDE-5) inhibitors, diuretics, and alpha adrenergic blockers for benign prostatic hypertrophy in men (see Table 3.14). The PDE-5 inhibitors include the well-known and marketed drugs Viagra and Cialis, used to treat erectile dysfunction. (Levitra is another drug in this category.) These drugs vary by onset and duration of action. Rare side effects include changes in blue/green color vision and priapism, or prolonged painful erection. As stated earlier, a life-threatening hypotension (drop in blood pressure) can occur if these agents are used with any nitrate, including nitroglycerin.

Diuretics used to treat high blood pressure and heart failure also fall into this classification. Diuretics work by eliminating excess salt and water from the body and by dilating (widening) blood vessels. Many antihypertensive drugs listed in Table 3.14 are available in combination with a diuretic.

Hydrochlorothiazide and furosemide act at different sites of the kidney, and their onset, duration of action, and potency differ. Diuretics should be taken in the morning or early evening. Most can cause a loss of potassium, which can cause muscle cramps, or, in severe cases, irregular heart rates. Diuretics that contain triamterene and spironolactone are considered potassium-sparing.

Diuretics must be used with caution with ACE inhibitors, digoxin, and lithium; the pharmacist should assess the potential for interactions for patients on these drugs. Potassium loss can be offset by consuming potassium-rich foods such as fresh citrus fruits and bananas or taking potassium supplements.

Tamulosin is a common alpha-adrenergic blocker used to treat benign prostatic hypertrophy (BPH). A common side effect is first-dose syncope (or drop in blood pressure causing fainting), so they are usually prescribed as a bedtime dose.

TABLE 3.14 Renal and Genitourinary Agents

Generic Name	Trade Name	Classification
Erectile Dysfunction		
sildenafil	Viagra	phosphodiesterase inhibitor
tadalafil	Cialis	phosphodiesterase inhibitor
vardenafil	Levitra	phosphodiesterase inhibitor
Heart Failure, Hypertension		
furosemide	Lasix	loop diuretic
hydrochlorothiazide	Esidrix, HydroDIURIL, Oretic	thiazide diuretic
spironolactone	Aldactone	potassium-sparing diuretic
triamterene-hydrochlorothiazide	Dyazide, Maxzide	combination, potassium-sparing

Hematologic Agents

Additional frequently prescribed medications are listed in Table 3.15 on the next page. Warfarin (Coumadin) is used both short and long term to prevent blood clots in high-risk patients. Patients on this drug are less likely to clot but more likely to bleed. Like digoxin, toxic levels are close to therapeutic levels. Patients are monitored on a routine basis with a blood test called an INR (international normalized ratio); a therapeutic level is between 2.0 and 3.5. Some prescribers may write "brand necessary" (DAW1) on prescriptions for blood thinners. Newer agents have been introduced in the past year to prevent clot formation, including dabigatran (Pradaxa) and rivaroxaban (Xarelto), that are faster acting and do not require regular blood testing. The disadvantage to these new agents is the lack of an antidote for treating an overdose.

Warfarin works by inhibiting vitamin K–dependent clotting factors. Vitamins and diets that are high in vitamin K (green vegetables) can impair the effect of the blood thinner. The key is to maintain a stable intake of greens. This drug is very susceptible to drug interactions, including aspirin and many herbal drugs. When other drugs are added to the regimen or dosages are adjusted, the pharmacist must assess the potential significance of the interaction.

Clopidogrel (Plavix) often works in concert with aspirin to further decrease the risk of blood clots. Plavix is a platelet inhibitor. When platelets clump together, the clotting process is initiated and a clot can form; Plavix (and aspirin) prevent the platelets from clumping together. Diet does not affect Plavix, but the use of omeprazole, a PPI, can interfere with its therapeutic effect.

Heparin is a parenteral anticlotting drug that is used intravenously and subcutaneously to treat and prevent blood clots in the lungs and legs, especially in a hospital setting. Frequent blood tests are required to prevent the major side effect: bleeding. Lovenox is used in both community and hospital settings as a subcutaneous (under the skin) injection to prevent blood clots during high-risk procedures, or to allow time for warfarin to take effect (usually one week). Lovenox, which has been shown to be as effective as heparin, can be administered subcutaneously, requires no blood tests, and causes less bleeding.

TABLE 3.15 Hematologic Agents

Generic Name	Trade Name	Classification	Indication
clopidogrel	Plavix	antiplatelet drug	prevent blood clots
enoxaparin	Lovenox	thrombin inhibitor	prevent blood clots
heparin	generic only	thrombin inhibitor	prevent blood clots
warfarin	Coumadin	blood thinner	prevent blood clots
rivaroxaban	Xarelto	factor Xa inhibitor	prevent blood clots
dabigatran	Pradaxa	thrombin inhibitor	prevent blood clots

Table 3.16 lists potent parenteral biotech agents used in the hospital or outpatient clinic to treat a variety of medical conditions: (1) anemias from chronic kidney disease or cancer chemotherapy; (2) low white and red blood cell count for those at risk of an infection or experiencing severe fatigue; and (3) inflammatory diseases. Remicade has a wide spectrum of uses, from severe rheumatoid arthritis to GI inflammatory diseases like Crohn's disease to severe psoriasis that is unresponsive to conventional therapy. However, technicians working in a hospital or servicing a cancer or dialysis clinic need to be familiar with colony-stimilating factors such as Aranesp, Procrit, and Neupogen. These are life-saving drugs for patients undergoing chemotherapy, which can depress the bone marrow and subsequent immune system function.

TABLE 3.16 Biological and Immunologic Agents

Generic Name	Trade Name	Classification
darbepoetin alfa	Aranesp	Anemias
epoetin alfa	Procrit	Anemias
filgrastim	Neupogen	stimulates WBC
infliximab	Remicade	Inflammatory disorders
pegfilgrastim	Neulasta	stimulates WBC

Miscellaneous Drugs

Triamcinolone is the most frequently prescribed topical drug. It is a corticosteroid and is available in different strengths in both a cream and an ointment form. It is more potent than hydrocortisone, which is available as an OTC. Topical corticosteroids are useful to treat skin conditions such as eczema, psoriasis, allergic reaction from bug bites, or dermatitis from poison ivy.

It is common for patients on long-term diuretics such as hydrochlorothiazide and furosemide to have muscle cramps from a low potassium blood level; even potassium-sparing diuretics may cause this side effect. Patients on the heart drug digoxin are also more susceptible to toxicity with a low blood potassium level. In addition to changes in diet, the prescriber may add a daily dose or two (10-40 mEq) of potassium chloride per day in tablet or capsule form. This medication should be taken with food and a glass of water so that it does not irritate the esophagus.

TABLE 3.17 Miscellaneous Agents

Generic Name	Trade Name	Classification	Indication
cholecalciferol	Vitamin D	fat-soluble vitamin	deficiency, osteoporosis
folic acid	many generics	B vitamin	heart disease, with MTX
potassium chloride	K-Dur, Klorcon	mineral	K+ replacement
triamcinolone	Kenalog	topical steroid	inflammatory skin disease, eczema

Vitamin D and folic acid are commonly prescribed vitamins. Both are available as an OTC; prescription dosages are much higher. For example, vitamin D is available as an OTC in doses of 400 to 2,000 international units (IU) per day; a common prescription dose is 50,000 IU once a week or more. Vitamin D improves the absorption of calcium (i.e., vitamin D-fortified milk) and is commonly prescribed or recommended for patients who have or are at risk for osteoporosis. The potent drug methotrexate (MTX) is commonly prescribed for rheumatoid arthritis. Folic acid may reduce some of the drug's toxicity. Folic acid is also recommended for females who may become pregnant to decrease the risk of spina bifida (a birth deformity) in the neonate. High doses are found in all prenatal vitamins. Some cardiologists may recommend taking folic acid to reduce blood levels of homocysteine, which is thought to be a risk factor for heart disease.

Over-the-Counter Drugs and Dietary Supplements

Over-the-counter (OTC) drugs are available for sale without a prescription for the treatment of self-limited illnesses. The FDA is responsible for the review and approval of OTC drugs. Many of these commonly used drugs, such as acetaminophen (Tylenol), ibuprofen (Advil), naproxen (Aleve), loperamide (Imodium), ranitidine (Zantac), omeprazole (Prilosec), lantoprazole (Prevacid), fexofedadine (Allegra), loratadine (Claritin), cetirizine (Zyrtec), meclizine (Bonine, Antivert), and hydrocortisone were once prescription-only products. Many require a prescription in higher doses.

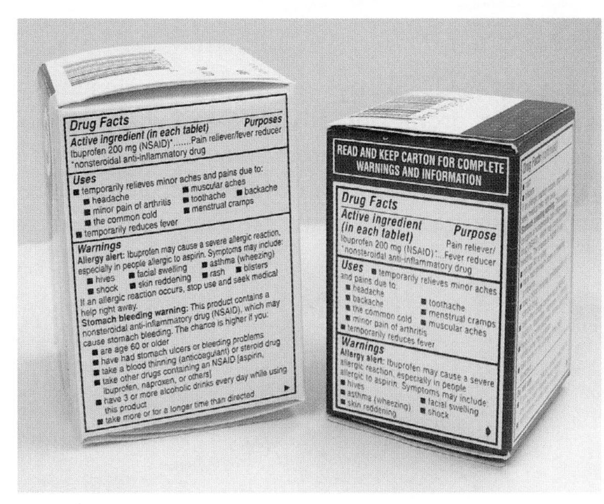

Both branded and generic OTC drugs must provide consumers with information on dosage, frequency of administration, precautions, and warnings.

It is the responsibility of OTC drug manufacturers to provide product label information on the safe and effective use of these drugs. OTC drugs are susceptible to the same side effects, adverse effects, and drug interactions as prescription drugs. Some OTC drugs, especially cough and cold products, may not be indicated for use in young children. Others may increase blood pressure. Antihistamines found in many cold medicines may not be appropriate for daytime use.

Dietary supplements, including vitamins, minerals, and herbal medications, are not as closely regulated by the FDA. Manufacturers are not required to provide consumers with complete information. Most labels include only a list of ingredients and a daily serving size (dose). Dietary supplement labels cannot make any disease claim. Natural herbal medications (see Table 3.18) are considered weak drugs and can cause side effects and interact with prescription drugs. For example, garlic, ginger, and gingko can interfere with the blood thinner warfarin.

TABLE 3.18 Indications for Common Dietary Supplements

Diet Supplement	Indications
calcium and vitamin D	osteoporosis
echinacea	boosts immune system
garlic	antibacterial and antiviral action; maintains healthy cholesterol
ginger	nausea, motion sickness
gingko	memory
glucosamine/chondroitin	osteoarthritis
melatonin	insomnia, especially in shift workers or time zone travelers
Policosanol	maintains healthy cholesterol
omega-3 fatty acids (fish oil)	lowers triglycerides
saw palmetto	benign prostatic hypertrophy or BPH
St. John's Wort	mild depression
vitamin C	common cold
zinc	boosts immune system, common cold

Table 3.19 on the next page lists many of the OTC drugs and dietary supplements the technician may be responsible for ordering, promoting, stocking, and checking expiration dates. Questions about drug product selection, indications, dose, frequency, side effects, and warnings and interactions must always be referred to the pharmacist. The technician may only highlight information written on the label for the customer.

TABLE 3.19 Common OTC Drugs and Indications

Generic Name	Brand Name	Indication(s)
ibuprofen	Advil	headache, pain
oxymetazoline	Afrin	nasal decongestant
naproxen	Aleve	headache, pain
fexofenadine	Allegra	allergy
diphenhydramine	Benadryl	allergy
loratadine	Claritin	allergy
hydrocortisone	Cortizone-10	itching, inflammation
clotrimazole	Lotrimin	topical antifungal
meclizine	Antivert, Bonine	vertigo, dizziness
miconazole	Monistat	vaginal antifungal
guaifenesin	Mucinex	expectorant
triple antibiotic	Neosporin	topical anti-infective
lansoprazole	Prevacid	heartburn
omeprazole	Prilosec	heartburn
ranitidine	Zantac	heartburn
cetirizine	Zyrtec	allergy

Skills Quiz

Reflect on the information presented in the chapter by answering the following questions.

1. The scientific study of drugs and how they work, including side effects, adverse reactions, and drug interactions, is called
   a. pharmacokinetics.
   b. pharmaceutics.
   c. pharmacognosy.
   d. pharmacology.
2. Which of the following agents might be used in a patient with BPH?
   a. metoprolol
   b. tamulosin
   c. verapamil
   d. vardenafil
3. Diabetes may be treated with oral agents or injectable agents. Which of the following is injected subcutaneously?
   a. metformin
   b. pioglitazone
   c. Lantus
   d. glyburide
4. A patient hands you a prescription for Viagra. When you check the patient profile, you see the patient also has a prescription for _________, which could cause severe hypotension if the two drugs are taken together.
   a. nifedipine
   b. furosemide
   c. losartan
   d. nitroglycerin
5. A patient has a prescription for alendronate 70 mg to be taken weekly (every Monday morning) and a calcium supplement to be taken twice daily. When should the calcium be taken on Monday?
   a. with the alendronate
   b. 30 minutes after the alendronate
   c. 30 minutes before the alendronate
   d. take a double dose of calcium Monday evening
6. Zolpidem is used to treat
   a. insomnia.
   b. ADHD.
   c. heartburn.
   d. high blood pressure.
7. Which drug may cause Plavix to be less effective at reducing platelet aggregation?
   a. digoxin
   b. omeprazole
   c. gemfibrozil
   d. warfarin
8. A patient comes to the pharmacy counter and asks for a refill on his prescription for his rescue asthma medication. Which agent will you refill and prepare?
   a. Advair
   b. Flovent
   c. albuterol
   d. Spiriva
9. ACE inhibitors cause retention of
   a. sodium.
   b. fluid.
   c. potassium.
   d. calcium.
10. A MedGuide is required to warn patients about the rare but serious adverse reaction of ruptured tendons than can occur with
    a. Cialis.
    b. Levaquin.
    c. carvedilol.
    d. Zetia.

Thinking Beyond the Exam

As a student of pharmacology, learning about all of the drugs on the market can be overwhelming. Most pharmacists have a favorite reference they turn to to answer a question outside of their expertise. Identify some common references used in pharmacies today, including books, journals, and websites that provide reliable and up-to-date information.

Pharmacology Practice Exam

Select the best answer to the following questions.

1. Which drug belongs to the class of drugs with the common side effect of a drug-induced cough due to build up of bradykinin?
   a. amlodipine
   b. benazepril
   c. diltiazem
   d. duloxetine

2. Which antimicrobial should have the auxiliary label "Do not drink alcohol" attached to the prescription vial?
   a. penicillin
   b. levofloxacin
   c. metronidazole
   d. azithromycin

3. Toxic levels of which drug will cause nausea, vomiting, decreased heart rate, visual disturbances, and death?
   a. digoxin
   b. acetaminophen
   c. levothyroxine
   d. fluconazole

4. A patient brings a new prescription to the pharmacy for meloxicam 7.5 mg po daily. Which of the drugs on the patient's profile should be stopped to prevent duplication of therapy and an increased risk of side effects, including GI bleed?
   a. furosemide
   b. escitalopram
   c. trazodone
   d. naproxen

5. To which class of drugs do valsartan (Diovan) and losartan (Cozaar) belong?
   a. HMG CoA reductase inhibitor
   b. angiotensin receptor blocker
   c. calcium channel blocker
   d. serotonin reuptake inhibitor

6. Which of the following medications is considered a maintenance anti-inflammatory drug to prevent the bronchospasm in asthma?
   a. Ventolin
   b. Flovent
   c. ProAir
   d. Xopenex

7. Which dietary supplement is indicated to lower triglyceride levels in the blood and has a prescription version called Lovaza?
   a. echinacea
   b. St. John's Wort
   c. ginger
   d. fish oil

8. A patient on Coumadin (warfarin) will need to have regular blood work to measure the level of
   a. anticoagulation.
   b. blood glucose.
   c. white blood cells.
   d. potassium.

9. A home-use urine dip stick test that measures HCG in the urine will detect
   a. urinary ketones.
   b. urinary tract infection.
   c. pregnancy.
   d. diabetes.

10. Many drugs may be absorbed through the skin from either a patch reservoir or a topical cream or ointment. Which drug is commonly administered through the topical route?
    a. levothyroxine
    b. insulin
    c. nicotine
    d. simvastatin

11. A common side effect of HMG CoA reductase inhibitors like atorvastatin is ______________ and requires referral to the physician for evaluation.
    a. muscle fatigue
    b. hiatal hernia
    c. severe diarrhea
    d. bradycardia

12. Because of the high risk of addiction and physical dependence, drug prescriptions are more likely to be forged for what drug category?
    a. corticosteroids
    b. narcotic analgesics
    c. COX-2 inhibitors
    d. anticonvulsants

13. Which group of drugs carries a black box warning for increased risk of suicidal thoughts and behavior in young children, adolescents, and young adults?
    a. CNS stimulants
    b. antidepressants
    c. anxiolytics
    d. antipsychotics

14. Which drug requires the following instructions to ensure absorption of the active ingredient and prevent esophageal erosion? "Must be taken first thing in the morning, with water only (not a caffeinated drink), at least 30 minutes before any other medication, and the patient must remain in an upright position."
    a. Lipitor
    b. Synthroid
    c. Fosamax
    d. Nexium

15. Although the side effects of this class of drug are rare, when taken with a vasodilator like nitroglycerin, a severe drop in blood pressure will occur and may be life threatening. Which of the following is a drug in the phosphodiesterase (PDE-5) inhibitor class?
    a. sildenafil
    b. spironolactone
    c. simvastatin
    d. sertraline

16. The drug methotrexate is used to treat rheumatoid arthritis. What vitamin can reduce the toxicity of methotrexate?
    a. vitamin B12
    b. riboflavin
    c. vitamin D
    d. folic acid

17. Which pair of drugs is known to have a 5 percent chance of cross allergenicity and could cause an anaphylactic reaction?
    a. penicillin and cephalexin
    b. simvastatin and propranolol
    c. glipizide and omeprazole
    d. erythromycin and gentamicin

18. A drug that is a Category X for use in pregnancy is
    a. Zofran.
    b. Xopenex.
    c. Accutane.
    d. Heparin.

19. The site of action of furosemide and hydrochlorothiazide is the
    a. liver.
    b. kidney.
    c. heart.
    d. lungs.

20. A patient who takes an overdose of warfarin would experience what reaction?
    a. vomiting
    b. bradycardia
    c. bleeding
    d. drowsiness

21. A newer class of drugs used to treat asthma decreases inflammation as a leukotriene receptor antagonist. Which drug is in this class?
    a. Xopenex
    b. Singulair
    c. Spiriva
    d. Symbicort

22. Anti-infectives are used to treat bacterial, fungal, and viral infections. Which drug is an antiviral agent used to prevent and treat herpes infections?
    a. fluconazole
    b. doxycycline
    c. valacyclovir
    d. cefdinir

23. Patients taking first generation antipsychotic drugs may experience side effects related to the lack of dopamine in the CNS, including tremors, rigidity, and involuntary movement similar to Parkinson's disease. Which drug is a first-generation antipsychotic?
    a. chlorpromazine
    b. risperidone
    c. quetiapine
    d. benztropine

24. Which antibiotic treats only infections of the GI tract caused by *Clostridium difficile* when given orally, but when given intravenously will treat methacillin resistant *Staphylococcus aureus*?
    a. erythromycin
    b. gentamicin
    c. clindamycin
    d. vancomycin

25. What OTC drug was once prescription only and is used to treat allergies and hay fever?
    a. Prilosec
    b. Claritin
    c. Pepcid
    d. Aleve

Pharmacy Law and Regulation

4

Learning Objectives

- Be familiar with landmark legislation pertinent to the practice of pharmacy.
- Identify legislation that affects patient counseling, confidentiality of health records, and sale of pseudoephedrine products.
- Know the definition of a controlled drug.
- Understand the difference between drug tolerance, and psychological and physical dependence.
- Identify the classes of controlled drugs.
- Know what DEA forms are required for ordering and destroying Schedule II drugs.
- Identify three characteristics that differentiate a Schedule II prescription from other prescriptions.
- Recognize situations that may indicate potential abuse or forged prescriptions.
- Know the refill and transfer limitations for Schedule III and IV drug prescriptions.
- Understand the restrictions and legal record-keeping requirements for Schedule V medications.
- Know DEA-mandated inventory and record-keeping requirements for Schedule II, III, and IV medications.
- Be familiar with nationally recognized professional standards that affect pharmacy operations.
- Define standard of care and ethics, and apply examples to pharmacy practice.

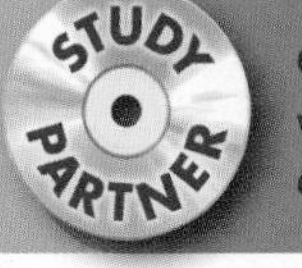

Continue your review with more than 1,000 exam-style questions.

The primary role of the pharmacy profession is to protect the health of the public. The pharmacy technician must be aware of the unique state and federal laws and regulations that further that aim. This chapter discusses special requirements for handling controlled drugs, including storage, recordkeeping, inventory control, safety, and abuse potential. It also outlines the professional standards for products, services, and personal behavior.

Law and the Pharmacy Technician

The practice of pharmacy is governed by numerous laws and regulations. The pharmacy technician needs to be familiar with these laws and regulations and their effect on issues such as patient privacy, product and patient information, and medication disposal.

Laws are created by the legislative branches of government (i.e., Congress and state legislatures). A regulation is a written rule with procedures that dictate how a law should be implemented. For example, Food and Drug Administration (FDA) regulations govern the approval process for new drugs and dictate when pharmacies must provide consumers medication guides for high-risk drugs. Drug Enforcement Agency (DEA) rules spell out procedures for ordering and dispensing controlled drugs, and the Center for Medicare and Medicaid Services regulates Medicare Part D prescriptions (discussed in Chapter 10).

Federal laws and regulations play an important role in pharmacy practice and are one of nine knowledge areas covered on the new Pharmacy Technician Certification Board (PTCB) exam. Several federal laws and regulations are discussed in detail in this chapter. Other areas of regulation, including those governing proper drug storage, hygiene, and infection control, are covered in subsequent chapters.

In addition to DEA laws and regulations governing the dispensing, inventory, and sale of controlled drugs (covered in depth later in the chapter), pharmacy technicians must be familiar with federal laws governing patient counseling, privacy, and the sale of over-the-counter (OTC) products containing pseudoephedrine.

The Omnibus Budget Reconciliation Act of 1990 (OBRA-90) mandated that pharmacies offer patient counseling to all patients on federally or state-funded programs. Private insurers adopted this policy and it has become the "standard of care" in all U.S. community pharmacies. The Health Insurance Portability and Accountability Act (HIPAA) is responsible for ensuring the confidentiality of all health records, including pharmacy, under penalty of law. The Methamphetamine Control Act contains provisions regarding the sale of over-the-counter products that contain pseudoephedrine, which can be used in the production of methamphetamine. The pharmacist can dispense only limited quantities of these OTC decongestant products and must assess and document their legitimate use.

Rather than present a lengthy review of all of the applicable laws and regulations, Table 4.1 lists the most pertinent points from federal law that are likely to appear on the certification exam.

TABLE 4.1 Timeline of Pharmacy-Related Federal Laws

Law	Year Passed	Significance to Pharmacy Practice
Pure Food and Drug Act	1906	first law to regulate the development, compounding, distribution, storage, and dispensing of drugs; no false or misleading information on label about drug strength or purity; no interstate transport or sale of adulterated or misbranded food or drugs
Food, Drug, and Cosmetic Act (FDCA)	1938	clearly defined adulteration and misbranding; created the federal Food and Drug Administration (FDA); required that products be safe for human use
Durham-Humphrey Amendments to FDCA	1951	distinguished between prescription (legend) and nonprescription drugs; required that all drug products have adequate usage directions or bear the legend "Caution: Federal Law Prohibits without Prescription"; allowed verbal prescription and refill requests to pharmacies by telephone
Kefauver-Harris Amendment to FDCA	1962	requires that drugs be not only safe but effective; requires that pharmaceutical manufacturers file an Investigational New Drug Application (INDA) before starting clinical trials on human subjects

TABLE 4.1 Timeline of Pharmacy-Related Federal Laws *(continued)*

Law	Year Passed	Significance to Pharmacy Practice
Comprehensive Drug Abuse Prevention and Control Act (Controlled Substances Act)	1970	established the federal Drug Enforcement Agency (DEA); created a schedule of drugs that has the potential for abuse and/or addiction and categorized them into five classes
Poison Prevention Packaging Act	1970	requires child-resistant containers for most prescription and over-the-counter (OTC) drugs to prevent accidental ingestion and poisoning.
Drug Listing Act	1972	requires National Drug Code (NDC) numbers be assigned to every marketed drug
Orphan Drug Act	1983	provides tax incentives for developing and marketing drugs used to treat rare conditions (orphan drugs); established life-long exclusive license for manufacturers that develop orphan drugs
Drug Price Competition and Patent Term Restoration Act	1984	streamlined the FDA approval process for marketing generic drugs; extends the term of patents for companies that develop new drugs
Prescription Drug Marketing Act	1987	prohibits the re-importation of drugs to the United States, except by the manufacturer
Anabolic Steroid Control Act	1990	redefined anabolic steroids as Schedule III controlled substances
Omnibus Budget Reconciliation Act (OBRA)	1990	requires pharmacist to engage in drug utilization reviews (DUR); requires technicians to offer patients the option of prescription counseling without charge
Dietary Supplement Health and Education Act (DSHEA)	1994	classifies herbal supplements as food products rather than drugs; prohibits manufacturers of herbs and dietary supplements from making claims that their products treat or cure any specific disease or illness
Health Insurance Portability and Accountability Act (HIPAA)	1996	addresses patient privacy concerns; allows employees to more easily move their health insurance from one job to another
Medicare Modernization Act	2003	provides a voluntary prescription drug plan for Medicare patients, for additional cost; created the health savings account (HSA)
FDA Modernization Act	2004	changed federal legend to "Rx Only"; allowed pharmacist to compound for individual patients for products not commercially available
Combat Methamphetamine Epidemic Act	2005	restricts sales of drugs used to manufacture methamphetamines, such as pseudoephedrine, ephedrine, and phenylpropanolamine, to behind the pharmacy counter; in some states, only a pharmacist may complete the sale
Patient Protection and Affordable Care Act (ACA)	2010	mandates universal health care coverage for U.S. citizens; provides catastrophic coverage for high-cost illnesses; prohibits insurers from refusing coverage to those with pre-existing conditions

Drug Enforcement Agency (DEA) Regulations

The Drug Enforcement Agency is the federal agency responsible for supervising and enforcing laws related to the use and sale of legal (and illegal) controlled substances. A controlled drug is defined as a substance that has the potential for abuse and physical or psychological dependence.

Three terms characterize the abuse potential of controlled drugs. Drug tolerance is defined as requiring higher and higher doses of a drug to achieve the desired pharmacological effect, such as pain relief or "getting high." Physical dependence occurs when a drug must be taken continuously in higher doses because of drug tolerance; if the drug is stopped, withdrawal symptoms occur. Physical dependence can occur while taking a drug that is necessary to treat a medical condition. In some cases, physical dependence can lead to addiction, which is a compulsive and uncontrollable use of a controlled drug. This type of dependence can result in drug-seeking behavior.

Psychological dependence occurs when a patient takes a controlled drug on a regular basis as a crutch or because it produces a sense of enhanced well-being, for example, a patient taking sleeping pills routinely, rather than as needed (p.r.n.). The patient fears that he or she will not be able to sleep without the medication. Many such medications interfere with normal sleep patterns if taken for several weeks and are then stopped abruptly.

Working in concert with state agencies, the DEA conducts unannounced physical inspections of pharmacies and investigates unsafe or improper prescribing and dispensing of controlled drugs. The DEA monitors the flow of controlled drugs from manufacturer to wholesaler to pharmacy to patient. Pharmacies, physicians and other prescribers, manufacturers, and wholesalers are required to register with the DEA to dispense, prescribe, produce, or distribute controlled drugs.

The DEA requires practitioners who dispense narcotic drugs used in the treatment of substance abuse (i.e., methadone clinics) to complete a separate registration annually. Suboxone (buprenorphine-naloxone) and Subutex (buprenorphine) are alternatives to methadone, used in the treatment of narcotic-addicted patients, and require a special X DEA number to dispense. Prescriptions for these drugs may be filled at the local community pharmacy. Methadone may be dispensed only for the treatment of narcotic addiction at properly licensed clinics. The hospital or community pharmacy is allowed to dispense methadone if it is prescribed for pain management.

Drug Classifications

In 1970, the federal Controlled Substances Act, as part of the Comprehensive Drug Abuse Prevention and Control Act, created a classification system for drugs that have the potential for abuse and categorized them according to medical use and the severity of the potential for abuse.

These categories, or schedules, are identified by the Roman numerals I through V (see Table 4.2). The lower the schedule number, the higher the risk of abuse. Schedule I drugs, such as heroin, are illegal and have the highest risk of abuse and dependence.

The DEA and individual states have the option to reclassify any drug that has the potential for abuse. When there is a disparity between state and federal regulation of a drug, the strictest regulation is applied. For example, many states classified carisoprodol (Soma) as a Schedule IV drug (or C-IV) before the DEA approved the change to C-IV in 2011.

Stock bottles of all controlled substances must be clearly marked with an uppercase Roman numeral with or without the uppercase letter C.

- II or C-II
- III or C-III
- IV or C-IV
- V or C-V

TABLE 4.2 Drug Schedules under the Controlled Substances Act of 1970

Schedule	Manufacturer's Label	Abuse Potential	Accepted Medical Use	Examples
Schedule I	C-I	highest potential for abuse	for research only; must have license to obtain; no accepted medical use in the United States	heroin, lysergic acid diethylamide (LSD)
Schedule II	C-II	high possibility of abuse, which can lead to severe psychological or physical dependence	dispensing severely restricted; cannot be prescribed by telephone except in an emergency or hospice; no refills on prescriptions	morphine, oxycodone, meperidine, hydromorphone, fentanyl, methylphenidate, dextroamphetamine
Schedule III	C-III	less potential for abuse and addiction than C-II	prescriptions can be refilled up to five times within six months if authorized by physician	hydrocodone with aspirin or acetaminophen, testosterone or other anabolic steroids
Schedule IV	C-IV	lower abuse potential than C-II and C-III; associated with limited physical or psychological dependence	same as for Schedule III	benzodiazepines, zolpidem, eszopictone (Lunesta), phenobarbital, carisoprodol
Schedule V	C-V	lowest abuse potential	some sold without a prescription depending on state law; if so, purchaser must be over 18 and is required to sign log and show driver's license	liquid codeine combination cough preparations, diphenoxylate/atropine

The C symbol is not required on the prescription label, but any controlled drug dispensed must include a transfer warning label that reads, "Caution: Federal law prohibits the transfer of this drug to any person other than the patient for whom it was prescribed." A controlled substance must be prescribed for a legitimate medical reason.

Schedule II

Schedule II (C-II) drugs are legally prescribed and dispensed but are carefully regulated because of the high risk for abuse and dependence. Many of the top 200 prescribed drugs are in this category, including morphine, Percocet (oxycodone-acetaminophen), OxyContin (oxycodone), Adderall (dextroamphetamine-amphetamine), and Ritalin (methylphenidate).

Schedule II drugs must be ordered and purchased by the pharmacist. The order must be submitted in triplicate on a DEA 222 form (see Figure 4.1). Some states permit electronic ordering of these drugs through a specially encrypted system, the Controlled Substance Ordering System (CSOS), administered by the DEA.

The pharmacist must verify the receipt of all Schedule II drugs, including type and quantity. Schedule II drugs must be stored in a safe or locked cabinet. Dispensing of Schedule II drugs is tightly regulated. In most pharmacies, the pharmacist is the only person allowed to dispense a Schedule II drug. In the hospital, narcotics are stored in a

FIGURE 4.1
DEA 222 Form

When ordering Schedule II controlled substances, the pharmacist must complete and sign this form.

See Reverse of PURCHASER'S Copy for Instructions | No order form may be issued for Schedule I and II substances unless a completed application form has been received, (21 CFR 1305.04). | OMB APPROVAL No. 1117-0010

TO: (Name of Supplier) | STREET ADDRESS

CITY and STATE | DATE | TO BE FILLED IN BY SUPPLIER

SUPPLIERS DEA REGISTRATION No.

LINE No.	No. of Packages	Size of Package	Name of Item	National Drug Code	Packages Shipped	Date Shipped
	TO BE FILLED IN BY PURCHASER					
1						
2						
3						
4						
5			VOID			
6						
7						
8						
9						
10						

LAST LINE COMPLETED (MUST BE 10 OR LESS) | SIGNATURE OF PURCHASER OR ATTORNEY OR AGENT

Date Issued | DEA Registration No. | Name and Address of Registrant

Schedules

Registered as a | No. of this Order Form

DEA Form -222 (Oct. 1992)

U.S. OFFICIAL ORDER FORMS - SCHEDULES I & II
DRUG ENFORCEMENT ADMINISTRATION
SUPPLIER'S Copy 1

FIGURE 4.2
Perpetual Inventory Record

A perpetual inventory record accounts for each unit of a Schedule II drug dispensed or received.

The Corner Drug Store – C-II Perpetual Log

Drug Name: *Methylphenidate 5mg Tabs* NDC: *0123-4567-10*

Prescription No.	Dispense Date	QTY Dispensed	Inventory	RPh Initials
Starting	*Inventory*	-----	*380*	-----
2001415	*01/22/20XX*	*−30*	*350*	*JPS*
2001423	*02/07/20XX*	*−90*	*260*	*RJA*
INV. 55874	*02/08/20XX*	*+200*	*460*	*RJA*
2001439	*02/10/20XX*	*−120*	*340*	*CA*
2001445	*02/15/20XX*	*−30*		
2001452	*02/27/20XX*			

locked unit at the nursing station. Access is limited to a nurse with the appropriate key or lock code.

In both community and hospital pharmacies, each dosage unit of a Schedule II drug must be accounted for by a manual, perpetual, or computerized inventory record (see Figure 4.2). A shortage of a Schedule II drug triggers an immediate investigation. Automated dispensing machine stations (i.e., Pyxis) automatically update inventory anytime a drug is dispensed.

The technician must review every prescription carefully for completeness and authenticity, and especially prescriptions for Schedule II drugs (discussed in Chapter 8).

A prescription for a Schedule II drug must be complete, written in indelible black ink, and signed by the prescribing physician. There may be no alterations. The pharmacist should recognize the prescriber's signature. The date on the prescription is important; some states limit the amount of time a Schedule II prescription is valid (e.g., from 72 hours to 30 days). No refills are allowed on Schedule II drugs, and most pharmacies are not allowed to store or file such prescriptions for future use.

Prescriptions for Schedule II drugs are the most commonly forged prescriptions. The pharmacy technician must be vigilant in reviewing narcotics prescriptions. It is not uncommon for a forged prescription to be presented by a new, supposedly out-of-state patient on a weekend or evening when the prescription cannot be authenticated. A patient who requests a brand name narcotic and offers to pay cash (instead of providing insurance information) should raise a red flag. Cash payment does not create a paper trail that could alert other pharmacies that receive a similar prescription. Table 4.3 provides a list of indicators that should alert the technician to check with the pharmacist.

Many children (and some adults) take methylphenidate (Ritalin, Concerta) and other stimulants such as dextroamphetamine-amphetamine salts (Adderall) daily to control attention-deficit hyperactivity disorder (ADHD). So that parents do not have to return to the pediatrician monthly for a new prescription, the DEA and most states allow the prescriber to prescribe for future use as long as the prescription includes the notation, "Do not fill until XX/XX/201X." The fill date cannot be more than 90 days from the date the prescription was written.

TABLE 4.3 Indicators of a Potentially Forged Prescription or Drug-seeking Behavior

- The prescription is altered (for example, a change in quantity).
- Prescription pads have been reported missing from local doctors' offices.
- The prescription is presented as a clever computerized fax and is not on tamper-proof safety paper.
- There are misspellings on the prescription.
- A refill is indicated for a Schedule II drug.
- A prescription from the emergency department is written for more than a #30 count or 7-day supply.
- A prescription is cut and pasted from a preprinted, signed prescription.
- A second or third prescription is added to a legal prescription written by a physician. More than one handwriting style is used.
- A patient presents a prescription containing several medications but wants the pharmacy to fill only the narcotic prescription.
- The prescription is signed with different handwriting or in different ink, or the prescription is not signed by the physician.
- The DEA number is missing, illegible, or incorrect.
- The prescription is written by an out-of-state physician or a physician practicing in an area far from the pharmacy. This event is particularly suspicious if the prescription is received at night or on the weekend, when it would be difficult to confirm the prescription.
- An individual other than the patient drops off the prescription. Pharmacy personnel should require a driver's license or other photo ID and document this information.
- A new patient specifies a brand name narcotic.
- A new patient wants to pay for the prescription with cash, even though he or she has insurance. Doing so avoids a paper trail.

Individual states may have additional regulations for Schedule II drugs. Some states allow a Schedule II prescription to be submitted by phone in an emergency, provided the prescriber mails a hard copy to the pharmacy within a specified amount of time (usually 72 hours to one week). The pharmacist must verify the authenticity of the prescriber's DEA number (see Chapter 2), reduce the verbal order to writing, and document the nature of the emergency on the back of the prescription. Some states also allow prescribers to order a Schedule II prescription for a hospice patient via fax or phone; most pharmacies treat this situation as an emergency and require the prescriber to mail a hard copy of the prescription within a week.

In the pharmacy, all prescriptions for Schedule II drugs must be filed separately from other prescriptions and must be readily retrievable. Each prescription must be signed and dated by the pharmacist. Federal law requires pharmacies to keep Schedule II prescriptions for a minimum of two years; state laws may require such prescriptions be kept on file for up to five years. In practice, most pharmacies keep all prescription records indefinitely for legal reasons.

Schedule III–IV

Schedule III and Schedule IV (C-III and C-IV) medications have less risk for abuse and dependence than Schedule II drugs, but the risk is clearly present, especially if these medications are used in high doses over a long period of time. The number one drug dispensed in community pharmacies is a combination of hydrocodone with acetaminophen (Lortab, Lorcet, and Vicodin).

Unlike Schedule II drugs, prescriptions for Schedule III and Schedule IV drugs can be refilled, but the DEA places limitations on these medications because of the potential for abuse and dependence. Prescriptions for these drugs can be refilled a maximum of five times, and refills must be dispensed within six months from the original date of the prescription.

The DEA also limits the transfer of Schedule III and Schedule IV medications between pharmacies. Patients may request the transfer of a prescription to another pharmacy for convenience, during a vacation, or if the patient has a second home in another community. In most states, only the pharmacist can legally transfer a prescription for a controlled drug. A patient may request that the receiving pharmacy call to request the transfer from the pharmacy that holds the hard copy of the prescription.

To minimize the possibility of abuse, a prescription for a Schedule III or Schedule IV drug that has been transferred to another pharmacy can only be transferred one time. The patient cannot refill the prescription at the original pharmacy but must request a new prescription from the prescriber. In transferring a prescription for a Schedule III or Schedule IV drug, the originating pharmacy must close the patient profile drug so that no additional refills can be obtained from that location. Documentation must include the name and phone number of the receiving pharmacy and the receiving pharmacist, as well as the DEA numbers of both pharmacies.

Prescriptions for Schedule III and Schedule IV drugs are less likely to be forged than Schedule II drugs, but are more likely to be refilled early. The pharmacy technician must review the date of the last refill and the days' supply. For example, a prescription for "Lorcet Plus #90 with Sig: 1 tab PO t.i.d. p.r.n." written on November 1, should last until around December 1. If the patient tries to refill the prescription on November 20th, the technician may have to tell the patient that the prescription cannot be refilled early. Each pharmacy has a policy regarding how far in advance (usually 24 to 48 hours) it will provide refills of Schedule III and Schedule IV drugs.

Schedule III and Schedule IV drugs do not have to be kept in a safe or locked cabinet and are generally stored with the inventory of nonscheduled drugs. No special DEA forms are needed to order or dispose of Schedule III and Schedule IV drugs, and a senior pharmacy technician may be responsible for ordering them. The pharmacist is often responsible for verifying and signing for the receipt of all Schedule III and Schedule IV drugs; these signed inventory receipts are kept on file.

After a prescription is filled for a Schedule III or Schedule IV medication, most pharmacies file the hard-copy prescription separately from both Schedule II and other non-controlled medications. Prescriptions must be readily accessible for inspection. If not separated from other prescriptions, Schedule III and Schedule IV prescriptions must be marked for easy identification with a large (at least 1 inch high) red C for control in the lower right corner.

Schedule V

These drugs have the lowest potential for abuse and dependence and include cough syrups that contain codeine (such as Cheracol or Robitussin AC), as well as diphenoxylate (Lomotil) for diarrhea, and pregabalin (Lyrica) for neuropathic pain.

Some states—and many pharmacies—require a prescription to dispense these medications. Insurance companies will not cover the cost of these medications without a prescription. Schedule V prescriptions are generally filed with the prescriptions for Schedule III and Schedule IV drugs for easy retrieval.

Federal law and many states allow pharmacists to dispense a Schedule V drug without a prescription if certain restrictions and record-keeping requirements are met. Restrictions for the sale of Schedule V medications include:

- Drugs must be stored behind the counter in the prescription area.
- The amount of cough syrup sold to a single customer is generally limited to a specific volume (such as 120 mL or 4 fl oz) within a 48-hour period.
- Only the pharmacist (or the pharmacy technician under direct supervision) can make the sale.
- The purchaser must be 18 years of age or older and have proof of identity.

If the state allows sale of Schedule V drugs without a prescription, it is the legal responsibility of the pharmacy technician or pharmacist to record all sales in a record book or computerized database and include the following information:

- name and address of the purchaser
- date of birth of the purchaser
- date of purchase
- name of the drug and quantity sold
- name and initials of the pharmacist handling or approving the sale

Controlled Drug Inventory

The DEA requires that all pharmacies complete a biennial (every two years) inventory that includes an exact count of all Schedule II drugs and an estimate of other controlled drugs. If a container designed to hold 1,000 doses or more has been opened, an exact count is necessary. The inventory record must contain the following information for each controlled medication:

- name of the drug
- dosage form and strength
- number of dosage units or volume in each container
- number of containers

Many community pharmacies have a policy or are subject to state law requiring them to perform an exact inventory of all Schedule II drugs monthly or according to some other regular schedule. In the hospital, inventories of narcotics are conducted at the start of each nursing shift, typically three times per day, or perpetually if an automated drug dispensing system is in use. Inventories of Schedule III and Schedule IV drugs are checked at least annually in most community and hospital pharmacies.

Disposal or destruction of any Schedule II drug must be recorded on a DEA 41 form and witnessed and signed by another pharmacist. Expired drugs and broken dosage units are generally saved until the next visit by a state drug inspector or until the pharmacist travels to a licensed destruction center. Disposal records must contain the following information:

- pharmacy DEA number, name, and address
- reverse distributor's DEA number, name, and address
- number of units (in finished forms and/or commercial containers) disposed of and the manner of disposal

Two copies of the form must be sent to the local DEA branch and one copy should be retained by the pharmacy for at least two years. The disposal record must be dated to reflect when the product was sent for destruction.

State Laws

In addition to knowledge of federal law, the pharmacy technician must be cognizant of state laws and regulations. Each state has a board of pharmacy, which is responsible for overseeing the practice of various professions, including pharmacy, within its state borders. Each state has different laws and regulations that affect the practice of pharmacy.

The pharmacy technician is responsible for registering annually with the state board of pharmacy (required in most states) and fulfilling all continuing education (CE) requirements. The state board of pharmacy may also require technicians to pass a certification exam within a certain period of time. If the technician is practicing in a specialty area such as sterile or nonsterile compounding or nuclear pharmacy, additional training and certification is required. In most states, the pharmacy technician may legally perform the following duties:

- dispensing medication, recordkeeping, pricing, and billing
- preparing doses of a premanufactured product
- compounding sterile and nonsterile medications according to protocol
- customer service for prescriptions
- transporting medications to patient care units in the hospital
- checking and replenishing drug inventory

In all practice locations, however, all duties must be carried out under the direct supervision of a licensed pharmacist. Some states may allow the technician to perform additional responsibilities, such as taking telephone refill requests from prescribers or assisting in drawing up medications for vaccine administration. It is important that you know what the state board of pharmacy allows. In some states, certified pharmacy technicians are allowed to check the work of other technicians, called "tech-check-tech."

Professional Standards

In addition to federal and state laws and regulations, the pharmacy technician is expected to observe accepted "standards of care" and ethical standards in carrying out his or her duties and responsibilities. A standard is a criteria established to measure product quality or professional performance against a norm. Standards exist for both drug products and professional behavior. The United States Pharmacopeia (USP) sets standards for compounding sterile and nonsterile products as well as standards for drug manufacturing. The Joint Commission (JC) establishes standards for hospital accreditation.

Standard of care is a legal term for the accepted level of care healthcare providers are expected to provide. When used to judge the quality or level of care provided to a patient, standard of care is measured against the actions of other healthcare professionals in the same situation; existing written guidelines, training programs, protocols, or policies and procedures; and expert testimony of health professionals provided by the plaintiff or the defense. If the standard of care was not met, and a patient was harmed as a result, a medical negligence lawsuit may result. OBRA-90, the federal law that requires all community pharmacies to offer patient counseling on prescriptions is an example of a standard of care.

When determining the appropriate standard of care, two criteria are considered: the level of training of the healthcare provider, and what is considered normal practice for the geographic area in which the healthcare provider works. A pharmacy technician would not be held to the same standard as a pharmacist unless the technician failed to follow proper procedure. The pharmacist is responsible for checking the pharmacy technician's work, so it is unlikely that a technician would be held liable if proper procedures were not followed. If a technician knowingly oversteps his or her role without the knowledge of the supervising pharmacist, the technician could be held liable. For example, if a technician performed a function not permitted under state or federal regulation—overriding an allergy or drug interaction alert or counseling a patient—that resulted in direct harm to the patient, the technician could be subject to a lawsuit and possible termination.

Ethics is the study of standards of conduct and moral judgment that defines the right or wrong of human conduct and character. Ethics is a process for reflection and analysis of behavior when the proper course of action is unclear. It is the basis on which to make judgments.

Many ethical dilemmas confront healthcare professionals in their daily activities. For example, some pharmacists and technicians have reservations about dispensing birth control, the "morning after pill," or other medication to terminate a pregnancy. Another ethical dilemma may involve post-dating drug insurance claims to "help out a patient." The "right" or "wrong" in situations such as these is a matter of individual conscience (rather than federal or state law) but must not be resolved to the detriment of patient care. If a pharmacist or technician is not comfortable dispensing a medication to terminate a pregnancy (or a potential pregnancy), there must be an alternative plan in place: Another staff member may dispense the drug and counsel the patient or the patient may be referred to another local pharmacy.

Skills Quiz

Reflect on the information presented in the chapter by answering the following questions.

1. A patient presents two prescriptions from a dentist, one for penicillin and the other for Vicodin 5/500. The patient wants to fill only the Vicodin prescription and will pay cash. You should
   a. update the patient profile, delete insurance information, and fill the prescription.
   b. give back the penicillin prescription and fill the Vicodin prescription.
   c. recognize the patient may be interested in the controlled substance alone and notify the pharmacist and dentist.
   d. fill both prescriptions, billing the patient's insurance, and dispense both to the patient.

2. A patient submits a handwritten prescription for morphine 15 mg #120, Sig: i PO q.i.d. p.r.n. pain, with two refills. All the physician information is correct, including the DEA number. What about this prescription raises questions?
   a. the quantity of morphine
   b. the number of refills
   c. the strength of the morphine
   d. the directions being p.r.n.

3. A patient picked up a new prescription for clonazepam 0.5 mg #90, Sig: i PO t.i.d. for anxiety on February 12. She is back on March 2 and wants a refill. You tell her that
   a. it is too early; the prescription cannot be refilled before March 12.
   b. the prescription has expired.
   c. you need to talk to the pharmacist and get approval to refill.
   d. you need to wait to fill it until the insurance will pay for the refill.

4. The pharmacist has asked you to collect all the outdated controlled substances and prepare them for destruction. What form will you need to fill out for an expired box of fentanyl patches?
   a. DEA 222 form
   b. CSOS
   c. DEA 41 form
   d. perpetual inventory

5. A community pharmacy may fill a methadone prescription as long as
   a. the prescriber's X DEA number is on the prescription.
   b. the patient is being treated for pain.
   c. the patient is being treated for heroin addiction.
   d. the medication is being used for drug tolerance.

6. The DEA differentiates the classes of controlled substances by the amount of
   a. abuse and dependence potential.
   b. abuse and cost.
   c. street value and drug-seeking potential.
   d. acetaminophen content and dependence potential.

7. An order arrives from the wholesaler containing a tote with C-II substances. The proper procedure for receiving includes
   a. signing the driver receipt of tote and storing the medication.
   b. storing the drugs in the safe and filing the invoice in the appropriate file.
   c. storing the drugs in inventory, signing receipt of tote, and filing invoice.
   d. signing receipt for driver, opening tote, and verifying content with invoice and DEA 222 form.

8. How often does the DEA require an inventory of all controlled substances?
   a. biennially
   b. annually
   c. twice per year
   d. three times per year

9. A patient submits a prescription for Robitussin AC. You should
   a. sell the patient a bottle from stock since it is a Schedule V, if your state law does not require a prescription.
   b. sell the patient a bottle of OTC Mucinex DM, as it does the same thing and is cheaper.
   c. counsel the patient about the abuse potential of the drug and encourage him or her not to fill the prescription.
   d. fill the prescription in the usual manner using the patient's insurance to bill for the medication.

10. A pharmacist in Florida contacts your pharmacy in Georgia and asks to transfer a patient's prescription for diazepam 10 mg with 5 refills. This prescription
    a. cannot be transferred because it is a controlled drug.
    b. can be transferred twice.
    c. can be transferred back to Georgia once the patient returns from vacation.
    d. voids all remaining refills if the prescription is transferred to Florida.

Thinking Beyond the Exam

The pharmacy technician has significant responsibilities when it comes to preparing a prescription for a controlled substance. You receive a prescription with one of the following issues. What would you do?

- The signature of a well-known doctor looks somewhat different than it has in the past.
- The prescription appears to be a well-manufactured or faxed copy.
- The quantity appears to have been altered.
- The prescriber's DEA number is missing.

Sterile and Nonsterile Compounding

5

Learning Objectives

- Understand the requirements for infection control, including hand washing, hand hygiene, and personal protective equipment.
- Define the role of OSHA and the NRC in the protection of healthcare workers.
- Understand the basic requirements for handling and disposing of pharmaceutical waste.
- Know the documentation requirements for sterile and nonsterile compounding.
- Determine product stability including beyond-use dating and signs of incompatibility.
- Identify the equipment and supplies for sterile and nonsterile compounding.
- Know how to use and maintain the equipment used in compounding.
- Discuss USP guidelines for sterile and nonsterile compounding processes.

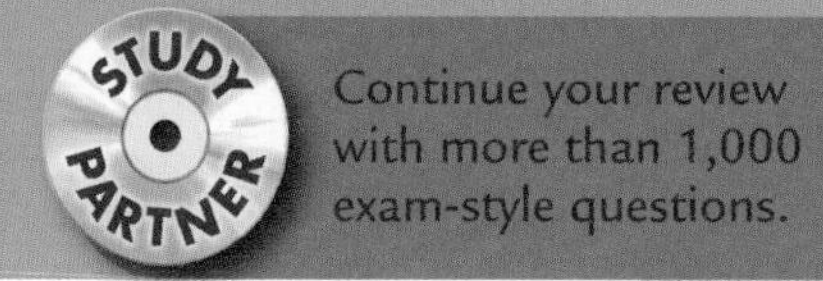

Sterile and nonsterile compounding make up the third knowledge domain covered on the revised PTCB exam. This domain also includes information on worker and patient safety, waste disposal, documentation requirements, product stability, and compounding equipment and facilities.

The practice of pharmacy today uses a high percentage of manufactured products dispensed directly to the patient. However, there are situations which require specially trained pharmacy personnel to prepare both sterile and nonsterile extemporaneous compounds pursuant to a prescription. Pharmacy technicians working in both community and institutional pharmacies need the knowledge and skills to ensure that compounding is performed according to strict regulations, and in a manner that ensures patient and worker safety.

Infection Control

The Food and Drug Administration (FDA) defines compounding as extemporaneous combining, mixing, or altering of ingredients by a pharmacist in response to a physician's prescription to create a medication tailored to the specialized medical needs of an individual patient. Following established guidelines ensures a

TABLE 5.1 USP Good Compounding Practices

Component	Standards
Facility	designated area with low traffic flow and adequate space for working and equipment storage
Personnel	compounding staff trained and proficient in the skills necessary to compound drugs and maintain equipment
Equipment	must be maintained and calibrated for accurate compounding and adequate for the products being compounded
Ingredient selection	USP/National Formulary-quality ingredients stored and used appropriately
Compounding	periodic and final check by the pharmacist process
Packaging and storage	product-appropriate containers that meet storage requirements for the product
Beyond-use dating	stability of preparation after compounding calculated by ingredients and dosage form
Controls	quality assurance programs established to guarantee equipment, staff, and product quality
Labeling of excess product	ingredients, lot, compound date, beyond-use date, and compounder information
Records and reports	records of ingredients, personnel, and equipment for compounding an individual product as well as for all the ingredients and equipment used for compounding processes
Patient counseling	patient education by the pharmacist to ensure appropriate use and storage of the medication

high-grade product. Quality-control measures, documentation, and recordkeeping are all important to ensure that professional standards are met.

When a product is compounded, whether sterile or nonsterile, it should be free of contamination and pathogens (an infectious agent, such as a virus or bacteria, that causes disease or illness to its host). To achieve this, a technician should be familiar with good compounding practices (GCP) outlined in United States Pharmacopeia (USP) and outlined in brief in Table 5.1. USP Chapter <795> discusses nonsterile compounding practices. USP Chapter <797> covers sterile compounding.

Hand Hygiene and Hand Washing

Basic hand washing is performed by healthcare workers at regular intervals including after eating, after using the rest room, and before and after caring for a patient. Hand washing prevents contamination of pharmaceutical products and transfer of pathogens to patients or equipment. Such contamination may compromise the health and recovery of patients in both inpatient and outpatient settings. Table 5.2 describes the accepted techniques for basic hand washing.

Example 5.1

While delivering medications to a patient care unit at the hospital, a nurse withdraws heparin from a vial for a subcutaneous dose. She washes her hands using an alcohol-based hand gel, an acceptable alternative to soap and water. Why is it important to clean hands before compounding or administering medication?

TABLE 5.2 Basic Hand Washing Techniques

Wet hands with warm water (avoid hot water; repeated exposure may increase the risk of hand irritation) and apply soap as recommended by the manufacturer.
Rub hands together vigorously for 20 to 30 seconds, covering all areas of hands and fingers.
Rinse hands with water.
Dry thoroughly with a disposable towel.
Use towel to turn off the faucet.

As long as hands are not visibly dirty, alcohol-based gels are an acceptable alternative to washing with soap and water. This is referred to as hand hygiene. Specially formulated gels have antimicrobial activity, are quick drying, and are available in convenient locations throughout institutions. Hand gels do not replace the need for periodic hand washing.

Both hand washing and hand hygiene minimize the transmission of infectious agents and are effective techniques for preventing touch contamination, the most common source of infection.

Aseptic Hand Washing

Pharmacy personnel who prepare compounded sterile preparations (CSP) must undertake a more thorough type of hand washing referred to as aseptic hand washing. In aseptic hand washing, IV technicians wash their arms (up to the elbow) and hands using an appropriate antimicrobial agent and following a specific sequence. Special attention should be paid to areas that harbor multiple microorganisms, such as under the fingernails and in the creases of skin. Proper aseptic hand washing takes a minimum of 30 seconds, and more commonly, two to four minutes to complete. To become proficient at aseptic hand washing, technicians need to practice the steps until the process becomes second nature. Learning this process is critical because the most common source of contamination in the preparation of parenteral products is touch contamination by a healthcare worker who has not practiced correct aseptic technique in hand washing. Sterile compounding technicians need to know not only the aseptic hand-washing process but also the circumstances under which the process must be performed or repeated. The following situations require the completion of aseptic hand washing:

- when first entering the sterile compounding area
- when reentering the sterile compounding area
- after eating
- after using the rest room
- after sneezing or coughing
- after a major contamination, such as a needle stick or a drug spill with a volume greater than 5 mL
- after the hands touch any item that is obviously contaminated, such as the floor, the waste receptacle or sharps container, or a visibly soiled item

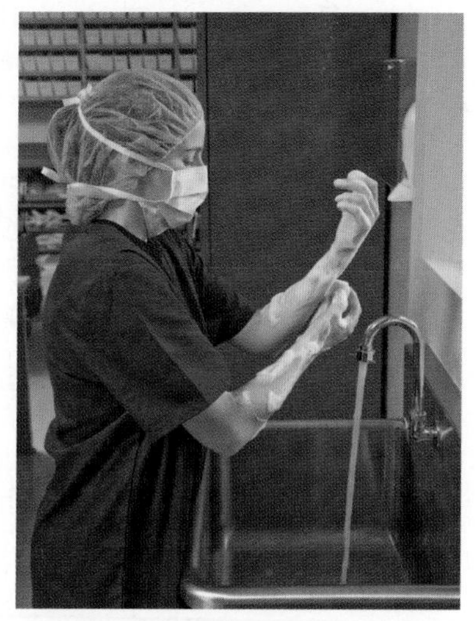

Aseptic hand washing is an important step in preventing touch contamination, the leading cause of contaminated parenteral products.

Personal Protective Equipment

The United States Pharmacopia (USP) has adopted the strict guidelines established by the Centers for Disease Control and Prevention (CDC) for protective garb worn by anyone involved in the manufacture of compounded sterile products (CSPs). The guidelines specify that individuals put on protective foot booties, a head covering, a gown, and a mask, in that order, in the anteroom. The gown must be clean, disposable, and nonshedding, with arms that fit snugly around the wrist. Goggles are recommended when making hazardous CSPs. Table 5.3 lists the required order of the steps for cleansing and garbing.

TABLE 5.3 CSP Garbing and Hand Washing

In the Anteroom
Remove all personal outer garments (i.e., sweaters, jackets)
Remove jewelry from hands, wrists, or other visible body parts
No artificial nails, nail polish, cosmetics, or perfume are permitted
Put on PPE, in the following order:
Shoe covers
Hair cover
Face mask (beard cover, if applicable)
Perform aseptic hand washing procedures
Nonshedding gown
In the Buffer Area or Clean Room
Apply foamed, sterile, 70% isopropyl alcohol antiseptic hand cleanser
Don sterile, powder-free gloves

Example 5.2

Today is the first day of training in the clean room. The instructor tells students to go to the anteroom to don aseptic garb and perform an aseptic hand washing. What personal protective equipment (PPE) should be worn when compounding sterile preparations?

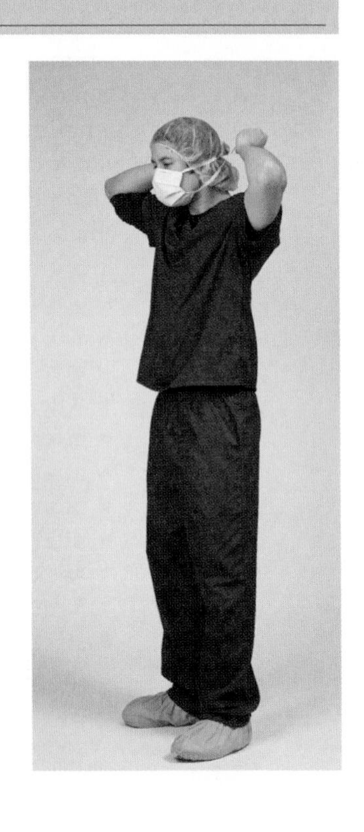

Universal Precaution

Universal precaution refers to the manner in which healthcare professionals, caregivers, and those who render first aid provide patient care in a safe manner that prevents the transmission of pathogens from blood or other body fluids. Healthcare workers should adopt universal precautions to protect themselves and others against infection. Universal precaution assumes any patient may carry an infectious pathogen.

Universal precautions include:

- washing hands before and after rendering patient care
- wearing gloves when handling bodily fluids
- wearing personal protective equipment (PPE), which may include a gown, eye protection and a facemask
- Proper disposal of all potentially infected nonreusable medical supplies in an appropriate biohazard container
- never recapping a hypodermic needles that have been used in patient treatment or medication administration, and use safety needles whenever possible
- disposing of sharps in the appropriate puncture-resistant container

Bloodborne and other infectious pathogens are not transmitted through normal social contact, such as shaking hands, drinking from a water fountain, or sitting on a toilet seat. A bloodborne pathogen is a microorganism capable of causing disease when transmitted from one individual to another through contact with contaminated blood. Pathogens may also be transmitted via other bodily fluids, such as saliva, semen, and sputum. Tuberculosis and pneumonia are examples of a pathogen transmitted by sputum. Table 5.4 lists possible transmission routes for bacteria, viruses, fungi, and other pathogens.

The most common bloodborne pathogens found in the healthcare setting are HIV/AIDs and hepatitis B. Other pathogens that can be bloodborne include hepatitis C, viral hemorrhagic fever, syphilis, and Creutzfeldt-Jakob disease.

All healthcare providers, including pharmacy technicians, should use universal precautions to protect themselves, other healthcare workers, and patients from the transmission of infectious pathogens.

TABLE 5.4 Pathogen Transmission

Transmission Paths
Needlestick injuries
Sharing hypodermic needles and syringes
Medical devices, such as scalpels and suture needles
Open wounds and skin abrasions
Blood and blood-product transfusions that have not been properly screened and tested
Transmitting Fluids
Seminal
Vaginal
Synovial
Pleural
Peritoneal
Pericardial
Amniotic
Cerebrospinal

Needle Safety

Universal precautions emphasize the importance of proper needle handling. During the compounding process, the technician should be careful to prevent cross contamination of products, contamination of ingredients, and needlesticks. Universal precautions specify that needles that are use in the patient care setting should not be recapped, and should instead, be placed uncapped into a puncture-proof sharps container. However, sterile compounding personnel are often required to perform compounding functions that require them to recap needles. Although there is no risk of exposure to patient blood or fluids during compounding, a needlestick could contaminate the final product with the healthcare worker's blood. If a needlestick occurs during compounding, the parenteral should be discarded and remixed once the wound is treated and covered. Follow the institution's policy and procedures for treating and reporting a needlestick.

When multiple vials of pharmaceuticals are compounded for medium- to high-risk parenterals, a different needle and syringe should be used for each vial. Total parenteral nutrition (TPN) is an example of a type of large volume parenteral that a pharmacy technician may be asked to compound. Multi-dose vials may be used to compound more than one TPN. Cross-contamination compromises the sterility of the final product.

In addition to cross-contamination, the pharmacy technician should also be aware that some ingredients when added together in high concentration will precipitate. For example, if calcium gluconate and potassium phosphate are added together or mixed into a TPN without proper dilution, a precipitant will form and white particles will be seen in the final product.

Two other sources of contamination are touch and aspiration of sputum. Touch contamination is the leading cause of pathogen transmission. In addition to the use of aseptic hand washing, antiseptic hand sanitizer, and sterile gloves to prevent contamination, the pharmacy technician needs to be proficient in needle and syringe manipulation to avoid touching the needle, syringe tip, or syringe plunger and potentially transmitting pathogens such as bacteria, viruses, or fungi from fingers, hands, and work surfaces. Wearing a face mask prevents expectorated sputum that may be expelled while talking or coughing from contaminating the compounding area.

Protecting Healthcare Workers

Pharmacists and pharmacy technicians need to be aware of, and adequately protected from, any potential side effects resulting from the preparation of hazardous substances or radiopharmaceuticals. A technician who is pregnant or may become pregnant should not count (or prepare) cancer chemotherapy drugs, including methotrexate (also used for rheumatoid arthritis), or drugs such as isotretinoin (Accutane) or finasteride (Proscar), due to the potential risk to the fetus.

Certain areas of the hospital utilize additional PPE, such as fitted respirators in respiratory isolation settings, chemical resistant garb and gloves for compounding and administering chemotherapeutic agents to cancer patients, lead-lined aprons and protection barriers for radiologic areas, and gowns, gloves, head coverings and masks in the operating suite or units with infectious patients.

The Occupational Safety and Health Administration (OSHA) and the Nuclear Regulatory Commission (NRC) both have regulations to minimize exposure to hazardous chemicals and radioactive materials that can adversely impact the short- and long-term health of pharmacists and technicians.

OSHA is the federal agency primarily responsible for ensuring employee health and safety in the workplace. In the field of pharmacy, OSHA establishes policies and requires training to prevent inadvertent needlesticks and the safe disposal of syringes to prevent the transmission of communicable diseases such as HIV/AIDS and hepatitis. Specially designed sharps containers are frequently used for the safe disposal of syringes and needles.

Hazardous Substances

In the hospital and in compounding pharmacies, OSHA establishes policies to protect pharmacists and technicians from unnecessary exposure to hazardous substances, such as cytotoxic drugs that can produce acute, chronic, and long-term effects when inhaled, ingested, or through contact with exposed skin. Adverse effects may include allergic skin rashes and an increased risk of cancer. In women of childbearing age, exposure may result in an increased risk of infertility, spontaneous abortions, low birth weight infants, and congenital birth defects.

USP Chapter <797> regulations require anyone handling or preparing hazardous agents, including chemotherapy drugs, to don protective garb and utilize special equipment and technique during the preparation of hazardous agents. In addition to standard shoe covers, hair cover, and face mask, personnel who compound hazardous agents must also don goggles, a gown made of impervious material, and must double glove. Upon completion of compounding activities, garb must be disposed of in a special hazardous waste container. In addition to protective clothing and good sterile techniques, compounding must be done in a biological safety cabinet (BSC) or compounding aseptic containment isolator (CACI) which filters potentially hazardous air away from the worker in order to minimize worker exposure.

USP Chapter <797> and OSHA regulations require that hazardous agent spills be dealt with immediately. Every hazardous substance has a Material Safety Data Sheet (MSDS), which outlines specific recommendations for responding to a hazardous exposure. Pharmacies that compound hazardous agents are required to have immediate access to a sink and an eye wash kit. Eyes or skin should be thoroughly flushed with water to dilute any contaminating substance.

Hazardous spill cleanup or decontamination should be undertaken using a spill kit while wearing full protective clothing. Use absorbent towels provided in the spill kit to clean up the spill from the outside edge and work inward. Pick up broken glass with care. Never use bare hands. Cleanup materials and protective clothing should be properly disposed of in labeled hazardous waste containers.

Radioactive Material

The federal Nuclear Regulatory Commission (NRC) regulates the medical use of radioactive materials to minimize radiation exposure to patients and medical staff. Radioactive materials may be used for diagnostic (e.g., imaging the thyroid gland) or therapeutic (e.g., cancer treatment) purposes. Directly and through agreements with state agencies, the NRC oversees the medical use of radioactive materials through licensing, inspection, investigation, and enforcement programs. The NRC licenses facilities, authorizes individuals to administer radioactive materials, and develops appropriate regulations and guidance for their handling and use.

This specialty field of practice is called nuclear medicine or nuclear pharmacy. Drugs that contain a small amount of radioactive material are called radiopharmaceuticals. A nuclear pharmacy technician works under the direct supervision of a nuclear pharmacist and receives special training and education on radiation safety.

Individuals authorized to handle radioactive materials must wear protective garments to reduce radiation exposure, and follow strict guidelines with regard to the receipt, handling, disposition, disposal, and transfer of radioactive materials. To avoid exposure to radiation, nuclear pharmacists do most of their hands-on work in contained workstations with lead glass screens and gloved ports.

Exposure to a small amount of radiation, like an X-ray, is not harmful. Pharmacists, technicians, and others working in a nuclear pharmacy wear monitoring badges and their exposure is monitored on a weekly, monthly, quarterly, annual, and lifetime basis. USP Chapter <823> provides further guidance for pharmacy personnel who prepare radiopharmaceuticals.

Waste Handling and Disposal

The discovery of residual pharmaceuticals in the surface, ground, and drinking water in the United States has raised concern about the environmental consequences of inappropriate disposal of pharmaceutical waste. Small concentrations of drugs can have detrimental effects on aquatic species and, potentially, on human health and development.

A pharmacy technician must be aware of disposal requirements for individual pharmaceuticals based on the employer's policy and procedures. The U.S. Environmental Protection Agency (EPA) and state governments monitor pharmaceutical waste disposal.

Example 5.3

Outside the pharmacy door there is a pool of red liquid; it may be blood. You call environmental services to help with the cleanup but to contain the liquid you cover it with absorbent towels. Where should the towels be disposed?

In healthcare institutions, many items can become contaminated with blood and other bodily fluids. Items that cannot be sterilized become biological waste. Proper disposal of contaminated items is important. Biological waste must be disposed of in a red bucket or bag clearly labeled "biohazard." Some institutions use red bags for disposal of contaminated sheets or towels. Sharp items such as needles or glass should only be disposed of in hard-sided containers called sharps containers.

During the admixture and administration of chemotherapy, any unadministered medication left in the IV bags and tubing, bottles, and vials must be disposed of in a hazardous waste container with a yellow label identifying it as hazardous waste.

Although chemotherapy agents provide substantial benefit to the patient, they pose a potential health risk to healthcare workers and others who may be exposed to them. Precautions should always be used when dealing with chemotherapy pharmaceuticals.

Should a "chemo spill" occur, retrieve a spill kit without delay. Table 5.5 lists the contents of a typical spill kit. Table 5.6 outlines proper handling and cleanup procedures in the event of a spill. The goal is to safely prepare chemotherapeutic agents while minimizing the hazard to all.

TABLE 5.5 Spill Kit Contents

- Two pairs of nitrile disposable gloves
- Pair of safety goggles
- Disposable shoe covers
- Respirator mask
- Tongs and/or forceps or dustpan and hand broom for picking up broken glass or other contaminated sharps
- Nonabsorbent gown
- Absorbent towels
- All-purpose disinfectant, such as normal household bleach (diluted 1 to 10)
- A copy of the spill cleanup protocol
- Sharps hazardous waste container(s)
- Biohazardous spill warning signs

TABLE 5.6 Proper Chemotherapy Handling and Cleanup Procedures

Proper Handling
Follow the institution's policy and procedure when handling chemotherapy drugs.
Always work under a vertical laminar airflow hood or in a glove box vented to the outside of the facility when preparing cytotoxic drugs.
Don PPE appropriate for working with hazardous agents.
Use chemotherapy venting pins in preparing chemotherapeutic medications.
Maintain negative vial pressure throughout compounding procedures to avoid aspiration. Do not fill syringe to more than 75% of maximum capacity to avoid dislodging the syringe plunger from the barrel.
If gloves are punctured, torn, or have some breach of integrity, change them immediately.
Know the location of a hazardous waste cleanup kit (spill kit) in the event of a spill or other accident.
Report spills or exposure without delay.
Use hazardous waste receptacles for used needles, syringes, vials, and ampules.
Have and review MSDS for chemicals used in the pharmacy.
In the Event of a Spill
Wear protective clothing, a nonabsorbent gown that fastens in the back, a mask, shoe covers, goggles, and chemo-block gloves (if unavailable, double glove using two pairs of latex gloves).

Hazardous Waste

Over the past several years, as the disposal of unused pharmaceutical products has come under review, new hazardous waste regulations have been established. Although biological and chemotherapeutic waste has been regulated for years, pharmaceutical waste was not, and unused medication was often flushed down the toilet or sink and then flowed into the wastewater system.

The EPA defines hazardous waste as waste that causes or contributes to an increase in mortality or an increase in irreversible or incapacitating reversible illness, or waste that poses a threat to human health when improperly treated, stored, transported, disposed of, or otherwise mismanaged. Table 5.7 lists examples of hazardous pharmaceutical waste based on the EPA's waste determination. Further information about hazardous waste is available on the EPA's website at www.epa.gov and from state environmental protection agencies.

TABLE 5.7 Hazardous Pharmaceutical Waste

Waste Determination	Example
Ignitable	flammable liquid or gas/aerosol or oxidizer, ethanol, ethyl chloride spray, silver nitrate swabs
Reactive	nitroglycerin
Heavy metals	products with thimerosol preservatives; burn ointments with silver compounds; m-creosol preservatives; selenium, mercury, silver sulfadiazine, and barium.
Corrosivity	acids and bases; acetic acid
Specifically listed drugs (P-list)	highly hazardous unused pharmaceuticals and chemicals; nicotine, physostigmine, chlorambucil, and warfarin

The pharmacy technician must know the correct policies and procedures for disposing of pharmaceutical and hazardous medical waste. There are significant fines for the inappropriate disposal of any waste. Black waste containers are used for pharmaceutical waste and must be labeled as to its contents. Storage and removal of filled containers must be handled in accordance with the federal hazardous waste regulations.

Outdated pharmaceuticals returned to the manufacturer for credit are exempt from waste disposal regulations. The manufacturer must treat the returned pharmaceuticals as hazardous waste and dispose of them according to federal regulations. If credit is not available, the pharmacy must dispose of outdated pharmaceuticals in accordance with hazardous waste regulations.

Nonsterile Compounding

USP Chapter <795> provides specific guidelines for nonsterile compounding procedures. The pharmacy should have a designated area for nonsterile compounding, also referred to as extemporaneous compounding. The area should be removed from excessive traffic and air flow that can interfere with the accuracy of the balance and disturb stock powders. The nonsterile compounding area is a separate area and, in most cases, a separate room from the sterile compounding area. The workspace should be of adequate size and have the necessary storage space for equipment and chemicals. The compounding area must be a defined area of the pharmacy free of products not essential to the compounding function. The area must be well-maintained, neat, clean, uncluttered, and dedicated specifically for nonsterile compounding. Equipment, including the scales, weights, and measures, should be inspected and calibrated as needed to ensure accuracy. If compounded pharmaceuticals are stored in a refrigerator or freezer, the temperature must be recorded at least daily to ensure proper storage conditions are maintained.

The nonsterile compounding technician should be trained and proficient in the skills necessary to compound pharmaceutical dosage forms in accordance with state and federal standards. The technician should wear a gown or lab coat. Competency should be documented periodically to ensure the technician is practicing good compounding skills.

Documentation

High-grade chemicals and ingredients that meet USP or National Formulary (NF) standards should be used for compounding. A Material Safety Data Sheet (MSDS) should be on file for every chemical stored in the pharmacy to facilitate safe clean up of accidental spills or contamination.

Water intended for the purpose of compounding must be purified. Sterile water is acceptable because it has been purified. Rinse equipment with purified water as required by the USP Chapter <795>. Compounding documentation should include the purified water source, lot, and beyond-use date.

When compounding, follow a master control record, similar to a recipe. The master control record is a computer record of all the ingredients, the quantities used, and the national drug code for each. The pharmacist should check product at various points in production. When compounding a product for dispensing, the technician should generate a dispensing log from the master control record, similar to the log for Magic Mouthwash shown in Figure 5.1.

FIGURE 5.1 Dispensing Log for "Magic Mouthwash"

Patient Name ________________ Date Prepared 12/2/20XX

Rx # ________________ Master Control Record # ________________

Compounding Formula for "Magic Mouthwash"

Ingredient Name	Amount Needed	Manufacturer	NDC #	Lot #	Expiration Date	Prepared By	Checked By
Lidocaine 2% viscous	60 mL	HiTech	50838-0775-04		12/10/20XX		
Diphenhydramine 12.5 mg/mL	60 mL	Walgreens	00363-0379-34		07/12/20XX		
Mylanta, generic	60 mL	Qualitest	00603-0712-57		03/12/20XX		
Nystatin suspension	60 mL	Qualitest	00603-1481-58		09/11/20XX		
Total quantity	240 mL						

Prepared by ________________

Approved by ________________

Date ________________

Beyond-use date ________________

Directions ________________

Auxiliary Labeling: SHAKE WELL

A dispensing log is printed each time a product is made and is unique for each prescription. It is a record of the calculations, any notes on special equipment used, ingredient lot numbers and expiration dates, the initials of the technician compounding, and the pharmacist who checked the technician's work.

Magic Mouthwash, used to reduce pain and inflammation of the mouth and throat, is one of the products often compounded in community and institutional pharmacies. A standard formula for Magic Mouthwash is equal parts viscous lidocaine 2%, diphenhydramine 12.5 mg/5 mL solution, generic Mylanta, and nystatin oral suspension. In the dispensing log, enter the ingredients, quantity, manufacturer, lot number, and beyond-use date in the appropriate columns.

As with other types of manufactured products, the stability of a nonsterile compounded product may be compromised if it is not stored correctly. The master control record should provide instructions for proper packaging and storage.

For Magic Mouthwash, the technician transfers 8 ounces of mixed ingredients to an 8-ounce brown bottle and labels the bottle with a computer-generated prescription label and a "Shake Well" auxiliary label to ensure that the patient gets equal amounts of each ingredient in every dose. The technician calculates the beyond-use date, marks it on the label, and notes it in the dispensing log.

The pharmacy technician is responsible for much of the documentation verifying the integrity of the pharmaceutical products dispensed. USP Chapter <795> outlines the documentation requirements to ensure adequate quality control for all processes and ingredients, as well as equipment maintenance.

To ensure a high-quality product is produced each time, it is necessary to document that the proper quantities and sequences were used. The pharmacy should maintain other records documenting equipment maintenance and environmental controls, such as room temperature, refrigerator temperature, and freezer temperature.

A community pharmacy is not allowed to manufacture bulk quantities of product for resale in the future, although occasionally a pharmacy makes more than the prescription requires. The excess can be stored for future use as long as it is adequately labeled as to the ingredients, beyond-use date, and store-assigned lot number.

USP guidelines for both sterile and nonsterile compounding determine the beyond-use or expiration date of compounded pharmaceuticals. If reliable scientific testing data is available, the beyond-use date may be adjusted based on that data.

For nonsterile compounded products, the beyond-use date identifies the time in the future when the stability and strength of the product can no longer be assured. USP Chapter <795> includes tables listing the estimated shelf life of nonsterile compounded products. The shelf life of liquids can be as short as 14 days; solids or nonaqueous dosage forms may have a shelf life of up to six months.

Nonsterile Compounding Equipment and Supplies

Community pharmacies must have the equipment necessary to compound prescribed nonsterile products. The state board of pharmacy lists the minimum equipment necessary for a licensed pharmacy, including a scale, spatulas, graduated cylinders, compounding slabs, storage containers, and mortar and pestle. A technician must be familiar with the proper use of each item.

Most pharmacies have a Class III (formerly called Class A) prescription balance. This is a two-pan balance used to weigh small amounts of materials. A counterbalance is used to weigh larger amounts up to 5 kg. A digital electronic analytical balance, which uses a single pan, is easier to use and more accurate, but it is expensive and may not be available in some community pharmacies.

Pharmaceutical weights are used with the two-pan balances. Typical weight sets include metric and apothecary weights. Metric weights vary in size from 10 mg to 100 g. Apothecary weights also come in various sizes. Weights should be stored in their original box and only handled with the forceps provided to prevent the transfer of oil deposits from hands that can result in inaccurate measurements. Pans should always be covered with weighing papers to prevent damage that could cause inaccuracies.

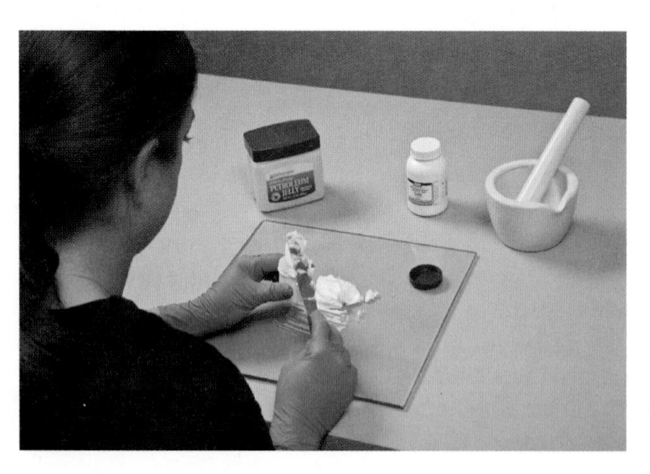

The spatula is used to transfer solid dosage forms to weighing pans and for other tasks, such as preparing ointments and creams or loosening material from the surface of a mortar and transferring to a container. Spatulas may be made of plastic, rubber, or stainless steel. Hard rubber is used for corrosive materials such as iodine or mercuric salts.

A compounding slab, or ointment slab, is a plate made of glass. The surface must be smooth, hard, and nonabsorbent. The slab is used to mix ingredients (spatulation) evenly for an ointment or cream. Ointments and creams are stored in ointment jars that range in size from 1 ounce to 1 pound, or put into tubes.

A mortar and pestle is used for grinding and mixing pharmaceutical ingredients. Both the mortar and pestle can be made of glass, porcelain, or Wedgwood. The coarser the mortar surface, the finer the triturating (grinding) of the powder or crystal. The glass variety is used to mix liquids, and the porcelain or Wedgwood type is used to grind crystals, granules, and powders. High-volume compounding pharmacies may have an electric mortar and pestle for grinding and mixing.

Made of glass or polypropylene, cylinders, pipettes, and beakers are used to measure liquids. Their shape can be conical or cylindrical. They are calibrated in metric and apothecary units. Graduated cylinders are more accurate and should be read from the bottom of the meniscus. Beakers are used to measure larger volumes, and pipettes are used to measure volumes less than 1.5 mL.

Depending on the amount of compounding done on site, the pharmacy may have other equipment, including a convection oven, single-punch tablet press, pellet press, or capsule machine. These facilitate making tablet, pellet, and capsule dosage forms. Empty hard-shell capsules are stocked for punching powder into capsules. Capsules are made of gelatin and range in size from 5 to 000. The smallest size, 5, can contain about 97 mg of aspirin; the largest capsule size, 000, can contain about 1040 mg.

Basic Nonsterile Compounding Steps

Although usually done in the community pharmacy setting, compounding of nonsterile products may also be done in institutions. Even the simple reconstitution of an antibiotic suspension signifies compounding and should follow the requirements outlined in USP Chapter <795>. Some basic steps in the compounding process are outlined here, but proficiency in nonsterile compounding will require further study.

1. A master control record (recipe) must be on file for any product the pharmacy compounds. This document establishes the standardization of ingredients and directions for compounding a specific pharmaceutical product.
2. When a pharmaceutical is made for a specific patient prescription from the master control record, the pharmacy will generate a dispensing log, also referred to as a compounding log, which is a unique, patient-specific document. The dispensing log includes a list of all of the ingredients, the quantity, date of compounding, source of drugs (manufacturer), NDC, the lot number and expiration date for each ingredient, and the initials of the compounder and pharmacist.
3. Double check calculations prior to any compounding.
4. Measure the quantity of all ingredients and have the pharmacist double-check.
5. Incorporate the ingredients as required for the dosage form and have the pharmacist double-check the end product. If at any time in the process you do not feel the product is correct, ask the pharmacist for assistance.
6. Package the pharmaceutical in the correct container such as an ointment jar, dropper bottle, or vial.
7. Label for patient use, including the beyond-use date. Make sure the dispensing log is complete.
8. Have the pharmacist perform a final check.
9. Have the pharmacist counsel the patient on the appropriate use and storage of the final product.

Sterile Compounding

Compounding sterile pharmaceuticals must be done in a facility designed to meet the requirements spelled out in USP Chapter <797> for an International Organization for Standardization (ISO) Class 5 environment, which is created through the use of a laminar airflow workbench (LAFW), also called an IV flow hood, or simply, a hood. The area must be separate from other activities not related to sterile compounding. An ISO Class 7 environment must be maintained for a buffer and clean room, and an ISO Class 8 environment is needed for the ante areas.

CSP Documentation and Regulation

As with nonsterile compounding USP Chapter <797> requires documentation of personnel training and competency, as well as the cleaning and maintenance of the equipment used in sterile compounding. Documentation provides proof that USP standards are being met.

Pharmacy personnel are evaluated for competency in compounding sterile products, including media fill testing, garbing, aseptic technique, achieving and maintaining ISO class conditions, and cleaning and disinfecting techniques. The pharmacy compounding supervisor must conduct a competency evaluation and documentation, both Sterile and Nonsterile Compounding, before allowing an employee to prepare CSPs. Based on the facility's compounding risk level (low, medium, or high), competency evaluations must be completed annually or semiannually. The sterile product compounding area (ISO Class 5 environment) must be cleaned and sanitized according to USP standards. Buffer area and ante area ceilings, walls and shelving must be cleaned monthly; counters, work surfaces and floors must be cleaned daily. At specified intervals, the supervisor of the sterile compounding pharmacy should visually observe and document the cleaning and disinfecting techniques used by pharmacy staff.

Routine environmental monitoring is required. Nonviable and viable airborne particle testing must be conducted at least every six months. Regular surface sampling is done to ensure cleaning and disinfecting procedures meet the required standards. If any area is out of compliance, corrective action should be taken and documented.

CSP Stability

Beyond-use dating of compounded sterile products is based on contamination risk or specific sterility testing provided by the hospital or manufacturer, as well as storage conditions (see Table 5.8). USP Chapter <797> provides the guidelines for product stability. Risk levels for CSPs may be low, medium, or high depending on the number and sterility of ingredients, the presence or absence of preservatives, the number of transfers from vials or ampules, and the use of automated dispensing devices. Since CSPs may be compounded in anticipation of use, if a compound is stored for an extended period of time, the risk of microbial and pyrogen formation increases. Information about the chemical stability of a CSP is obtained from the manufacturer's literature or from specific product testing.

TABLE 5.8 Beyond-Use Dates for Compounded Sterile Products

Risk Category	Room Temperature	Refrigeration	Frozen (<+10 °)
Immediate use	1 hour	1 hour	n/a
Low risk	48 hours	14 days	45 days
Low risk with <12 hour BUD*	12 hours	12 hours	n/a
Medium risk	30 hours	9 days	45 days
High risk	24 hours	3 days	45 days

* BUD = beyond-use date.
Adapted from USP Chapter <797>.

Incompatibility in CSP

The process of compounding, whether sterile or nonsterile, requires knowledge of product compatibility. Although some incompatibilities are obvious, such as precipitation, others, such as invisible complexes formed between drug and container, are only detectable with advanced testing.

Whether the pharmaceutical will be drawn up in the same syringe, added to a small- or large-volume parenteral, or introduced through a Y-site on an intravenous line, compatibility should be known before a drug is administered to the patient.

Example 5.4

The pharmacy technician has completed compounding a TPN. Before labeling the bag, she holds it up to the light and sees white particles floating in the solution. Is there a problem, and, if so, what can be done to correct the final product?

There should never be visible particles floating in the final parenteral solution. The precipitant is a nonsoluble salt that forms a complex the body cannot utilize. A precipitant may clog an IV site or form a thrombus, occluding the vein. A common cause of TPN precipitation is a mixture of calcium gluconate and potassium phosphate in too high of a concentration, or too close together without adequate mixing. Use a handbook on injectable drug compatibilities, such as *Trissel's Handbook of Injectable Drugs*, to verify ingredient compatibility.

It is not possible to correct drug incompatibility and the product should be discarded. Never filter the parenteral and dispense it. The concentration of one or more of the ingredients will not be as ordered, which can potentially compromise the therapy. If ever in doubt, throw out the product and start over.

Equipment and Supplies for CSP

For all CSPs, the supplies, equipment, and ingredients must be sterile, and all equipment must be properly calibrated, set up, and maintained. Documentation of all facets of the facility and equipment must be meticulously kept. Tables 5.9 and 5.10 list items that may be used in sterile compounding. The pharmacy technician must be proficient in the use of all of these items and trained in compounding techniques.

TABLE 5.9 Sterile Compounding Equipment and Supplies

Equipment	Description
Horizontal Laminar Airflow Workbench (LAFW)	the aseptic work area within the dedicated compounding area
Automated compounding device (ACD)	programmable machine for making complex parenterals
Closed system transfer device	needleless system to mix parenterals, i.e., add-a-vial, ADD-vantage
Syringes	1 mL, 5 mL, 10 mL, 20 mL, 50 mL calibrated device
Isopropyl alcohol	for cleaning hoods and vial tops and opening ampules
Needles	18 to 21 gauge or 1 to 1½ inch length for manipulating ingredients (Always use a needle with safety shield to prevent needlesticks.)
Dispensing pins	facilitates multiple entry into a vial without a needle
IV sets	for transferring large volumes between containers
Filters	to remove contaminants such as glass, paint, fibers, rubber cores, and bacteria from IV fluids: 5 microns, 0.45 micron, and 0.22 micron
Sterile absorbent pads	for cleaning hood or for spills
Personal protective equipment	gowns, goggles, gloves, hair and shoe covers, face masks

TABLE 5.10 Products used in Sterile Compounding

Small-volume parenterals	25 mL, 50 mL, 100 mL normal saline or dextrose 5%
Large-volume parenterals	250 mL, 500 mL, 1000 mL saline or dextrose solutions
TPN solutions	amino acid solutions, dextrose solutions, fat emulsions
TPN additives	electrolytes, trace elements, vitamins
Diluents	sterile water for injection, lidocaine, sodium chloride, bacteriostatic water for injection
Pharmaceuticals	antibiotics, chemotherapy, proton pump inhibitor, H2 blockers, etc.

The pharmacy technician should be trained in the steps necessary to produce a compounded sterile preparation. Entire manuals are written to teach the steps necessary to compound sterile products. This chapter highlights only the major steps. The technician should have adequate time to practice technique in an appropriate training environment prior to making CSPs for patient administration.

1. Aseptic hand washing
   - At least 30 seconds, and preferably 2 to 4 minutes, of hand washing using an acceptable soap, and in a manner prescribed in USP Chapter <797>.
2. Garbing, according to USP guidelines outlined in Chapter <797>.
3. Hood cleaning
   - The hood should be cleaned, first with sterile water, and then with sterile 70% isopropyl alcohol (IPA) at the interval, and in a manner prescribed by USP Chapter <797>. (Figure 5.2 shows the cleaning order and directions of the surfaces in a laminar airflow workbench.)
4. The technician should use proper aseptic technique and work at least 6 inches inside the laminar airflow workbench and 3 inches away from the sides.
5. Properly swab vial tops, ampule necks, and injection ports with sterile 70% IPA prior to needle insertion.
6. Avoid touch contamination of the CSP by employing correct aseptic technique throughout the compounding procedure.
7. Seal IV bags and vials. Label for use and with beyond-use date.
8. Have pharmacist double-check work.

Whether sterile or nonsterile, compounding requires knowledge and skills to ensure that the patient receives a safely compounded product, at the correct dose or strength, administered via the correct route as prescribed by the practitioner.

FIGURE 5.2
Laminar Airflow Workbench and Hood Cleaning Order

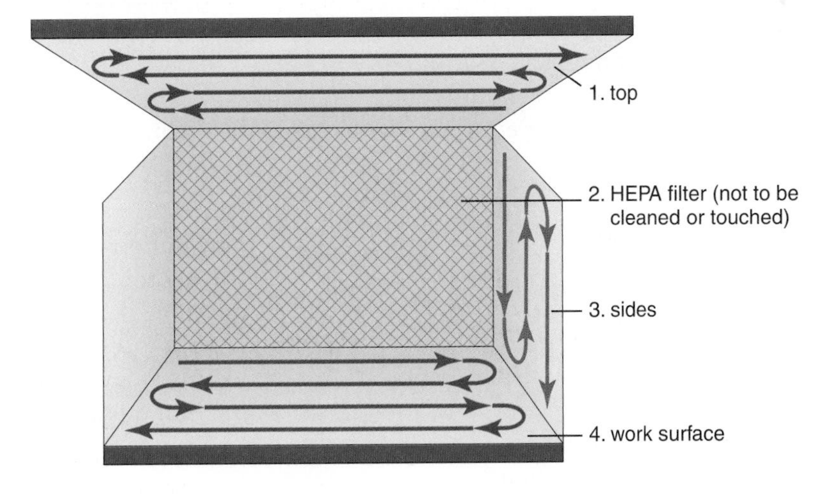

Skills Quiz

1. What organization defines good compounding practices for pharmacies?
   a. OBRA
   b. USP
   c. FDA
   d. HIPAA

2. When working with a two-pan balance in nonsterile compounding, always
   a. work in a ventilated area
   b. use a spatula to place the weights on the pans
   c. cover the pans with weighing papers
   d. pipette liquids onto the pans carefully

3. The master control record for Magic Mouthwash calls for equal quantities of viscous lidocaine 2%, liquid antacid, diphenhydramine liquid 12.5 mg/5 mL, and nystatin oral suspension. To make an 8-ounce bottle for a prescription, how much viscous lidocaine 2% will be entered in the dispensing log?
   a. 10 mL
   b. 40 mL
   c. 60 mL
   d. 80 mL

4. Calculate the beyond-use date of a liquid cough syrup if promethazine syrup 25 mg/5 mL expires in 12 months and guaifenesin syrup 100 mg/5 mL expires in 4 months.
   a. 30 days
   b. 90 days
   c. 14 days
   d. 180 days

5. OSHA is responsible for protecting healthcare workers from exposure to
   a. unfair work practices.
   b. hazardous substances.
   c. workplace discrimination.
   d. category X drugs.

6. What is most commonly used for hand hygiene in hospitals by staff and visitors?
   a. alcohol-based gels
   b. water
   c. soap and water
   d. isopropyl alcohol

7. The average amount of time the hands should be rubbed together with soap for proper hand washing is
   a. 5 seconds.
   b. 10 to 15 seconds.
   c. 20 to 30 seconds.
   d. 1 minute.

8. What is the most common cause of transmission of infectious agents in the healthcare setting?
   a. touch
   b. airborne
   c. blood
   d. sputum

9. Which of the following is the correct order for garbing for sterile product compounding?
   a. face mask, shoe covers, gown, hand wash
   b. shoe covers, hair cover, face mask, hand wash, gown
   c. hand wash, gown, hair cover, shoe covers, face mask
   d. gown, hair cover, shoe cover, hand wash, face mask

10. Before donning sterile gloves in preparation for sterile compounding, where should antiseptic hand cleansing be done?
    a. main pharmacy
    b. anteroom
    c. clean room
    d. bathroom

11. Which of the following is not considered personal protective equipment (PPE) used in compounding nonhazardous sterile products?
    a. goggles or face shield
    b. fitted respirator
    c. chemo-block gown
    d. powder-free gloves

12. Exposure to radioactive material is possible in what area of pharmacy practice?
    a. institutional
    b. community
    c. industrial
    d. nuclear

13. The concept of universal precaution assumes
    a. all patients have infectious pathogens.
    b. all patients will sue the facility.
    c. all healthcare professional make mistakes.
    d. all sterile products contain pathogens.

14. Universal precautions help to protect the patient and healthcare professional from what common bloodborne pathogen?
    a. hepatitis B
    b. tuberculosis
    c. pneumonia
    d. meningitis

15. ________ help(s) to prevent needlesticks.
    a. safety needles
    b. never recapping a needle
    c. biohazard waste containers
    d. all of the above

16. Hazardous pharmaceutical waste has been identified in
    a. ground water.
    b. surface water.
    c. drinking water.
    d. all of the above.

17. Which pharmaceuticals should be discarded in a container for hazardous pharmaceutical waste to prevent contamination of the waste system?
    a. acetaminophen
    b. warfarin
    c. diphenhydramine
    d. atorvastatin

18. How long may a low-risk compounded sterile pharmaceutical be stored at room temperature before it must be discarded?
    a. 1 hour
    b. 2 days
    c. 14 days
    d. 45 days

19. What document is needed to prove that an ISO class 5 environment is free of particles and contaminants?
    a. master control record
    b. temperature log
    c. environment testing record
    d. competency record

20. Which piece of equipment most accurately measures the volume of liquid used to compound an antibiotic suspension with purified water?
    a. beaker
    b. pipette
    c. graduated cylinder
    d. Class III balance

Thinking Beyond the Exam

You want to become more involved in preventing environmental contamination from pharmaceutical waste. What programs are currently in place to help prevent medical and pharmaceutical waste from contaminating the water supply or washing up on public beaches? What could you do in your community to help reduce pharmaceutical waste? Discuss with your local hospital their plan for disposing of unused pharmaceutical waste.

Medication Safety

6

Learning Objectives

- Define medical error and medication error.
- Differentiate between generic, trade, and chemical drug names.
- Identify strategies to prevent data entry errors.
- Know the FDA source for assessing the bioequivalence of drugs.
- Define the components of the NDC number and its significance in medication error prevention.
- Identify FDA-mandated sources of information on medications for healthcare professionals and patients.
- Recognize when pharmacist intervention should occur.
- Explain FDA categories for use of drugs in pregnancy.
- Recognize look-alike/sound-alike medications and techniques to prevent errors.
- Identify high-risk/alert medications.
- List innovations and techniques to reduce medication errors.
- Know the restrictions on the use of the morning-after pill, Accutane, and thalidomide.
- Understand the provisions of the Poison Prevention Packaging Act of 1970.

Continue your review with more than 1,000 exam-style questions.

When used safely and stored properly, medications can effectively treat and cure illnesses and control symptoms for conditions such as high blood pressure, diabetes, and high cholesterol. The goal of the profession of pharmacy is to get the right drug in the right strength by the right route safely to the right patient at the right time. These five rights (the five Rs) are an important means of preventing medication errors.

Medical and Medication Errors

Government and professional organizations have created laws, regulations, and standards to guarantee the quality of pharmaceutical products, ensure that potent medications are used correctly, and minimize medication errors. A medical error is any instance in health care—regardless of the cause—that contributes to an unintended response. There are multiple sources of medical errors and all healthcare

TABLE 6.1 Categories of Medication Errors and Causes

Category	Definition	Example
Omission	The prescribed dose is not given/taken.	A patient forgets to take the medication.
Wrong dose	The dose given is 5% greater or less than the dose prescribed.	A nurse gives one tablet but the order is for two tablets.
Extra dose	The patient receives more doses than prescribed.	Instead of 7 days of antibiotic therapy, the patient is dispensed 10 days' supply and takes all 10 days supplied.
Wrong dosage form	The formulation is not the accepted interpretation of the physician's order.	The patient has an order for Ondansetron oral disintegrating tablets but is dispensed oral swallow tablets.
Wrong time	The medication is given too early or too long after the intended time of administration.	A patient in the hospital is to receive an intravenous antibiotic at 8 a.m. but does not receive the medication until noon.
Human failure	An error caused by an individual.	A technician pulls a bottle of medication from the shelf to fill a prescription from memory and does not read the label. Stores frequently relocate medication.
Technical failure	Equipment is not working properly.	The pharmacy's automatic dispensing machine is malfunctioning.
Organizational failure	The rules, policies, or procedures are not adequate.	An outdated policy on sterile compounding leads to compromised sterility of an admixture.

providers must be alert to the circumstances, decisions, actions, or inaction that may lead to a medical error. The National Coordinating Council for Medication Error Reporting and Prevention defines a medication error as a preventable event that occurs while the medication is in the control of the healthcare professional, patient, or consumer that may cause or lead to inappropriate medication use or patient harm. Medication errors fall into several categories, including omission error, wrong dose error, extra dose error, wrong dosage form error, and wrong time error. Medication errors may be the result of human failure, technical failure, or organizational failure. See Table 6.1 for definitions and examples of error and failure categories.

Protecting the Public

The primary mission of the profession of pharmacy is to promote and protect the safety of the public. The U.S. Food and Drug Administration (FDA), the Drug Enforcement Administration (DEA), the Consumer Product Safety Commission (CPSC), and state boards of pharmacy have drafted laws and regulations to support this mission. These laws and regulations have reduced medical mistakes, medication errors, accidental childhood ingestions, and drug diversions, and have expanded patient education.

The FDA has the primary responsibility and the regulatory authority to create and enforce regulations that ensure the safety of pharmaceutical products. The FDA is responsible for the review and approval of all prescription and over-the-counter (OTC) medications, including generic drugs. Although the manufacture of vitamins and herbal and diet supplements is not under FDA control, the FDA does monitor adverse reactions and marketing claims.

Each drug approved by the FDA has a chemical name, a generic or nonproprietary name, and a brand or trade name. Table 6.2 lists the different names for a commonly used pain medication. A chemical name describes the chemical structure of the drug molecule. A generic or nonproprietary name is developed to provide a name that is not patent protected. The brand name is owned by the company that develops and markets the drug. Once the original patent of an FDA-approved drug expires (usually 17+ years after the patent is filed), any manufacturer can market a generic version of the drug, which usually sells for a reduced price.

TABLE 6.2 Drug Names

Name Category	Drug Name
Chemical	2-(4-isobutylphenyl) propionic acid
Generic	ibuprofen
Brand	Advil, Motrin, Motrin IB

Generic vs. Brand Name Drugs

To earn FDA approval for a generic drug, the manufacturer must demonstrate that the generic drug is bioequivalent—comparable in pharmacologic activity, efficacy, and safety—to the brand name drug. Bioequivalence data considers how the drug is absorbed, the blood and tissue levels, and how the drug is eliminated from the body. The FDA is also responsible for publishing the *Orange Book* (www.paradigmcollege.net/certexamreview3e/fda_orangebook), which lists FDA-approved drug products and their therapeutic equivalents. When in doubt, the pharmacy technician can refer to the *Orange Book* to determine whether a given generic drug and dosage form can be safely substituted for a brand name product.

A pharmacy may dispense a generic drug unless the prescriber writes "dispense as written" (DAW), "brand name necessary," or similar wording on the prescription. Most pharmacy software programs default to a generic drug when available because the cost is less for both the patient and the insurer. A patient may request a brand name drug.

NDC Number

Once the FDA approves a brand or generic drug, the drug is assigned a National Drug Code number (NDC). The NDC number (and barcode) must appear on all manufacturer labels of drug stock bottles and boxes (see Figure 6.1). The NDC is a 10- or 11-digit number provides several pieces of information: the identity of the manufacturer or wholesaler (first four or five numbers); the drug product (middle three or four numbers); and the packaging size and type (last two numbers). Table 6.3 explains the parts of an NDC number.

The NDC number plays a crucial role in the prevention of medication errors. In many community pharmacies, the barcode on the manufacturer stock bottle must be scanned to ensure the correct drug, dose, and dosage form are dispensed. For example, if the prescription is for the antibiotic clarithromycin 500 mg but the technician inadvertently selects clarithromycin 500 mg XL, the drug NDC barcode will be different. The computer will indicate the error and will not print a prescription label.

FIGURE 6.1 NDC Numbers and Bar Codes

All stock medication labels include a unique, product-specific National Drug Code (NDC) number in both numeric and bar code form. The first four digits of the NDC number identify the manufacturer, the second four digits indicate the product code, and the last two digits show the packaging size and type.

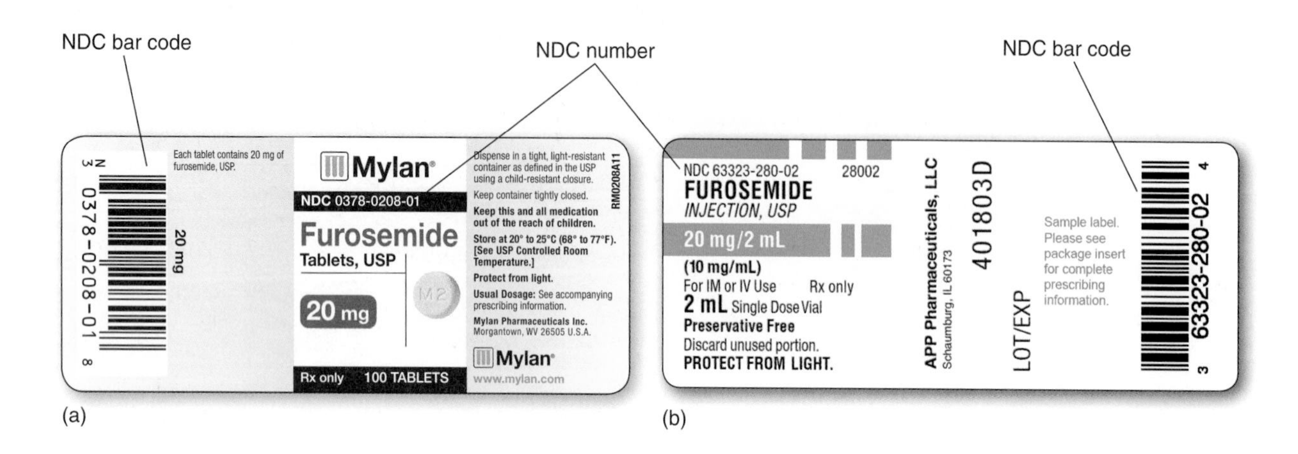

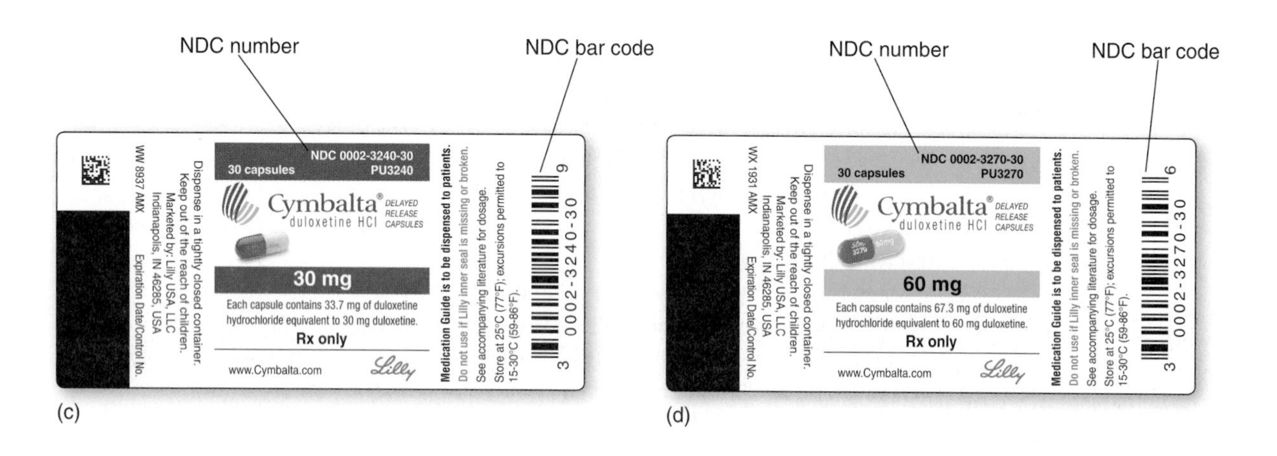

TABLE 6.3 Reading NDC Numbers

	Manufacturer		Product Code		Packing Size and Type	
	NDC	*Name*	*NDC*	*Product*	*NDC*	*Size*
(a)	0378	Mylan Pharmaceuticals, Inc	0208	furosemide 20 mg tablet	01	100 tablets
(b)	63323	APP Pharmaceuticals, LLC	280	furosemide injection 20 mg/2mL	02	2 mL vial
(c)	0002	Lilly	3240	Cymbalta 30 mg	30	30 capsules
(d)	0002	Lilly	3270	Cymbalta 60 mg	30	30 capsules

Patient Education

The FDA imposes strict guidelines on the packaging and labeling of medications. The agency requires manufacturers to include safety information in the product package insert (PPI) attached to each stock bottle. This document is for medical and pharmacy staff and includes information on precautions, contraindications, warnings, and adverse reactions. This information is also published in the *Physician's Desk Reference* (PDR).

Through a program called MedWatch (www.paradigmcollege.net/certexamreview3e/fda/MedWatch), the FDA monitors drugs for any incidence and the severity of adverse reactions that may require additional warnings. VAERS is a similar program that monitors adverse reactions from vaccines (www.paradigmcollege.net/certexamreview3e/hhs/vaccine_monitoring). Drug manufacturers are required to report any serious side effects or adverse reactions to the FDA. Depending on the frequency and severity of the reactions, the FDA may require additional labeling or warning statements or may require the manufacturer to withdraw the product from the market.

Avandia, Paxil, Adderall, Accutane, and Coumadin are examples of drugs that require additional strict warnings (called black box warnings) and communications to pharmacists and prescribers. Black box warnings are the most significant warning assigned to a product regulated by the FDA. Warnings must be observed and followed when dispensing these products. For select high-risk drugs, such as those listed in Table 6.4, the FDA requires the pharmacy to provide the consumer with additional written information, called a medication guide, or MedGuide. This information is provided to the patient to promote the safe and effective use of a high-risk drug and to minimize the risk of serious adverse reactions. By law, the pharmacy must provide a MedGuide to patients when dispensing these medications.

TABLE 6.4 High-Risk Drugs Requiring Medication Guides

Drug	Risk Factor
Accutane	causes birth defects; women must be on some form of birth control or be advised not to get pregnant while taking this medication
Adderall	may cause insomnia, loss of appetite, and changes in pulse and blood pressure; monitor symptoms and vital signs
Antidepressants	may be associated with an increase in suicide risk, especially in adolescent patients; watch for changes in behavior
Estrogen/ progesterone	may cause an increased risk of heart attack or stroke among smokers; the patient taking this type of drug should not smoke
Concerta	similar to Adderall
Coumadin	reduces blood clotting; patients must be careful when working with sharp objects, shaving, and participating in contact sports while taking this drug; interacts with many drugs
NSAIDs*	may cause an increase in risk of stomach ulcers; take with food and no longer than necessary
Ritalin	similar to Adderall
Serevent	not as effective as a rescue drug in reversing acute shortness of breath
Strattera	an increase in suicidal thoughts or actions in children and teens
Symlin	may cause hypoglycemia in diabetics; eat a well-balanced diet

*Nonsteroidal anti-inflammatory drug.

High-Risk/Alert Medications

As discussed previously, the Institute for Safe Medication Practices (ISMP), the Joint Commission, and the FDA have declared some pharmaceuticals high risk because of the potential for dispensing errors. The community pharmacy is required to provide consumers with a MedGuide each time a high-risk medication is dispensed. In institutions, accreditation standards require adoption of warning lists of high-risk/alert medications, look-alike/sound-alike medications, and a list of medications and abbreviations to avoid. The ISMP has created a list of categories (classes) of medications used in both institution and community pharmacies that have a high incidence of error (see Table 6.5). Technicians and pharmacists should be familiar with the list and perform extra verification before dispensing any medication on the list. Failure to comply may cost the institution its accreditation.

TABLE 6.5 ISMP Categories of High-Risk/Alert Medications

Category	Examples
adrenergic agonists, IV	epinephrine
adrenergic antagonists, IV	metoprolol
anesthetic agents	propofol, ketamine
antithrombotic agents	warfarin, low-molecular-weight heparin
antiarrhythmics	lidocaine, amiodarone
chemotherapeutic agents	methotrexate, fluorouracil
hypertonic dextrose (20% or greater)	total parenteral nutrition solutions
epidural and intrathecal medications	lidocaine, preservative-free methotrexate
inotropic medications, IV	digoxin, milrinone
insulin	Humalog, Novalog, regular insulin
liposomal forms of drugs	amphotericin B
moderate sedative agents, oral and IV	midazolam
narcotics/opioids	morphine, meperidine, oxycodone
neuromuscular blocking agent	succinylcholine, rocuronium, vecuronium
hypertonic sodium chloride, IV	sodium chloride greater than 0.9% concentration

Safe Use of Drugs during Pregnancy

The FDA is also responsible for classifying fetal risk for prescription and OTC drugs based on human and animal research studies. There is often limited data on the safety of drug use during pregnancy, so the benefits and risks must always be assessed. Table 6.6 lists the FDA drug classifications for drug use during pregnancy.

Safe Use of Drugs in Women of Child-bearing Age

The FDA has approved over-the-counter sale of morning-after birth control pills, such as Plan B, One Step, and Next Choice, but with restrictions. At most pharmacies these products are available without a prescription if the customer can prove he/she is 17 years of age or older; younger patients must present a prescription. The pill(s) are taken in split doses, 12 hours apart, within 72 hours of unprotected sex when there is a risk of pregnancy. Newer versions are available as a one-tablet dose.

TABLE 6.6 Drug Risk Classifications for Pregnant Women

Category	Recommendation for Use
Category A	safe for use in pregnancy
Category B	shown to be safe in animal studies and presumed safe in humans
Category C	insufficient information to judge level of safety
Category D	should not be used in pregnancy due to results in animal studies demonstrating fetal risk, but benefits may outweigh risk; use extreme caution
Category X	absolutely contraindicated during pregnancy

The pharmacy technician must be aware of special risk evaluation and mitigation strategies (REMS) for women of childbearing age mandated by the FDA to promote patient safety. IPLEDGE is a REMS intended to reduce the risk of fetal exposure to Accutane (isotretinoin), which is used to treat severe acne. A similar program, STEPS (System for Thalidomide Education and Prescribing Safety), is intended to mitigate the risks for both men and women taking Thalomid (thalidomide) for the treatment of leprosy or severe nerve inflammation and pain. Prescribers, pharmacies, and patients must be preenrolled and preapproved to prescribe, dispense, or receive these medications.

Both of these drugs are classified as Category X drugs, indicating a very high risk for birth defects. Prescribers, pharmacists, and patients must register with the associated programs before the drug can be dispensed and complete follow-up reports. Patients must sign an informed consent before the medication can be prescribed.

Women of childbearing age should not get pregnant one month before or one month after taking these drugs. They must have two negative pregnancy tests, undergo required birth control counseling, and sign a pledge to use two forms of contraception while taking either drug. A maximum 30-day supply of medication can be prescribed and dispensed, with no refills, and the medication must be picked up at the pharmacy within seven days of the date of the prescription.

Drug Registry Programs

In addition to isotretinoin and thalidomide (both Category X medications), a few other medications are closely monitored by the manufacturer or governmental oversight agencies. Clozapine is an antipsychotic medication that can cause agranulocytosis. Clozapine registry requirements state that the patient must be registered with the dispensing pharmacy and the prescribing physician. There must be appropriate laboratory monitoring of the patient's white blood cell (WBC) and absolute neutrophil count (ANC) at intervals determined by the length of therapy (usually weekly but may be required more often if levels drop substantially). Clozapine is prescribed infrequently today because of its potential adverse side effects and because there are safer alternative drugs on the market.

Before the long-acting injectable formulation of the antipsychotic medication olanzapine can be administered to a patient, the prescriber, healthcare facility, patient, and pharmacy must be enrolled in the Zyprexa Relprevv Patient Care Program. Postinjection delirium/sedation syndrome (PDSS) may occur in patients after administration. Patients must be monitored for at least three hours after every monthly injection. Everyone in the pharmacy involved with the process must be aware of the high risk associated with olanzapine injection.

Utilization Review and Pharmacist Intervention

At what point should a technician filling a prescription or medication order consult the pharmacist? Sometimes while entering a prescription into the pharmacy computer, a popup alert may appear (also referred to as utilization review) to warn the technician there might be a problem with the prescription—a drug interaction with another medication or a duplication of therapy—that requires review by a pharmacist or the prescriber. When an alert appears, the pharmacy technician must stop entering the prescription and notify the pharmacist.

A prompt for a utilization review may also appear when the pharmacy submits a prescription claim to an insurance provider. During the review, the insurance provider will have a list of all medications the patient has filled at any pharmacy in which a medication claim was sent for online adjudication. Examples include drug-drug interactions in which the combination might harm the patient by increasing or decreasing one drug's action, drug combinations that prolong the QT interval leading to potentially life-threatening arrhythmias, or a duplicate therapy warning. These will result in a rejection of the prescription claim, and the technician should notify the pharmacist who will review the information and handle the follow-up with the prescriber or insurer.

The technician may also receive an alert regarding known drug allergies and adverse drug reactions (ADR) based on the patient profile, history of allergies, and ADRs. The technician should consult a pharmacist before proceeding. A patient's allergy list should be updated every time he or she presents a new prescription as new allergies may have occurred since the last update. Common allergies include penicillin, sulfa, codeine, and allergies to foods such as eggs or nuts. Some pharmaceuticals, including vaccines, are grown in egg cultures and should not be dispensed to patients with egg allergies. Atrovent contains soy lecithin and should not be dispensed to patients with peanut allergies. The pharmacist will use his or her professional judgment to decide whether to contact the prescriber or fill the prescription.

Insurance companies sometimes require pharmacies to get prior authorization before dispensing specific brand name or high-cost medication. The insurer may also refuse reimbursement for some medications and recommend a therapeutic substitution. Commonly, insurance companies require therapeutic substitution for such medications as proton pump inhibitors, antihyperlipidemic-like statins, antidepressants, and nonsteroidal anti-inflammatory drugs such as naproxen. When prior authorization is required, it is up to the prescribing physician to justify the use of the more expensive drug. The technician or pharmacist will need to fax the insurance company requirement to the practitioner for review; the pharmacist may be able to expedite the clarification process by telephone, particularly if a delay would harm the patient (waiting for an antibiotic needed to treat an infection, for example). Often, the prescriber will change to a comparable medication that is covered by insurance.

A pharmacist should always be consulted if a patient requests counseling on a prescription or OTC product. If counseling is not requested, the technician is bound by law to offer counseling from the pharmacist. If specifically asked, the technician may point out the location of a product. In some states, pharmacy technicians are allowed to consult with patients on OTC medications. In other states, technicians are permitted only to read the medication label to the patient and then refer the patient to the pharmicist for more information. Pharmacists are allowed to recommend an OTC product for a self-limited condition. Pharmacists do not diagnose, however, so if the patient is unsure what is wrong, the pharmacist may advise the patient to see a physician.

Patients often have questions at the time they pick up medications or after beginning a medication. A pharmacy technician is permitted to answer questions about the price or what a tablet looks like, but the technician should not advise the patient about issues such as missed doses or improper use of a medication. Patient counseling is the responsibility of the pharmacist.

Techniques to Reduce Errors

Some simple techniques may be used to help the pharmacy staff identify and prevent errors when dispensing certain pharmaceuticals. When dealing with look-alike/sound-alike names, the pharmacy should first separate the inventory so that similar-sounding and -looking products are not next to each other on the shelf.

Individual pharmacies and drug manufacturers also use tall man lettering to distinguish between two products with similar names. A portion of the drug name will be written in capital letters, and often in bolder type. Figure 6.2 shows the use of tall-man lettering to distinguish between vinBLAStine sulfate and vinCRIStine sulfate. Capitalizing the letters in names that are similar attracts the eye and makes it easier to distinguish one product from its look-alike.

When writing a prescription, practitioners are encouraged to avoid using certain error-prone abbreviations, such as those listed in Table 6.7. Although this is difficult to enforce outside of the hospital setting, use of these abbreviations in an institutional setting may affect the institution's accreditation.

The technician also should be familiar with the correct way to write numbers with decimal points. Any whole number (1 or greater) should never be written with a decimal point and trailing zero. If the decimal point is misread, it could lead to a tenfold increase in dose. Any number less than 1 should be preceded by a zero and a decimal point.

FIGURE 6.2 Tall-Man Lettering

Tall-man lettering helps distinguish between vinBLAStine sulfate and vinCRIStine sulfate.

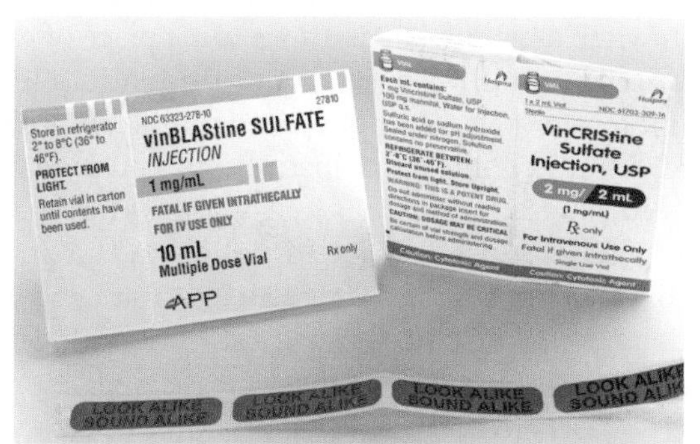

TABLE 6.7 Error-Prone Abbreviations to Avoid

Abbreviation	Meaning	Abbreviation	Meaning
cc	cubic centimeter (mL)	gr	grain
HS	bedtime	QD	daily
QOD	every other day	AU	both ears
AS	left ear	AD	right ear
OU	both eyes	OS	left eye
OD	right eye	MgSO4	magnesium sulfate
MSO4	morphine sulfate	U, or IU	units

Example 6.1

Using Decimals and Whole Numbers

Warfarin 5.0 mg is incorrect; it should be written as warfarin 5 mg.

Clonidine .1 mg is incorrect; it should be written as clonadine 0.1 mg.

Innovations

In the past few years, many new technologies have been developed to reduce medical errors. Barcode scanning, used for years in retail sales, is now being used by both hospitals and pharmacies as a means to identify patients and drugs. Most institutions now issue patient barcode identification wrist bands at admission. Before every treatment the patient is identified by name, date of birth, and barcode. Medications have individual barcodes for institutional use as do manufacturer bulk bottles for pharmacy stock. When a prescription is entered into the computer, the product barcode is scanned to verify the product matches the prescription. Prescription refills are also selected by barcode. Before administering a medication in the hospital, a nurse will scan the patient, the patient profile, and the medication barcode to be sure they match. Barcodes have reduced selection errors.

As medicine becomes more computerized, more physicians are transmitting prescriptions electronically. In the retail pharmacy this is called e-prescribing. E-prescribing eliminates problems created by illegible handwriting and assumption errors—errors that occur when a technician assumes some piece of essential information on a prescription instead of calling to verify the information. In institutions, electronic prescribing is referred to as a computerized physician order entry (CPOE).

In addition to electronic prescribing, many institutions and individual practices have begun to replace paper recordkeeping with the electronic health record (EHR). Physician notes, medication orders, laboratory orders, nursing notes, and all other patient information can be accessed online by authorized users. An electronic medication administration record (eMAR) documents the type of medication and time of administration. Studies have shown that these automated systems decrease medication errors; however, healthcare workers need to be aware that technology may create new errors.

Pharmacy automation systems are also helping to reduce errors in medication administration. Mail-order and high-volume community and hospital pharmacies are increasingly filling prescriptions using robotic automation to scan barcodes and deliver the medication to the pharmacist, who then performs the final check. Automated compounding is being used to prepare commonly used, complex IV products such as total parenteral nutrition (TPN).

Computer software and hardware enables nurses to select medication based on the patient's electronic medication administration record (eMAR). A computerized medication storage cabinet (like an Omnicell or Pyxis) will direct the nurse to select the medication from a specific storage area or drawer in the drug cabinet. Additionally, barcode scanning is used to match the patient's wrist band to the unit dose package, helping to ensure that the five Rs are followed.

One of the most important components of medication error prevention is the communication between healthcare provider and patient. The Joint Commission Medication Reconciliation Process has made the recognition of patient medications a priority for institutions. When a patient is admitted to the hospital, the hospital creates a computerized list of any medications the patient is taking, including OTC products. During hospitalization, any medication changes are updated in the electronic health record. Upon discharge, the patient receives a list of all medications, including any medications stopped or changed. A copy of the list is sent to the patient's primary care physician, and to all other healthcare providers, including home health agencies, social workers, or hospice providers.

Reporting Medication Errors and Adverse Reactions

There are various systems in place for reporting medication errors. These systems are not intended to be punitive but to help institutions develop a better understanding of the causes of medication errors and to reduce or eliminate them. Even in the community pharmacy, documenting near misses helps to identify changes that can improve workflow and reduce errors.

A number of agencies tracks and/or works to minimize medication errors, including:

- **The American Society of Health-System Pharmacists** (ASHP) publishes comprehensive guidelines on the prevention of medication errors in hospitals.
- **The Institute for Safe Medication Practices** (ISMP) is a nonprofit healthcare organization whose members include pharmacists, physicians, and nurses. This organization disseminates information to healthcare personnel regarding safe medication practices. The ISMP also maintains lists of error-prone abbreviations that contribute to medication errors.
- **Medication Error Reporting Program** (MERP) is a voluntary medication error reporting program administered by the ISMP. It allows healthcare providers who have made a medication error to self-report anonymously. The confidential information submitted to MERP may be used as part of future case studies and for the education and training of healthcare professionals.
- **MedWatch** is a voluntary program administered by the FDA. This program allows for the reporting of adverse events related to drugs and medical devices. Reporting can be done by filling out a one-page form (FDA 3500) in print, online, or by phone or fax. The information is used to detect unsafe trends related to particular drugs and medical devices so that timely action may be taken.

Consumer Product Safety Commission

The Poison Prevention Packaging Act of 1970, enforced by the U.S. Consumer Product Safety Commission (CPSC), is intended to prevent or minimize accidental ingestion of toxic substances by children. The incidence of childhood deaths, emergency room visits, and calls to poison control centers has been considerably reduced since the law was enacted.

Toxic substances include both drugs and common household products. Common medications covered by this act include aspirin, acetaminophen (Tylenol), iron, most OTC products, and all prescription drugs, including controlled medications. These products must be dispensed by the technician or pharmacist in special child-proof packaging.

A child-resistant container is defined as one that cannot be opened by 80 percent of children but can be opened by 90 percent of adults. Most pharmacies stock safety lids for prescription containers that must be pressed down and then turned to open. Reuse of plastic prescription vials and lids on refills is not recommended and is prohibited by the Poison Prevention Act. In the interest of patient safety, certain medications, such as sublingual nitroglycerin for chest pain, are exempt from these childproof cap requirements. Prescriptions that are sent from a community pharmacy to either a nursing home or hospital are exempt from these special packaging requirements as well because the medication will be administered by a nurse and stored in a locked area. Certain drugs, such as metered dose inhalers (MDIs), birth control pills, and Medrol dose packs are also exempt because specialized packaging limits access by children.

The Poison Prevention Packaging Act allows elderly patients or patients with certain disabilities, such as rheumatoid arthritis, to opt out of special packaging requirements. In those cases, the technician may dispense the medications using a non-safety lid. Although not required by law, it is recommended that such a request be documented in the patient profile. Many pharmacies stock reversible lids with safety and nonsafety options.

The goal of the profession of pharmacy is to protect and safeguard the health of the public. It is the responsibility of all pharmacy personnel to minimize medication errors, such as failing to treat a diagnosed illness, unintended side effects or adverse effects, or in rare cases, death. Every pharmacy strives to fill all prescriptions accurately.

Among the main principles that govern the practice of pharmacy technicians, ensuring the 5 rights of medication safety (the 5 Rs) are followed every time is paramount. The pharmacy technician, as a member of the healthcare team, works to deliver the right drug, at the right dose, in the right route of administration, with the right frequency and time of administration to the right patient with 100 percent accuracy. The pharmacy technician has a moral and ethical obligation to raise questions to protect patient safety. Pharmacy technicians work closely with healthcare professionals in a variety of settings and should never be afraid to ask a question when patient safety is at stake. It is better to err on the side of caution than make a hasty decision and risk harming or killing a patient. Table 6.8 outlines questions technicians should consider when preparing medications.

The pharmacist is ultimately responsible for the accuracy and dispensing of prescriptions, but the pharmacy technician plays an important role in ensuring safety. The work area should be well lit and not cluttered, and drug stock bottles should be returned to inventory after dispensing. Actions must be focused—even while multitasking—to prevent errors. Personal calls or cell phones may distract attention and compromise safety. The technician should check the original prescription for completeness and legibility; many drugs have sound-alike or look-alike names. Prescribers often continue to use unapproved abbreviations, which can cause medication errors. When in doubt, the prescriber should be contacted for clarification and the correct information documented on the original prescription. Technicians must also verify patient identity, both when prescriptions are received and dispensed. Allergy history to medications must be updated. In the hospital environment, the pharmacy technician should never assume an error will be detected by a nurse or other healthcare professional if the technician forgets to follow good medication preparation procedures.

TABLE 6.8 Questions to Ask to Avoid Medication Errors

Question	Technician Action
Was the correct patient entered into the computer database?	Check the patient's date of birth or other identifying information.
Has the correct patient (or his or her representative) picked up the medication(s) at the pharmacy?	Verify the patient's address or date of birth.
Has the correct drug been dispensed?	Double-check look-alike and sound-alike drugs, and immediate vs. extended-release medications, such as metoprolol 25 mg and metoprolol ER 25 mg. Scan NDC numbers on Rx and stock bottles.
Is the dose correct?	Double-check the dosage, especially when a drug is prescribed for a pediatric or geriatric patient. Watch for identical drugs with similar packaging, such as azithromycin 100 mg/5 mL and azithromycin 200 mg/5 mL.
Has the correct amount been prepared and dispensed?	Select the right stock bottle from the shelf, such as amoxicillin 75 mL or amoxicillin 100 mL.
Is the route of administration correct?	Select an oral tablet or a sublingual tablet depending on prescription.
Is the dosage form correct?	Select regular tablet or quick-disintegrating tablet, whichever is called for on prescription.
Are the correct storage conditions maintained?	Ask the patient if he or she knows how to properly store nitroglycerin; if not, notify the pharmacist.
Is the administration time correct, and are the appropriate auxiliary labels provided?	Type the correct administration time into the computer database: to be given in the morning, at bedtime, or not specified. Attach any necessary auxiliary labels; if not sure, ask the pharmacist.

Skills Quiz

Reflect on the information presented in this chapter by answering the following questions.

1. Clopidogrel is the ________name for Plavix.
   a. trade
   b. brand
   c. generic
   d. chemical

2. The FDA online publication that lists approved drug products and their therapeutic equivalents is called the
   a. Blue Book.
   b. Red Book.
   c. Orange Book.
   d. Black Book.

3. Accutane is a Category X medication, which means __________for use in pregnant women.
   a. it is safe
   b. it is absolutely contraindicated
   c. there is insufficient data
   d. it is safe in animals and presumed safe

4. Thalomid (thalidomide) causes birth defects. Patients using this drug must register with _____to protect patient safety.
   a. iPLEDGE
   b. STEPS
   c. Plan B
   d. the FDA

5. The Poison Prevention Packaging Act requires child-resistant containers that________ % of children cannot open but _______% of adults can open.
   a. 100, 100
   b. 90, 90
   c. 80, 90
   d. 90, 80

6. You are asked to relocate stock in the pharmacy to prevent medication errors. Which technique will you use to complete this task?
   a. tall-man letters
   b. trailing zeros and leading zeros
   c. e-prescribing and CPOE
   d. look-alike/sound-alike inventory separation

7. Which of the following category of agents requires patients to receive a medication guide?
   a. penicillin
   b. naproxen
   c. prednisone
   d. loratidine

8. During the prescription entering process, an alert pops up warning the technician there is a drug-drug interaction. What should the technician do?
   a. tell the patient
   b. call the physician
   c. notify the pharmacist
   d. fill the prescription

9. Which of the following medication errors can be prevented by not using a trailing zero?
   a. missed dose
   b. overdose
   c. underdose
   d. extra dose

10. A patient picking up a prescription for Singulair requests information. The technician should
    a. refer the patient to the printed handout given with the prescription.
    b. counsel the patient.
    c. ask the pharmacist to counsel the patient.
    d. provide the patient with the manufacturer's website.

11. Incorrect admixture of a total parenteral nutrition by a malfunctioning automated compounding device would be an example of which type of medication error?
    a. human failure
    b. technical failure
    c. wrong-time error
    d. omission error

12. You receive a prescription from a patient for Adderall 20 mg tablets. You notice that the prescription is dirty and appears to be on regular paper. What do you do?
    a. fill the prescription
    b. fill and give a medication guide
    c. call the police
    d. notify the pharmacist

13. Which of these drugs requires registration before dispensing and periodic documentation of WBC/ANC to make sure the patient is not developing agranulocytosis?
    a. clozapine
    b. olanzapine
    c. isotretinoin
    d. thalidomide

14. A medication order for the antibiotic levofloxacin 500 mg po is received with directions "QD." What agency is responsible for safeguarding patients by issuing a list of error-prone abbreviations?
    a. FDA
    b. DEA
    c. ISMP
    d. ASHP

15. What is the name of the program established by the FDA to monitor medication reactions and adverse drug reactions?
    a. MERP
    b. MedWatch
    c. Poison Prevention Act
    d. ADR Reporter

16. Which of the following abbreviations is on the list of error-prone medications?
    a. QID
    b. QOD
    c. BID
    d. TID

17. In a retail pharmacy, what technology would help prevent selection of the wrong drug if the drug is a look-alike/sound-alike drug?
    a. barcode scanning
    b. drug utilization review
    c. CPOE
    d. e-prescribing

18. The NDC number for Humulin R 10 mL vial is 0002-8215-01. The middle number, 8215, represents the
    a. manufacturer.
    b. product.
    c. page size.
    d. dosage form.

19. Which of the following is not a look-alike/sound-alike name?
    a. guanfacine/guaifenesin
    b. Xanax/Zantac
    c. Prozac/fluoxetine
    d. MS Contin/OxyContin

20. A technician filling a new prescription should check the prescription for
    a. completeness.
    b. accuracy.
    c. authenticity.
    d. all of the above

Thinking Beyond the Exam

Medication errors can happen even in the best circumstances. From your experience, write a list of all the steps a prescription or medication order goes through before dispensing the final drug. Identify where potential medication errors might occur and what should be done to prevent errors from happening. Discuss whether these changes could be implemented at your work site and what barriers exist to making changes that may reduce errors.

Pharmacy Quality Assurance

7

Learning Objectives

- Define the meaning of quality assurance as it relates to health care.
- Explain how the National Drug Code is used to reduce errors.
- List the basic steps in continuous quality improvement (CQI).
- Discuss the need for communication as it relates to drug recalls.
- Identify areas of communication to decrease medication errors.
- Discuss advantages of a nonpunitive system of error reporting.
- Identify areas monitored by the infection control committee.
- Discuss ways to identify satisfaction as it relates to the patient, the employer, and the employee.

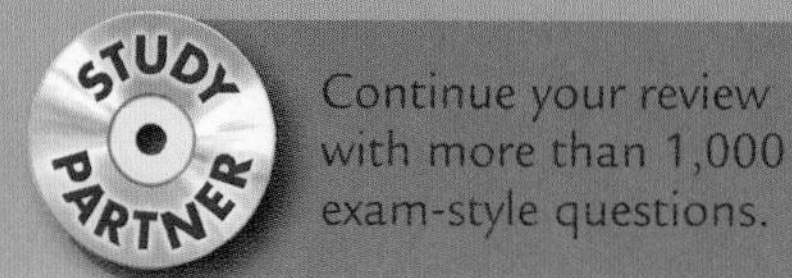

What does "quality assurance" mean? In 1999, the Institute of Medicine (IOM) published the report, "To Err Is Human: Building a Safer Health System," which broke the old rule of "don't tell" with regard to medical and medication errors. Medication errors occur in the best of systems equipped with the latest technology and best-trained healthcare providers. Although a small percentage of errors cause injury or harm, healthcare workers must strive to prevent error. Quality assurance means working continuously to review policies and procedures, educate staff, and provide patients with the best health care possible. Healthcare workers are only human. Mistakes happen. It is essential to remain vigilant to identify causes, reduce errors, and fix the system. In evaluating errors, the *how* and *why* are more important than the *who*.

Employee Quality

The quality of the workforce is an essential component of any quality-run business. To ensure that pharmacies and institutions employ the best-qualified people, the human resource department investigates all potential employees' credentials and past employment history. Credentials are the education and licensing required for the job. For example, a registered pharmacist must graduate from an accredited college of pharmacy and pass a licensing exam. Most states have a board of pharmacy that oversees the licensing of pharmacists. Each state board of pharmacy looks to the National Association of Boards of Pharmacy (NABP) for guidance on state requirements. As discussed in Chapter 1, state pharmacy boards also establish criteria for certifying pharmacy technicians. Technicians who pass a certification exam may be called a Certified Pharmacy Technician (CPhT).

Medication Selection

Before computers and barcodes were commonplace in the pharmacy, a technician would carefully read a product label and check it against a handwritten prescription. In today's pharmacy, technicians can scan the barcode on a stock bottle of a prescription drug. Barcodes help to ensure the prescription is filled correctly and refilled using the same product.

The national drug code (NDC), discussed in Chapter 6, plays an important role in preventing medication errors. Each brand and generic drug is assigned an NDC number that appears on all labels and barcodes. When the pharmacy receives a product from the manufacturer, the barcode, encrypted with the NDC number, is scanned into the computer system, which records the item as in stock.

The pharmacy technician uses the same barcode when filling or refilling a prescription. The computer matches the barcode on the package to the NDC stored in the prescription file. If the drug barcode does not match, the computer issues an alert to prevent the technicians from filling the prescription with the incorrect medication. If the pharmacy has purchased a generic drug from a different manufacturer, the technician will need to scan the new barcode and have the pharmacist verify it before filling the prescription. Any change in the stock or barcode should be double-checked by the pharmacist, as should the final prescription, before the medication is dispensed to the patient.

FDA Approval

Food and Drug Administration (FDA) approval is another important element in assuring the quality of pharmaceutical products. To earn FDA approval and be marketed in the United States, a drug must meet the FDA's requirements for safety and efficacy. A pharmacy technician can check the FDA website to see if a drug has received FDA approval and whether it is a generic or brand name product. Some drugs can be dispensed on a limited basis before receiving FDA approval. Investigational or experimental drugs do not have FDA approval. If an institution is working with a pharmaceutical company on an investigational drug, the institution will need to seek approval from its Investigation Review Board (IRB) before it can be used in a study or clinical trial. The IRB plays a critical role in reviewing all study data on investigational and experimental drugs to make sure that patients' rights are protected.

Infection Control

Chapter 5 discussed infection control as it relates to sterile and nonsterile compounding. For the pharmacy technician, it is important to use personal protective equipment (PPE) and follow compounding policies and procedures to ensure the final product is free of contaminates. A patient who develops an infection from a compounded sterile product administered in a hospital is said to have a nosocomial infection. Nosocomial infections may be life-threatening. The institution where the error occurred may be penalized, and insurers may refuse payment for treatment.

Properly documenting the compounding process verifies the technician has followed procedures correctly and ensures the integrity of the final product. Regular review of the technician's work by the supervising pharmacist, including testing for contamination, provides additional protection from error and helps to document the technician's competency. Quality review reports are kept on file with human resources and reviewed by the accrediting board when evaluating the pharmacy's performance.

In the hospital setting, an Infection Control Committee reviews the pharmacy's sterile compounding area for cleanliness, proper storage of pharmaceuticals, environmental and employee safety, and appropriate policies and procedures. The committee provides feedback on areas that need improvement and makes suggestions about training or retraining pharmacy staff or the environmental service staff that cleans the pharmacy.

Training is an important function in health care. Staff must be trained before a new drug or device is introduced into the healthcare environment. Example 7.1 looks at the proper use of safety needles and how training is documented in the employee's personnel file.

Example 7.1

In the past, nurses and other healthcare workers administered shots using needles with detached caps. Recapping needles and improper needle disposal resulted in unnecessary needlesticks, which can transmit bloodborne infections such as hepatitis and HIV. Institutions now use safety needles—a needle with a cover that slides down over the sharp end after use, to protect against needlesticks. All staff must be properly trained in the use of safety needles, and the training must be documented in the employee's personnel file.

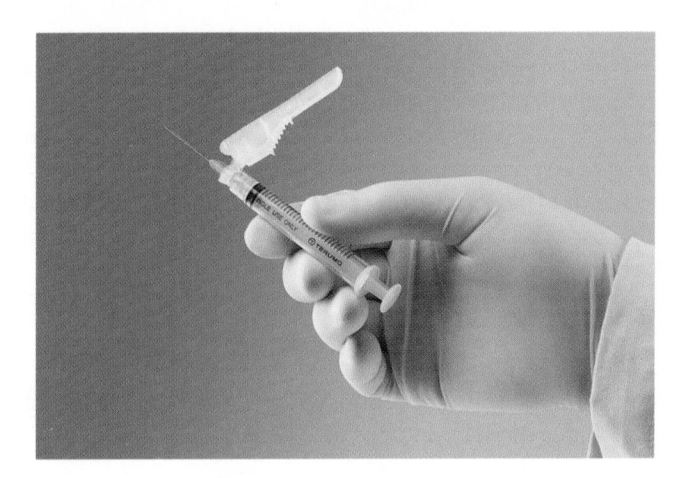

Risk Management

With all the training, documentation, policies, procedures, and technology now in place in health care, it seems that errors should not happen. Unfortunately, they do. Like any industry, health care must be on the lookout for practices, systems, and techniques that can cause errors. In health care, errors can harm patients and healthcare workers, and have consequences for institutions. The specialty area that monitors and works to improve systems is called risk management.

Risk management involves employees documenting errors, and even near misses (errors that did not reach the patient), to identify problems before they happen. Looking at the whole process step-by-step can help to identify areas of weakness that could result in patient harm.

A risk manager will always be on the lookout for ways to do a job better. Part of a pharmacy technician's job is to help identify areas of weakness or problems in the pharmacy setting. For example, the BigPharma Company introduces a new product, ABCocide. The company also has a product called ABCastatin. The company uses a white bottle with a beige label for all of its products. A technician stocking the new product on the shelf might notice the sound-alike name and look-alike packaging of the two products. To reduce the chances of a medication mix-up, the technician might take proactive measures, placing the two products on different shelves and updating the name in the pharmacy's computer record using tall-man lettering to make each product label look unique. The technician would then educate other pharmacy staff about the new product, caution them about potential look-alike/sound-alike problems, and explain the steps taken to prevent a medication error. Unfortunately, the causes of medication errors are not always so obvious.

So what if the technician took no steps to prevent an error? The ABCocide drug was stocked on the shelf next to ABCastatin. It was not labeled with tall man lettering. The next prescription refill for ABCastatin was filled with ABCocide instead. Hopefully, the error was caught before the medication was dispensed. In case of such an error, however, the individual who identified the error would generate an error report. The risk manager would use the report to prevent the error from happening again.

The process of investigating medication errors is not about finding blame with any one individual. Blame is counterproductive; many healthcare workers would feel uncomfortable filling out an error report knowing that someone would get in trouble. No one makes an error on purpose. Extenuating circumstances need to be evaluated and reviewed. It is important to learn from mistakes. And rarely is just one individual responsible for a mistake. By focusing on process instead of blame, it is possible to improve the system and prevent future errors.

Continuous Quality Improvement

Continuous quality improvement (CQI) is a process used to evaluate systems and errors. It includes these basic steps:

1. Describe the process and the sources of variation from the intended outcome.
2. Conduct a team analysis to clarify the source of variation and the extent of problem.
3. Discuss alternatives and make decisions on how to reduce variations.
4. Implement a plan and measure its effectiveness.

A full discussion of CQI is beyond the scope of this chapter, but it is important to note that it is a team process. Cooperation is needed at all levels to effectively manage errors and prevent future errors. The failure of a hospital or employer to change work practices that may cause errors and harm to patients is called organizational failure.

Communicating Recalls, Shortages, and Changes

The FDA is responsible for the safety and efficacy of the drugs produced and distributed within the United States. When a problem is identified with a drug or durable medical equipment, it is important for the FDA, the manufacturer, and the pharmacy to communicate to protect patient safety and ensure the drug or product is not sold.

In Chapter 9, a section on drug recalls discusses the different levels of recalls and the responsibility of pharmacy personnel based on the level of recall. The FDA posts information on recalls online at paradigmcollege.net/certexamreview3e/fda_safety_recalls. Notification of a drug recall is made by the manufacturer and/or wholesaler to the pharmacy. All pharmacies must respond to a drug recall even if the product is not in stock. The pharmacy is responsible for keeping a copy of all recall correspondence and isolating and documenting the stock on hand. If the recall, is a Class I, it is the pharmacy's responsibility to contact all patients who received the drug or product.

Communication is also important when there is a drug shortage. A wholesaler will identify an item in short supply and may even allocate or restrict the quantity available for purchase to prevent a pharmacy or purchaser from stockpiling the item. The pharmacy technician responsible for ordering and receiving should keep the pharmacy staff apprised of shortages and "outs," items that are not available. Often, if the pharmacist is aware of a shortage, he or she can change patient prescriptions to a more available product, thus ensuring there is no interruption in therapy.

It is also important to alert the pharmacy staff about any new products or changes in product packaging or location. Reading the label is the best way to identify a drug, but it is not uncommon for someone to think, "it is always in this spot on this shelf," or "the package always looked like this" when in a hurry. Many companies use the same package design for their entire line of pharmaceuticals, so it is essential to review the NDC number and the written information on the label before dispensing. By informing staff of new products and relocated products with sound-like names or look-alike packaging, the pharmacy technician is taking effective steps to prevent errors.

Measuring Job, Pharmacy, and Patient Satisfaction

Satisfaction can be viewed from the perspective of the healthcare provider, the pharmacy, and the patient. Personal satisfaction is an important aspect of a career as a pharmacy technician. Job satisfaction is about more than just earning a paycheck, although that may be one incentive. Satisfaction comes from doing the best job possible every day. This includes showing commitment to the profession by continuing to improve one's skills and knowledge through training and by becoming a certified pharmacy technician.

The employer's satisfaction with a technician's job performance is also an important aspect of a pharmacy technician's career. The director of pharmacy or supervising pharmacist will evaluate job performance by reviewing orders processed and proficiency in sterile or nonsterile compounding. The annual job review offers an opportunity to discuss any other contributions the technician has made. It is important to accept feedback and look for ways to improve any area identified as less than satisfactory, and to take advantage of classes offered to improve one's skills and knowledge.

Accreditation

There are a number of accrediting agencies that evaluate hospital and institutional pharmacy performance through on-site visits and performance reviews, including the Joint Commission and the federal Centers for Medicare and Medicaid Services (CMS). Facilities that receive an unsatisfactory rating will be given opportunities to implement improvement strategies and then be re-evaluated. If an institution with a pharmacy department fails to achieve accreditation, it may no longer be able to bill for reimbursement from insurance companies or federal or state agencies.

Patient Satisfaction

How can a healthcare provider or institution know if the patient is happy with the care provided? Many hospital and healthcare institutions use surveys (e.g., Press Ganey) to measure patient satisfaction. Surveys look at such things as wait time, staff professionalism, food quality, and other issues. Survey results can identify trends, areas that work well, and areas that need improvement. Institutions can also use survey results to compare their own performance over time, and compare their institution's performance against others. Such analysis can lead to improvements.

In community pharmacies, satisfaction is less likely to be measured by a formal survey. Repeat business is one measure of satisfaction. Patients that return again and again are usually content with the level of service. Magazines and newspapers in many areas can offer another means of assessing consumer satisfaction through annual "Best of" contests and surveys. These offer positive reinforcement that the institution is satisfying its clientele.

Quality assurance is an ongoing activity, and one in which the pharmacy technician has an important role to play. Only by identifying areas of weakness can pharmacy professionals and the institutions they serve become better at serving patients and protecting workers.

Skills Quiz

Reflect on the information presented in the chapter by answering the following questions.

1. What drug label information can be scanned to ensure the correct drug has been selected?
   a. manufacturer
   b. drug name
   c. barcode
   d. wholesaler sticker
2. What item used in the hospital will prevent needlesticks when used correctly?
   a. lancet
   b. safety needle
   c. calibrated syringe
   d. nonlatex gloves
3. The role of the Infection Control Committee in the hospital is to
   a. make sure patient care areas are sterile.
   b. provide patients with antibiotics.
   c. safeguard patients against nosocomial infections.
   d. make policy and procedures for cleaning the laminar airflow workbench.
4. To demonstrate that you have followed the policy and procedures for monitoring the pharmacy's refrigerator temperature, you should
   a. document the temperature on the appropriate log sheet.
   b. have another technician check the temperature with you.
   c. call the director of pharmacy and report the temperature.
   d. report the refrigerator temperature to risk management.
5. What is a commonly used technique to evaluate medication errors and prevent the same errors from happening again?
   a. IRB assessment
   b. FDA website
   c. satisfaction survey
   d. CQI process
6. Which of the following is *not* a step in the CQI process?
   a. fire the individual who made the error
   b. weigh alternatives and decide what to do
   c. implement the plan and measure success
   d. analyze the variables causing the error
7. You are moving some drugs around to make room for new products. What should you do when you are done?
   a. move on to the next job
   b. communicate the changes to the pharmacy staff
   c. document the job done in your personnel file
   d. order more stock to fill the shelves
8. A wholesaler identifies a drug recall. Some of the drug is on the pharmacy shelves. Until you get more information you should
   a. file the notice and wait.
   b. disregard the notice and throw it away.
   c. send it to the accounts receivable so they can file for credit.
   d. isolate the drug and fill out any form included.
9. The wholesaler is having difficulty getting the antihypertension drug metoprolol succinate. They have decided to allocate their limited supply and will release only half of what is ordered. You should
   a. file a grievance with the board of pharmacy.
   b. inform the pharmacist of the shortage and allocation.
   c. call all the patients taking the drug and tell them that you will not be able to fill their prescriptions.
   d. put it on backorder.

10. How can a hospital tell if patients are satisfied with the care they received?
    a. the patients return repeatedly
    b. the patients pay their bills on time
    c. the hospital receives positive responses to a satisfaction survey
    d. the hospital passes the accreditation survey
11. You are new to a community and looking for a job in a hospital pharmacy. How will you know if the hospital provides quality care?
    a. check the hospital accreditation standing
    b. ask to read the policy and procedure manual
    c. check with your area newspaper
    d. look at the latest satisfaction survey
12. To ensure the patient safety, what agency must review an investigational drug protocol before a hospital can participate in a drug trial?
    a. U.S. Pharmacopeia
    b. the hospital's chief executive officer
    c. the hospital's Investigation Review Board
    d. the U.S. Drug Enforcement Administration
13. Whose job is it to report medication errors?
    a. pharmacy director
    b. prescriber
    c. pharmacy technician
    d. everyone
14. What technology has decreased the number of selection errors?
    a. automatic dispensing machines
    b. barcode scanning
    c. online insurance billing
    d. computerized perpetual inventory
15. Nosocomial infections are infections that occur
    a. outside the hospital.
    b. in the community.
    c. in the hospital.
    d. in the upper respiratory tract.
16. When checking the will-call section you notice that the vial for a prescription of lovastatin is large. You identify the contents as Lovasa, not lovastatin. What should you do?
    a. notify the pharmacist of the error
    b. document the error
    c. correct the prescription
    d. all of the above
17. What is the purpose of recording your supervisor's assessment of your technique in sterile compounding in your human resources file?
    a. to document your level of skill
    b. to prove the hood room is not clean
    c. to ensure you do not make errors
    d. to check the integrity of the final product
18. What technique would a receiving pharmacy technician use to ensure the quality of the inventory?
    a. only stock brand name products
    b. relocate look-alike packages
    c. address recalls immediately
    d. communicate shortages to the pharmacist
19. If the pharmacy changes suppliers for the generic equivalent of Risperdal, the pharmacy technician selecting the drug for refills should
    a. use the brand name product for the refill.
    b. scan in the new NDC number and verify the product with the pharmacist.
    c. override the computer warning of selecting the wrong NDC and fill the prescription.
    d. tell the patient you need to order the product and send them away.

20. A prescription error is made and you were involved in filling the prescription. The director asks you to be on the CQI group evaluating the error. Why?
    a. You work in the system in which the error happened and can help analyze the process.
    b. You made the error, thus you have to account for fixing it.
    c. Your job is on the line if the committee feels you should not have made the error.
    d. Only you have ever made this kind of error.

Thinking Beyond the Exam

The Institute of Medicine's 1999 report "To Err Is Human..." has opened the lines of communication between healthcare providers and the patient in situations in which an error may have occurred. How are errors handled with regard to notifying patients? If you made an error that affected a patient, would you tell the patient? As a patient, how would you like a healthcare professional to handle the situation?

Medication Order and Entry Process

8

Learning Objectives

- Interpret common abbreviations used by prescribers in community and hospital settings.
- Explain the differences between a prescription and a medication order.
- Identify the components of a prescription, a medication order, and a patient profile.
- Review a prescription or medication order for completeness and accuracy.
- Review a prescription for authenticity and legality.
- Review the process for filling, labeling, and verifying a prescription or medication order.
- Identify five mechanisms for transferring medication information to a patient.

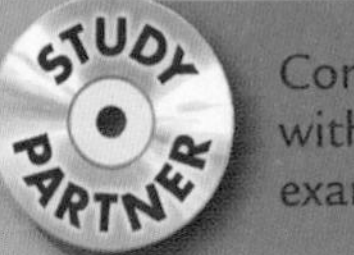

Continue your review with more than 1,000 exam-style questions.

In preparing for the exam, there is no substitute for course work and experience. As explained in Chapter 3, there are many drugs and much to learn in both the community and hospital pharmacy environments. This chapter reviews the components of a prescription and a hospital medical order, and common abbreviations used by prescribers. In both community and hospital pharmacies, the pharmacy technician is responsible for assessing the prescription or medication order for completeness and accuracy. In the community pharmacy, the technician has the added responsibility of checking the prescription for authenticity and legality. This chapter also discusses methods for providing medication information to patients, the process of filling, packaging, and labeling prescriptions, and the final check by the pharmacist.

The Prescription

In the community pharmacy, medications are dispensed to the patient based on information written by a prescriber on a prescription. A prescription is commonly presented by the patient to the technician after a visit to the doctor or emergency department, or after being discharged from the hospital. A prescription may be submitted by phone, fax, or computer (e-script). Table 8.1 lists the parts of a prescription. The prescription is a privileged communication from the prescriber to the technician and pharmacist, and is subject to The Health Insurance Portability and Accountability Act of 1996 (HIPAA) privacy laws.

The goal of the profession of pharmacy is to get the right drug and right strength by the right route safely to the right patient at the right time to prevent medication errors (the 5Rs). The role of the pharmacy technician is to greet customers; review new prescriptions; process refill requests; enter new prescription/refill information into the pharmacy database; update patient profiles; submit drug claims to insurance providers; retrieve, fill, and prepare medications for pharmacist verification and approval; dispense prescriptions; and complete any necessary transactions for copayments or cash payment.

In the community pharmacy, almost 50 percent of all prescriptions are submitted electronically. E-scripts have several advantages, including speed, accuracy, improved billing, and decreased potential for forgeries and medication errors. E-prescribing can minimize the risk of potential medication errors resulting from failure to understand a prescriber's handwriting, misinterpretation of abbreviations, and illegible faxes. Electronic prescribing of controlled substances must be approved by each state board of pharmacy.

TABLE 8.1 Parts of a Prescription

Prescriber	name, address, telephone number, and other information identifying the prescriber, including state license number, DEA number, and NPI
Date	date on which the prescription was written (may not be the same day the prescription was received)
Patient information	patient's full name, address, telephone number, and date of birth
℞	stands for the Latin word *recipe*, meaning *take*
Inscription	medication prescribed, including generic or brand name, strength, and amount
Subscription	instructions to the pharmacist on dispensing the medication
Signa	directions for the patient (commonly called the "sig")
Additional instructions	any additional instructions that the prescriber deems necessary
Signature	signature of the prescriber

The Medication Order

Medication orders are used to order pharmaceuticals in institutional settings such as hospitals, nursing homes, long-term care facilities, and psychiatric hospitals. Information is usually conveyed via a hard-copy medication order sent to the pharmacy from the nursing unit. In fully computerized institutions, the medication order will be transmitted online. The pharmacy technician is involved in placing or preparing individual oral unit doses. The pharmacy technician may also compound intravenous solutions, intravenous admixtures, and total parenteral nutrition and hazardous cancer chemotherapy drugs. The pharmacist must verify the accuracy of all compounded products. The technician works on the nursing unit to update inventory, check for expired drugs, and deliver needed medications. Automation and use of barcode scanning technology have been widely adopted in many institutions to reduce medication errors.

FIGURE 8.1 Elements of a Hospital Medication Order

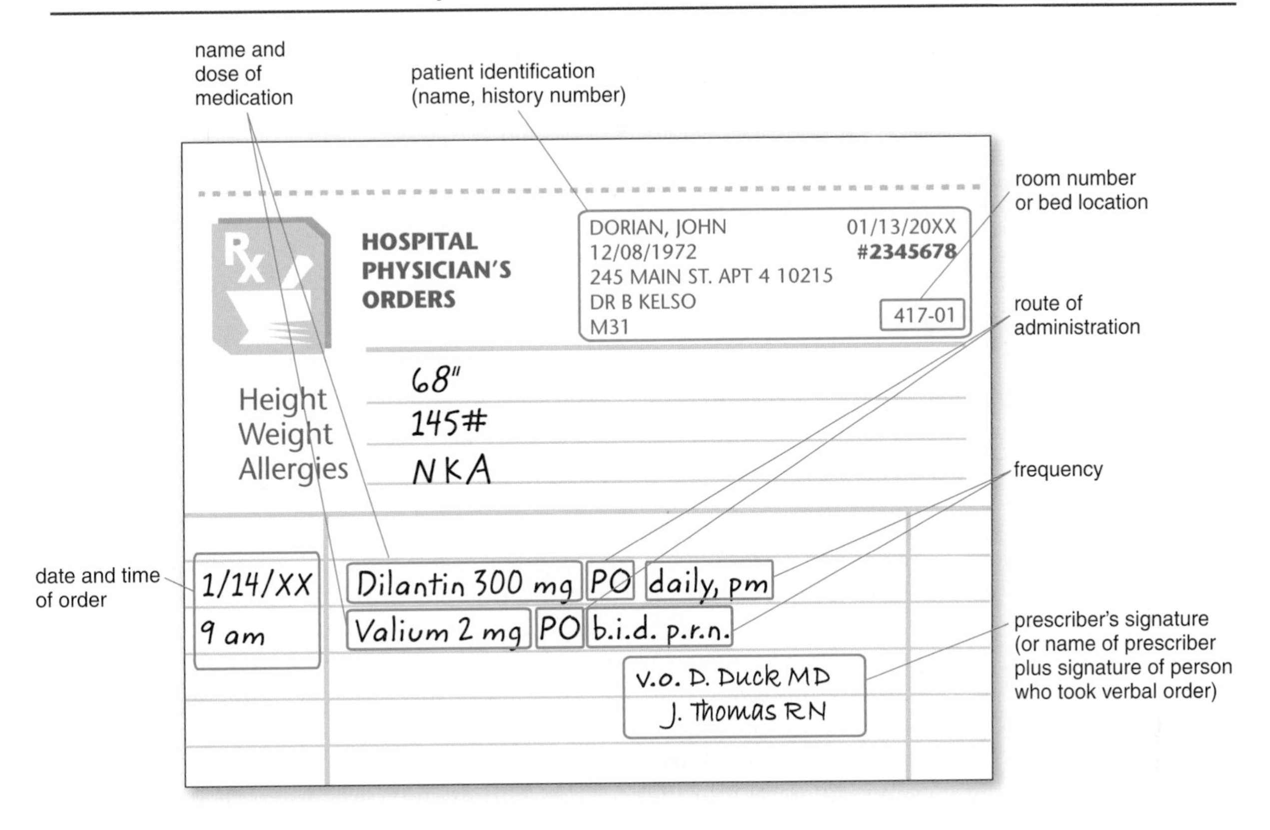

Figure 8.1 is an example of a hospital medication order. There are several differences between a prescription and a medication order, including:

- Prescriptions are directly dispensed to the patient; medication orders are filled and delivered to the unit and administered by nursing personnel in the hospital, nursing home, or other medical facility.
- Hospital orders are often for medications administered intravenously (IV), such as parenteral and nutritional solutions, antibiotics, or other medications.
- Prescriptions are for a defined amount of medication; medication orders, with the exception of narcotics, are dispensed until the order is changed or discontinued, or the patient is discharged.
- In addition to the pharmacist, nurses provide an extra layer of professional review and expertise that helps minimize medication errors.

In the institutional setting, the pharmacy more freely substitutes a generic medication for a brand name drug. Brand name drugs are dispensed only if no generic drug is available. If a nonpreferred or nonformulary medication is ordered in a hospital, the pharmacy (with medical staff approval) can institute automatic directives to substitute/interchange the approved formulary item without specific physician approval (for example, dispensing pantoprazole when omeprazole is ordered). Increasingly, hospital pharmacies employ robotic devices to assist the pharmacy technician in retrieving and packaging drugs for unit dose use, filling carts, stocking nursing units, and sterile compounding. Robotic systems can operate 24/7 with nary an error.

In the hospital (skilled nursing facility or home health care), medication orders often include IV solutions. Large-volume parenterals (LVPs) are intravenous (IV) infusions in which the volume of the infusion is more than 100 mL, but typically 500 mL to 1,000 mL. LVPs are most often used for fluid replacement and fluid maintenance for patients who cannot maintain adequate oral intake or need rapid replacement of fluids to treat dehydration. Patients who require additional nutrients intravenously receive a special LVP called total parenteral nutrition or TPN. Small-volume parenterals, often used to piggyback medications onto an LVP and IV set, are discussed in Chapter 5.

Common Abbreviations

For a pharmacy technician to fully review and transcribe a prescription or medical order, he or she must also understand and recognize the shorthand abbreviations used in medicine and pharmacy. Table 8.2 lists common prescription abbreviations for amounts, dosage forms, time, and site of administration. Most of these abbreviations are derived from Latin. Note that weight and volume amounts borrow heavily from the measurement systems discussed in Chapter 2. Table 8.2 also lists several common abbreviations that the Institute of Safe Medication Practices (ISMP) recommends should NOT be used because of the increased risk of medication error.

Focus and attention to detail are critical when reviewing a prescription. Note that when the units are abbreviated, there is a minimal visual difference between gram (g) and grain (gr), but 1 grain is equal to 65 mg and 1 g is equal to 1000 mg, so there is a potential for a dosage error. Remember that 1 mL is equal to 1 cc and is used interchangeably for parenteral solutions or oral solutions and suspensions. The IMSP recommends not using "cc" as it is easily misread.

If the amount of medication taken by the patient varies each day, the prescriber may use the abbreviation "q.s." This abbreviation is interpreted as "quantity sufficient" to fill the prescription. The technician will need to calculate the amount of medication needed, as in the example for Orapred.

℞ Orapred 15 mg/5 mL

Sig: 15 mg PO twice daily with food on Day 1 (5 mL twice daily or 10 mL)

10 mg twice daily on Day 2 (3.3 mL twice daily or 6.6 mL)

7.5 mg twice daily on Day 3 (2.5 mL twice daily or 5 mL)

5 mg twice daily on Days 4–5 (1.7 mL twice daily for 2 days or 6.8 mL)

Quantity: Add sufficient (q.s.) 28.4 mL is the exact quantity (rounded to 30 mL)

A stock bottle of Orapred is labeled 15 mg/5 mL. If a pediatrician writes a prescription as shown in the example, what quantity of medication should the technician enter into the computer and dispense?

Abbreviations for dosage forms are usually fairly straightforward. Many generic medications are available in both capsule and tablet formulations and can be used interchangeably if they are in the same dosage form. In some cases, the prescriber may write tablet but the capsule is available in stock; it can generally be substituted if approved by the prescriber. Pay attention to formulations: Wellbutrin SR (12 hour) is not equivalent to Wellbutrin XL (24 hour). Prescriptions written for the eyes and ears may be solution or suspension; there is a subtle difference between these dosage forms, and they should not be interchanged without the approval of the prescriber. Remember, sterile eye drops can be used in the ear, but ear drops cannot be used in the eye!

TABLE 8.2 Common Prescription Abbreviations

Abbreviation	Meaning	Abbreviation	Meaning
Amount/Dosage Form		***Time of Administration—Continued***	
cc*	cubic centimeter (mL)	p.c.	after meals
cap	capsule	P.M.	evening, after noon
g	gram	p.r.n.	as needed
gr*	grain	q6h	every 6 hours
gtt	drop	q.i.d.	four times a day
mg	milligram	stat	immediately
mL	milliliter (cc)	t.i.d.	three times a day
q.s.	a sufficient quantity	t.i.w.	three times a week
tbsp	tablespoonful	***Site of Administration***	
tsp	teaspoonful	AD*	right ear
MDI	metered-dose inhaler	AS*	left ear
sol	solution	AU*	each ear
supp	suppository	NPO	nothing by mouth
susp	suspension	OD*	right eye
tab	tablet	OS*	left eye
ung	ointment	OU*	each eye
Time of Administration		PO	oral, by mouth
a.c.	before meals	PR	per rectum
A.M.	morning, before noon	SL	sublingual (under the tongue)
b.i.d.	twice a day	TOP	topical (skin)
hr	hour	VAG	vaginally
h.s.*	at bedtime		

* Do NOT use these abbreviations. The Institute for Safe Medication Practices (IMSP) lists these as dangerous abbreviations because they are easily misread.

Time of administration is important. For instance, if a prescriber writes the following antibiotic prescription

> ℞ Augmentin 875 mg
>
> Sig: 1 tab PO q12h

the technician should transcribe it exactly this way in the computer. Entering "b.i.d." (twice a day) is not quite the same as q12h because the patient may take the medication six or eight hours apart.

Failure to differentiate the directions q.d. (daily) from q.i.d. (four times a day) could result in serious harm to a patient; often the tail of the q in q.d. (or a period between the q and d) may look like an i because it loops back. For this reason, the ISMP recommends avoiding the use of the lowercase abbreviation q.d.; either use QDay or daily or every day.

Some medications, like acid reducers and diabetic medications, are best taken before meals, and this direction will be abbreviated "a.c." Some medications that can cause stomach ulceration (like ibuprofen) are taken with food. If the prescriber writes "p.c.", the medication should be taken after meals.

Site of administration is usually PO or "per oral" for tablets, capsules, and many liquid solutions or suspensions. A few medications, such as nitroglycerin, work faster if placed under the tongue or sublingually (SL). If a patient is vomiting continuously, the prescriber may order a drug administered rectally.

℞ Phenergan 25 mg

Sig: 1 supp PR q6h p.r.n.

In the example above, the dosage form "supp" (suppository) and the "PR" designation indicate that the drug is to be administered per rectum. Creams and suppositories can also be prescribed vaginally or intravaginally (VAG).

As noted in Table 8.2, abbreviations for drug administration to the eye and ear, although common, should not be used because of the increased risk of medication error. Often, a prescription may not clearly state whether the left or right eye (or ear) is involved; in that case, it is appropriate for the technician to type in the sig field of the medication label "instill into the affected eye(s)". The pharmacist can then counsel the patient or parent when the prescription is dispensed.

It is important to remember that although the pharmacy technician is often the person who reviews a prescription, interprets the abbreviations in the directions, calculates the quantities, makes any necessary measurement conversions, and transcribes the information into the computer, the pharmacist is responsible for reviewing and approving all work and comparing the entry with a hard copy of the prescription. This is called the final check.

Completeness

To be complete, a prescription must contain all of the following information:

- patient name
- date written
- drug name, strength, and quantity
- directions for use
- special instructions (substitution permitted) and refills (if any)
- prescriber signature

A hospital medication order (Figure 8.1) will include patient name, drug name, strength, directions, and the prescriber's signature. In addition, it will be stamped with

FIGURE 8.2 **A Complete Prescription**

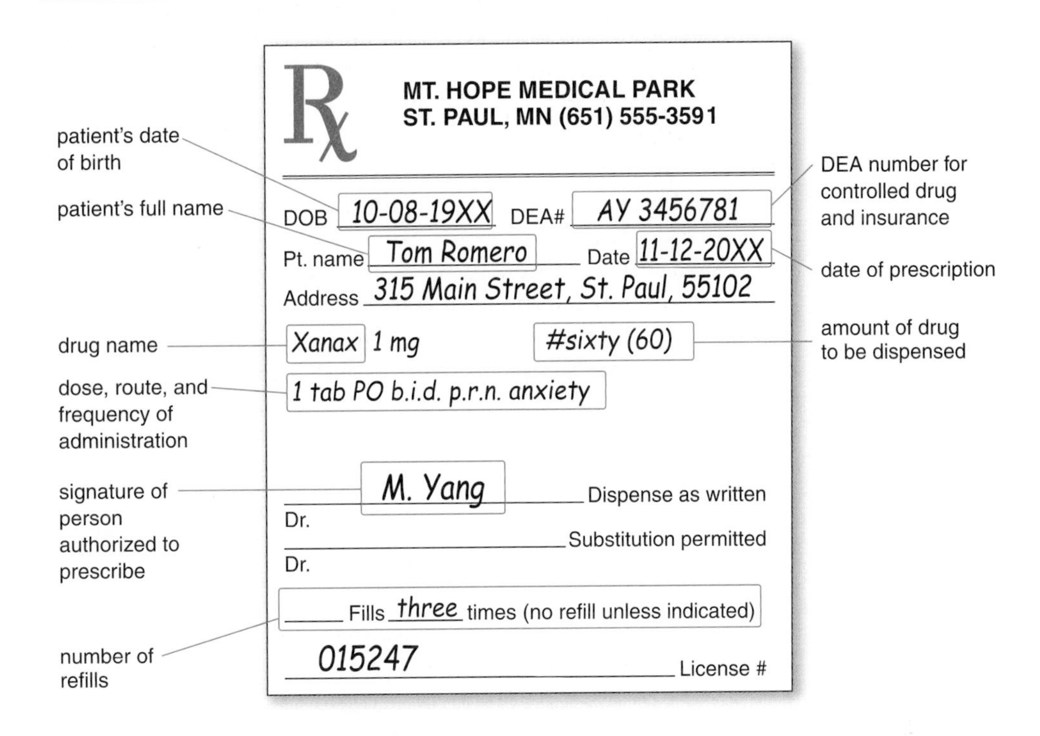

the time and date. Quantity, special instructions, and refills are usually not necessary in the hospital environment.

Patient name is obviously important. If the patient has recently married, divorced, or moved, it may be necessary to update the patient profile in the computer with any changes. Some patients may prefer their middle names instead of their first names, making locating the record in the database a challenge. Third-party payers require claims to be submitted under the name listed with the insurer.

If the drug name or directions are illegible, or the drug strength or quantity is missing, a call to the prescriber is necessary. Depending on the state and pharmacy's regulations, the pharmacist may need to verify any change. It is always good practice to verify information to minimize potential medication errors. If refills are not stated or circled on the prescription, assume that no refills were ordered.

Prescribers within the hospital are usually doctors (MD, DO) or residents or interns in training under direct supervision. In the community pharmacy, prescribers include not only doctors but dentists (DMD, DDS), veterinarians (DVM), podiatrists (DPM), optometrists (OD), physician assistants (PA), nurse practitioners (NP), advanced practice nurses (APN), and naturopaths (NP). Physician assistants must practice under the direct supervision (and license) of a practicing physician. A registered nurse may write a prescription, but it must be signed by a licensed prescriber. Nurse practitioners have prescriptive authority and can write or sign prescriptions according to the defined protocol in their states, even for controlled substances.

If the prescription is for a controlled drug, such as a narcotic pain medication, nerve medication, sleeping pill, or diet pill, the prescriber must have a federal DEA number on file in the pharmacy database and on the prescription. This number is required for anyone prescribing controlled drugs (discussed in Chapter 4) and differs from a state license number or national provider identifier (NPI). If this number is not listed or available, the technician may have to call the prescriber or his/her nurse and request the DEA number. A valid NPI number is usually required by insurance for reimbursement. The NPI is a national database of prescribers.

The information on the medication order is reviewed by the pharmacy technician (or nurse/unit clerk and pharmacist in the hospital) and entered into the patient profile in the computer. If the hospital has a computerized physician order entry, the prescriber will enter orders in the patient's profile and the pharmacy will verify the orders for accuracy and patient safety before dispensing. Nurses acknowledge the new order on the electronic medication administration record (eMAR) before administering the first dose.

A pharmacist is required to check all prescriptions entered by a pharmacy technician to decrease the potential for transcription errors. The trend to computerize order entry in hospitals and electronic prescribing in community pharmacies has reduced the potential for transcription errors and the need for pharmacy staff to interpret physicians' handwriting.

Accuracy

In addition to checking for completeness, the technician must review prescriptions for accuracy. Is the patient name correct? Is the patient's married or given name on the prescription? Is the prescription written using the patient's middle name rather than first name (e.g., J. Robert Williams instead of Jay Williams)? To ensure accuracy and reduce the potential for medication errors, the technician often requests the patient's date of birth and writes it on the prescription. It is not uncommon for two patients to have the same first and last name (e.g., Rhonda Taylor and Rhonda S. Taylor).

The pharmacy technician reviews the date the prescription was written. Do not assume that the prescription was written on the same day the pharmacy received it. If no date is written, it is commonly assumed that it was written on the date presented. If the prescription is for a controlled drug, the date is extremely important and the prescription cannot be filled without it. If there is no date on the controlled substance prescription, a follow-up call to the prescriber is necessary and the patient may need to get a new prescription.

The technician should also verify that the drug name, strength, and quantity are correct and legible. There are many drugs with look-alike and sound-alike names, so focus and attention to detail are important. Does the prescription say tramadol or trazodone, Trileptal or Trilipix, metformin or metformin ER? Many drugs come in various dosage forms—extended release and sustained release, inhalers and nebulizing solutions, and so on—so it is critical that the correct medication is entered into the patient profile in the computer. Is the drug strength and quantity familiar? It may be necessary to review various measurement systems of weight and volume. Drug strength may be stated in grams, grains, milligrams, or micrograms, and volume may be stated in cubic centimeters or milliliters. The technician must be able to convert measurements in the metric and avoirdupois systems of measurement (see Chapter 2).

Is the prescribed drug strength available as written? If the prescription reads

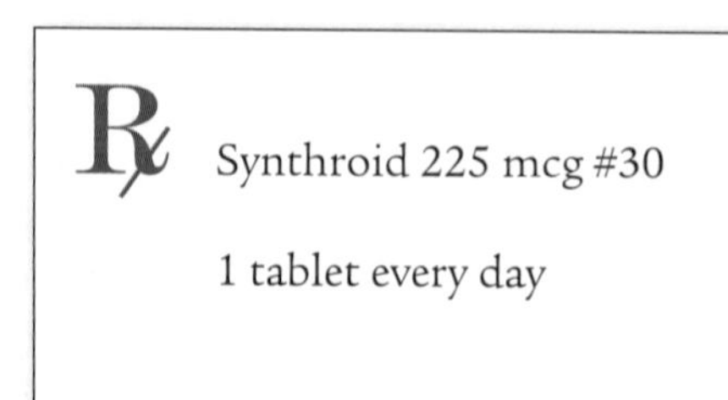
℞ Synthroid 225 mcg #30

1 tablet every day

but the drug is not available in that strength, how should the technician enter the drug in the computer? One option is to enter two prescriptions—one for 200 mcg and one for 25 mcg—but that would result in a higher cost to the patient and the insurer. Another option is to fill the prescription with the 150 mcg tablet and change the directions to "1.5 tablets per day." A pharmacy technician should not make any changes to a prescription, especially a prescription for controlled drugs, without first checking with the pharmacist. Usually such changes are initialed by the pharmacist.

Many medications are available in multiple doses and dosage forms. Metoprolol tartrate 25 mg is different from metoprolol succinate 25 mg; one is immediate release and one is controlled release. The same is true for metformin 500 mg and metformin ER 500 mg. It is important that the technician enter the correct drug into the computer from the original prescription.

The quantity to be dispensed is usually stated on the prescription. Sometimes, however, the prescriber may indicate a one-month or three-month supply instead. In such cases, the pharmacy technician must calculate the quantity to be dispensed. For example, the technician would enter #180 for the following prescription:

℞ Glipizide 10 mg PO b.i.d.

#90 days' supply

In some states, if a prescription is written for a 30-day supply with two refills, the pharmacy technician/pharmacist is allowed to fill a three-month supply. In other states, the medical office must be contacted for approval and the approval documented on the prescription. A prescription for simvastatin 40 mg #30 2 refills could be filled (in some states) with simvastatin 40 mg #90. The pharmacy may do this to reduce the patient's out-of-pocket costs. Many insurers charge the equivalent of two monthly copayments for a three-month supply.

The *Sig*, or directions for use, should be legible and clear on the prescription. Abbreviations are commonly used in directions. For the medication label, the technician should translate the information from the prescription into clear language the patient can understand. The instructions are printed on the label and reviewed and approved by the pharmacist before the medication is dispensed to the patient.

Most prescriptions have a preprinted statement from the prescriber's office indicating "substitution permissible." Drugs are often available as both a brand name and a lower cost generic. Most patients (and their insurance providers) prefer that the pharmacy dispense the lower-cost generic drug. For example, the cholesterol-lowering drug Lipitor is a brand name for the generic drug atorvastatin.

If the prescriber indicates "dispense as written" (DAW) or "brand medically necessary," then the brand name drug must be entered into the computer and dispensed. When billing the insurance provider, it is important to enter a DAW1 in the appropriate field. The patient may also request a brand name drug be dispensed (usually referred to as DAW2 for billing purposes), although this often requires a higher copayment. Brand name drugs are commonly ordered for Coumadin, Dilantin, and Synthroid because of the narrow therapeutic index of these medications.

The number of refills allowed is usually written or circled on the prescription. For a maintenance drug such as birth control pills, the prescriber may indicate p.r.n. or "as needed" refills. Refills for noncontrolled medications are generally approved for one year after the prescription is written. Schedule III and IV drugs can be refilled up to five times or six months from the date written. Schedule II drugs are subject to stricter laws that vary from state to state. Remember, refills are not allowed on any Schedule II medications, such as morphine, methadone, oxycodone, methylphenidate (Ritalin), Adderall, and Concerta.

Depending on state regulations and site policies, medication orders in a hospital are usually renewed every seven days. Orders on antibiotics and narcotics often have automatic stop orders (ASO) after a given period of time, as per hospital policy. The ASO requires the physician to continually review medications for each patient.

When reviewing the prescription, the technician should confirm that the prescriber's signature is legitimate. Often the prescriber's name is preprinted on the prescription at the top with address, phone number, and pertinent licensing numbers. If not legible or preprinted, the name may be identified in the computerized database by telephone number, DEA number, or NPI. Many insurance companies require a prescriber DEA and/or NPI number to process the prescription for reimbursement.

Many prescribers practice in more than one physical location or clinic; in such cases, it is important to identify both the correct name and phone number of the medical office in which the prescription was written. This is necessary to clarify prescription information or request future refills on medications. If the name or location cannot be identified, the technician should call the medical office or check with the patient for the correct office location.

Authenticity

The authenticity (and legality) of a medication order written in a closed system like a hospital is rarely an issue. However, in a community pharmacy setting, the technician as well as the pharmacist must verify the authenticity of the prescription, especially in the case of controlled medications.

It is important for the technician to verify the authenticity of all prescriptions. In rural areas, a technician may become familiar with all local prescribers, but in an urban area this will not be possible. Technicians need to learn common techniques for spotting illegal prescriptions. Has the prescription been altered in any way, especially in quantity or number of refills? No alterations can be made on a Schedule II prescription. Is the prescription written on tamper-proof paper with a visible watermark? Some prescriptions may be photocopies or facsimiles cleverly produced with a laser printer.

Prescription blanks are sometimes stolen from doctors' offices and prescriptions forged, especially for narcotics. Be wary of prescriptions written for unusual quantities for new, out-of-state patients, especially on weekends and nights when the prescription cannot be verified with the prescriber. Such "patients" often request expensive brand name drugs and pay cash so there is no paper trail.

It is important to know how to verify the prescriber's DEA number. This number consists of two letters (the second letter is the same as the first letter of the last name of the prescriber) plus seven numerals. (To review the steps, see Example 31 in Chapter 2.) Remember, even if the DEA number is correct, the prescription could be forged.

Legality

As already stated, state and federal regulations limit the number and timing of refills for controlled drugs and for copies of prescriptions transferred from other pharmacies. Prescriptions for Schedule II medications, which have the highest abuse potential of commercially available medications, require a hard copy; the prescriber may not fax or phone in such prescriptions unless permitted by state law. In the case of hospice care for terminally ill patients, most states allow the pharmacist to fill a Schedule II prescription based on a phone call if the prescription is immediately written out; some states require the prescriber to mail a hard copy of the prescription to the pharmacy within 72 hours.

Whenever state and federal regulations of controlled drugs conflict, apply the more stringent regulation. For example, some states may allow the pharmacist to dispense an emergency supply of Schedule II medications, but only if the prescriber mails or delivers a hard copy within a stated period of time (usually 48 to 72 hours). Most, but not all, states allow the dispensing of Schedule V drugs, such as cough syrups, without a prescription. However, many states (and pharmacies) do require a prescription (or evidence of diabetes) to dispense syringes.

Each state is responsible for regulating health professionals within that state, including pharmacists and pharmacy technicians. Know the regulations in your state. Can a physician assistant prescribe narcotics without the signature of his or her supervising physician? Can a nurse practitioner prescribe narcotics? Does a fax for a controlled drug require an electronic signature? Can a prescription for controlled drugs be submitted electronically? What are the state requirements for tamper-proof prescriptions?

The prescriber must also practice within his or her specialty. For example, a veterinarian cannot prescribe medications for humans, an optometrist is limited to eye medications, and a dentist is restricted to prescribing appropriate medications, such as antibiotics and pain medications, in a quantity limited to the needs at the time of prescribing. Physicians can prescribe medications for themselves and for family members in some states, but this privilege does not apply to controlled drugs.

Patient Profile

Each time a patient presents a prescription at the pharmacy, the technician must create or update the patient profile to track and fill prescriptions. All components of the profile should be updated, including physical address, prescription billing, and allergies (see Table 8.3 on the next page for the components of a patient profile). The pharmacist uses the data in the profile to counsel patients. The computer profile can also alert the pharmacist or technician to allergies or potential medication conflicts. The patient profile also includes an area for patient comments that help the pharmacy honor patient requests for a bottle without a child-resistant cap, a generic substitution when available, a 90-day supply, as well as notes about foreign language or sign language needs, or accommodations for visual impairment. When a patient requests a refill and does not have the previous medication container, the technician will retrieve the prescription information from the patient's medication history in the patient profile.

TABLE 8.3 Components of the Patient Profile

Component	Content
Identifying information	patient's full name (including middle initial), street address, telephone number, birth date, and gender; increasingly, pharmacy databases enter email addresses so refill notifications and other communications can be made electronically
Insurance information	information necessary for billing (see Chapter 10 for insurance and billing information)
Medical and allergy history	information concerning existing conditions (e.g., diabetes, heart disease), known allergies, and adverse drug reactions; pharmacy software reviews patient medical history to make sure the prescription is safe.
Medication and prescription history	Most databases list any prescriptions filled at the individual pharmacy location; some list OTC medications, as well. The new prescription is compared to previously filled prescriptions; pharmacy software reviews this information to check for adverse interactions with drugs or food.
Prescription preferences	patient preferences (e.g., child-resistant or non–child-resistant containers, generic substitutions, large-print labels, foreign language preference, etc.)
HIPAA and confidentiality	Pharmacies are required by law to provide new patients with a statement outlining patient confidentiality; the action must be documented. (This statement is for the protection of the pharmacy.)

Filling a Prescription or Medication Order

After checking the prescription for completeness, authenticity, accuracy, and legality, the technician enters and updates information in the patient profile (submitting a claim for drug insurance in real time), and the pharmacist verifies the information. The technician files the medication(s), scanning the barcode of the national drug code (NDC) number to aid in identifying the exact drug, dose, and package size. The NDC consists of 10 characters that identify the manufacturer or distributor, the drug formulation, and the size and type of packaging. After the technician confirms the NDC on the stock bottle with the printed medication information sheet, the computer prints a patient- and drug-specific medication container label. The label is affixed to the appropriate plastic or glass medication container. The label's instructions must read exactly as indicated in the signa on the original prescription.

Medication orders may also be for parenteral medications, including large volume parenterals with or without medications. LVPs usually consist of water with salt (saline, or NaCl) and/or glucose (dextrose). It is not unusual for an LVP to have additional additives, such as potassium chloride (KCl) or multivitamins, depending on the patient's requirements. LVPs may be sent to the nursing unit or may be available at the nursing unit via a Pyxis workstation. Table 8.5 lists the most common IV fluid products and their typical abbreviations.

TABLE 8.4 Steps for Filling a Medication Order

The following list outlines the typical steps involved in filling a medication order in the hospital.

1. Physician writes the medication order(s) on the patient chart or enters the order(s) in the computerized physician order entry system (CPOE).
2. The order is transmitted via computer or transported to the pharmacy by a tube system, transportation department, or pharmacy personnel making regular rounds.
3. The medication order is reviewed for accuracy and safety by the pharmacist and either entered into the patient's medication profile or verified in the medication profile from the CPOE system.
4. The medications are supplied to the nursing unit by various routes depending on the facility's system. A fill list is generated from the medication profiles, and a medication drawer is filled for each individual patient in a unit dose cart. The medication order may be filled by the technician, checked by the pharmacist for accuracy, and placed in a patient-specific drawer in a unit dose cart.
5. Pharmacy technicians are then responsible for delivering the medication cart to the nursing unit. This is usually done once a day in a large acute care hospital. The cart may carry more than one day of medication in a smaller hospital or long-term care facility.
6. A Pyxis or other automated dispensing system may also be used to fill a medication order. Once the pharmacist approves a medication order, the nurse may retrieve it from the medication station and administer it.
7. *Stat* orders are processed in a similar manner but given top priority. They are dispensed and delivered immediately for the nurse or doctor to administer. In a Pyxis system, some emergency medications, like nitroglycerin sublingual tablets, are available to the nurse before the pharmacist checks the order.

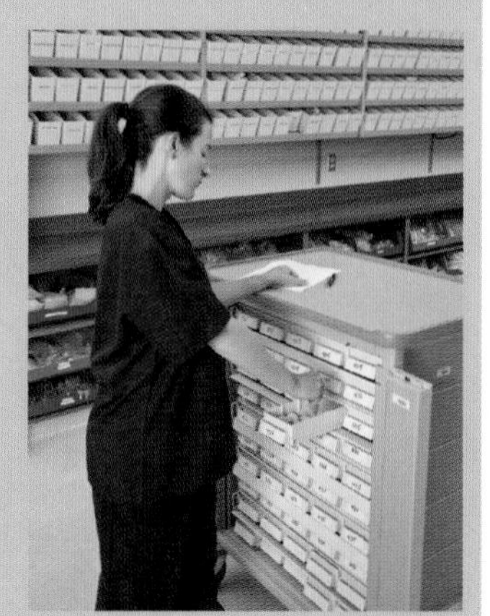

Medication cart

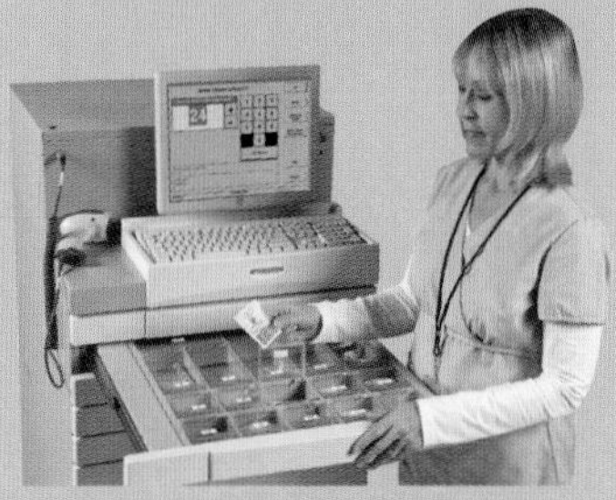

Omnicell automated dispensing system

A medication label for an IV contains the following information:

- patient's name and identification number
- room number
- fluid and amount
- barcode with drug name and strength (if appropriate)
- infusion period (e.g., infuse over 30 minutes)
- flow rate (e.g., 100 mL/hour)
- beyond-use date (or expiration date) and time
- additional information including hazardous drug warning, auxiliary labeling, storage requirements, and device-specific or drug-specific information, such as filters

TABLE 8.5 IV Fluids and Abbreviations

IV Fluid	Abbreviation
normal saline (0.9% NaCl)	NS
½ normal saline (0.45% NaCl)	½ NS
5% dextrose	D_5W
10% dextrose	$D_{10}W$
5% dextrose and normal saline	D_5NS
Lactated Ringer's solution	LR or RL

FIGURE 8.3
Steps for Filling a Prescription

Although each step in this process can be a source of medication error, each step also offers an opportunity for pharmacy personnel to correct errors.

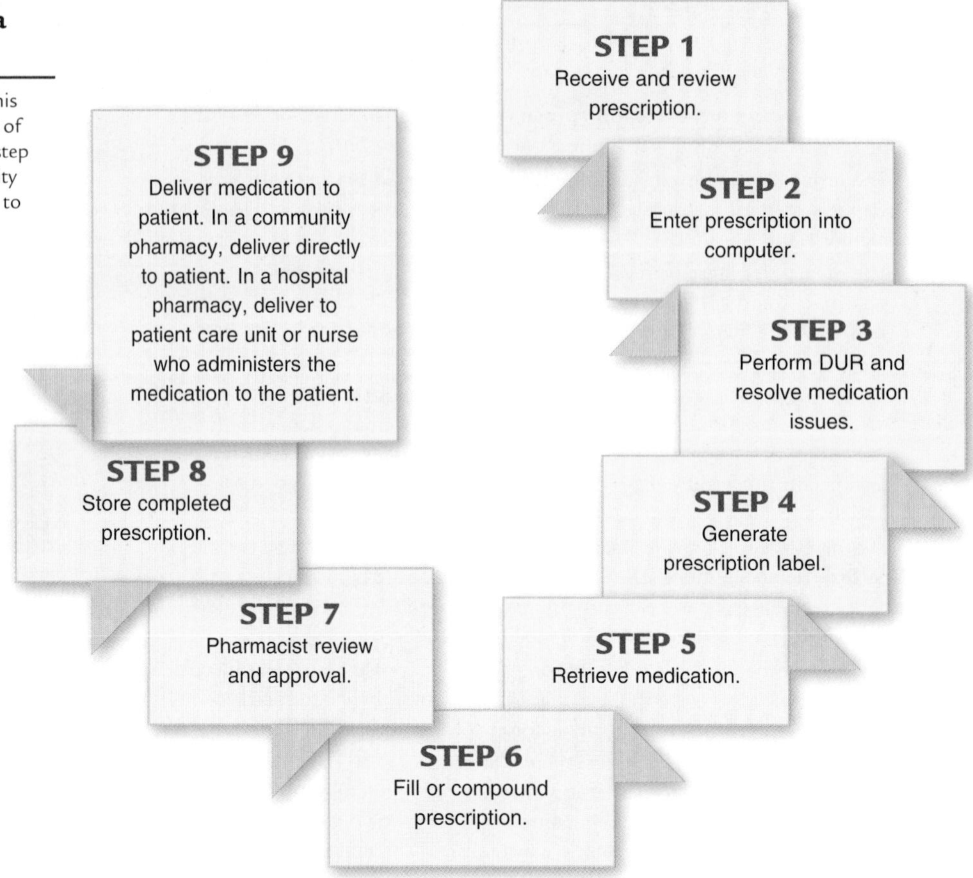

Packaging

Most pharmacy containers, called vials, used for tablets, capsules and liquids, are amber-colored plastic or glass to prevent ultraviolet (UV) light exposure and subsequent degradation of the medication. Product packaging from the manufacturer ensures stability and potency until the listed expiration date.

To comply with the Poison Prevention Packaging Act of 1970, all medications should be dispensed in child-resistant containers unless specifically requested by the patient. The caps on these containers are designed to be difficult for children to open. Certain drugs in original packaging are exempt from this requirement, including nitroglycerin sublingual tablets. Most OTC medications are available only in child-proof and tamper-proof packaging. Most reconstituted antibiotics require refrigeration and expire after 14 days. Vials of insulin at room temperature have an expiration of 28 days before they lose some potency. Insulin and many eye drops, suppositories, and injectable medications may require refrigeration in the pharmacy and at home. The shingles vaccine (Zostavax) is stored in a freezer and is stable for only 30 minutes after it is reconstituted.

In the hospital, parenteral medications, such as amphotericin B, are sensitive to light and may be protected by an amber-colored UV protected plastic wrap. Some drugs, such as IV nitroglycerin and amiodarone, may be absorbed by the plastic polyvinyl chloride (PVC) coated IV tubing, thus reducing the amount delivered intravenously to the patient. Such infusions require special plastic sets that are made of non-PVC film and contain no latex.

When dealing with hazardous cancer drugs in the hospital setting, a closed system transfer device (CSTD) is the preferred medication delivery system to minimize exposure—both for the pharmacy technician and hospital staff. The closed system circumvents pressurization issues with the vial and prevents the escape of toxic vapors. After barcode scanning, the drug is activated at the patient's bedside. Protective garb must be worn by nurses at the bedside, even in the case of preparing and administering a chemotherapy drug in a CSTD system.

Patient Medication Information

There are five distinct ways of communicating necessary medication information to the patient: (1) medication container label; (2) auxiliary labels; (3) medication information sheet; (4) an FDA-mandated MedGuide for select medications; and (5) counseling by the pharmacist.

After review and verification by the pharmacist, the computer generates a medication container label. The label is affixed to the container/bottle/box of prescribed medication and includes the following: the date dispensed; name, address, and phone number of the pharmacy; Rx number; patient name; number of refills; prescriber name; drug name; dose; directions; and manufacturer. Medication container labels for Schedule II–V drugs must contain a transfer warning that reads, "Caution: Federal law prohibits the transfer of this drug to any person other than the patient for whom it was prescribed."

Auxiliary labels are small, colorful labels that may be added to supplement the directions on the medication container label (see Figure 8.4). Auxiliary labels include warnings such as "caution with alcohol," "wear sunscreen," or "take with food." These labels are commonly affixed to the container by the pharmacist or an experienced technician.

FIGURE 8.4

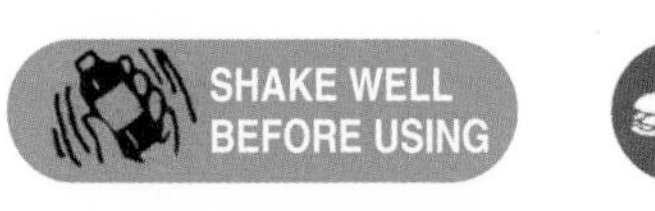

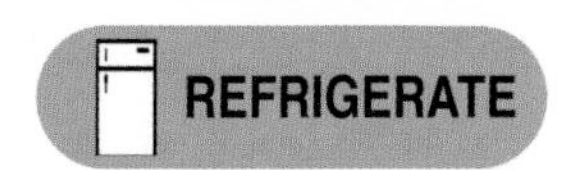

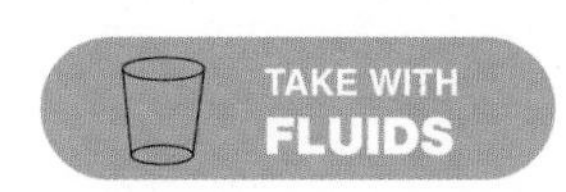

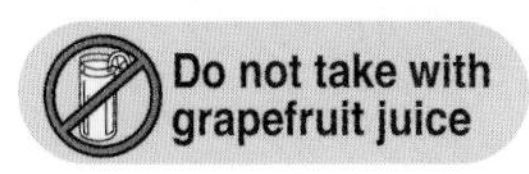

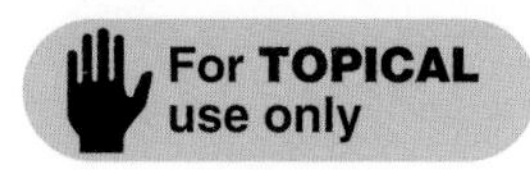

Auxiliary labels are placed on dispensed medications to help inform patients about how to take and store their medications safely and effectively.

A medication information sheet is a computerized printout that provides details on how to safely take the prescribed medication. The information sheet is automatically printed after the pharmacist has verified the prescription. After the pharmacist conducts a final check of the prescription and medication, the information sheet is attached to the bag containing the medication, which then is ready for patient pick-up.

The MedGuide (discussed in Chapter 6) is basically a black box warning advising consumers about potential adverse reactions or the proper use of selected high-risk medications. Birth control pills are commonly packaged with a MedGuide; other MedGuides are printed for the patient at the time of the pharmacist's final check.

Finally, by law, the technician must offer the patient counseling by the pharmacist. In some cases, especially with first-time medications or potential drug interactions, the pharmacist will take the initiative to counsel the patient. At other times, the patient may have a question and request counseling. The pharmacy technician is never allowed to counsel a patient.

Final Check by the Pharmacist

It is extremely important—and required by law—that the pharmacist checks every prescription to verify its accuracy before it is dispensed to the patient or sent to the nursing unit. Typically in a community pharmacy, the pharmacy technician will present the original hard copy prescription (if available), the medication information sheet, and the labeled container with the prescribed medication to the pharmacist for final check. The pharmacist reviews the original prescription, compares it with the patient profile, confirms that the medication information sheet has been printed, verifies that the drug selected by the technician (from the stock bottle) is correct, and checks the accuracy of the medication container label.

In the hospital, the medication order, label, compounding procedure, preparation records, and all materials used to prepare or make a compounded sterile product must be inspected by the pharmacist before the medication is sent to the nursing unit. The inspection should include verification of the identification and amount of ingredients, technique for aseptic mixing and sterilization, packaging, labeling, and physical appearance. A pharmacist may provide a physical check to look for incompatibilities between the additives and an IV solution.

Skills Quiz

Reflect on the information presented in this chapter by answering the following questions.

1. A medication order will include which of the following information?
   a. number of refills
   b. prescriber's DEA number
   c. drug name and dose
   d. the Rx symbol
2. In what part of a prescription would you find directions for the patient?
   a. inscription
   b. subscription
   c. superscription
   d. signa
3. What do you do when a prescriber writes "no substitution" on a Coumadin prescription?
   a. use a DAW2 code to bill the insurance
   b. ask the patient which he or she prefers, brand or generic
   c. dispense warfarin anyway; insurance wants generic
   d. use a DAW1 code to bill the insurance
4. Which of the following medications should be stored in the freezer?
   a. NovoLog
   b. Azithromycin suspension
   c. Zostavax
   d. nitroglycerine sublingual
5. The pharmacy receives a prescription that reads "Penicillin 250 mg tablets, i PO q.i.d. a.c." What should the instructions on the medication label say?
   a. Take 1 tablet by mouth 4 times a day, after meals.
   b. Take 1 tablet by mouth 4 times a day, before meals.
   c. Take 1 tablet by mouth daily, before meals.
   d. Take 1 tablet by mouth daily, after meals.
6. Which abbreviation might appear on a prescription for ciprofloxacin ophthalmic solution?
   a. SL
   b. OU
   c. PO
   d. PR
7. A patient hands you a prescription for Adderall and the quantity has been altered. What should you do?
   a. contact the prescriber
   b. notify the pharmacist
   c. fill the prescription
   d. give it back to the patient
8. A patient presents a prescription for Prednisone 10 mg i PO q.i.d. x 4 days, i PO t.i.d. x 4 days, i PO t.i.d. x 3 days, i PO b.i.d. x 2 days, then i PO qd x 1 day, then stop. How many tablets will you dispense?
   a. 10 tablets
   b. 20 tablets
   c. 30 tablets
   d. 40 tablets
9. A medication order is usually seen in a(n)
   a. acute care hospital.
   b. community pharmacy.
   c. chain pharmacy.
   d. outpatient hospital pharmacy.
10. The fill list is used by the technician to
    a. reorder drugs from the wholesaler.
    b. refill a used code cart.
    c. fill a patient's medication drawer.
    d. compound a sterile product.
11. A large-volume parenteral has at least ____ of fluid.
    a. 50 mL
    b. 100 mL
    c. 250 mL
    d. 500 mL

12. To prevent medication errors, the ISMP recommends that the ____ abbreviation not be used.
    a. TID
    b. QID
    c. QD
    d. BID

13. The prescription is for the Schedule II drug OxyContin. How many refills may the prescriber legally order?
    a. 0
    b. 1
    c. 2
    d. 5

14. What information is not required on the label of an intravenous infusion?
    a. number of refills
    b. infusion rate
    c. additives
    d. patient's name

15. Which is more characteristic of a medication order than a prescription?
    a. drug is dispensed directly to the patient
    b. a large volume parenteral for fluid replacement
    c. order contains quantity to dispense with number of refills
    d. physician's contact information is on the written document

16. In what situation is a technician allowed to dispense a prescription to a patient without a final check by the pharmacist?
    a. a double-check has occurred by a certified pharmacy technician
    b. a refill of a previously filled prescription
    c. a sterile compounded intravenous solution
    d. never; all prescriptions must be checked by a registered pharmacist

17. Which abbreviation would be used to indicate the route of administration is rectal?
    a. po
    b. pr
    c. pv
    d. sl

18. Transfer warnings are used on
    a. prescription labels for C-II to C-V medications.
    b. prescription labels to indicate this is a transferred prescription.
    c. prescriptions for topical medications.
    d. medication orders for intravenous solutions.

19. Amber or light-blocking vials are used to store medications to prevent
    a. contamination of the medications.
    b. privacy violations.
    c. degradation of the medication.
    d. leaching of the drug into vial plastic.

20. When should a patient profile be updated in a community pharmacy?
    a. only when a new patient is added to the computer
    b. every time a new prescription is filled
    c. once a year on the patient's birthday
    d. never; the physician keeps all the patient information up-to-date

Thinking Beyond the Exam

There are many pieces of information to consider when processing a prescription or medication order. A single mistake can have dire consequences. Think about all of the information presented in this chapter. What steps and precautions can you take to ensure a prescription is prepared accurately and safely every time?

A pharmacy technician has many legal and ethical responsibilities in the institutional pharmacy. During a busy day, a nurse knocks on the pharmacy door and demands a medication right away for a patient emergency. The pharmacist is away consulting on a chart and you are alone in the pharmacy. What do you do?

Pharmacy Inventory Management

9

Learning Objectives

- Identify components in profitable inventory management.
- Discuss the advantages and disadvantages of a formulary.
- Become familiar with purchasing concepts.
- Understand the receiving process.
- Explain stock rotation.
- Discuss storage requirements.
- Discuss the beyond-use date for insulin.
- Identify product removal requirements.

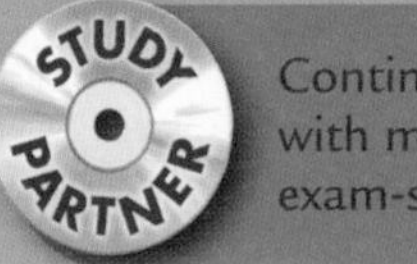

Continue your review with more than 1,000 exam-style questions.

One of the responsibilities of a pharmacy technician is inventory management. Inventory is one of the pharmacy's largest investments, and a busy retail pharmacy may have $300,000 or more in inventory on the shelves. While other factors can affect the pharmacy's profitability, proper inventory management of pharmaceuticals and over-the-counter products is important to the pharmacy's bottom line. The pharmacy needs to keep sufficient drug stocks on hand to meet customer needs while minimizing costs, including the cost of inventory on the shelf and waste generated when pharmaceuticals pass the beyond-use date. In a community pharmacy, insufficient inventory can cost the pharmacy individual and future sales if the pharmacy is not able to fill customers' prescriptions. In an institutional pharmacy, stock shortages may force the pharmacy to purchase products at a higher price. Inventory management, purchasing, and receiving are integral parts of the practice of pharmacy.

Inventory Considerations

The pharmacy technician is often responsible for ordering and receiving medications, durable medical equipment, and over-the-counter (OTC) products. The entire stock of pharmaceuticals on hand at a given time is referred to as inventory, and it is a major source of expense for the pharmacy. It is important for the pharmacy to maintain sufficient (but not excess) inventory to reduce waste and overhead while still meeting the needs of the community or hospital.

Ordering and Purchasing

With the exception of Schedule II drugs, ordering and purchasing often are initiated by the pharmacy technician. Medications are frequently ordered daily to minimize inventory costs and promote stock turnover. Most of the time, drugs are ordered from a wholesaler or corporate warehouse and are delivered to the pharmacy the following day. Chain pharmacies may receive warehouse orders only once a week and rely on a wholesale dealer to cover potential shortages during the week. This is known as "just-in-time" ordering—receiving medications just in time to sell.

In the past, it was common for pharmacies to order drugs directly from the manufacturer or pharmaceutical company. That practice is no longer as common. Pharmacies had to purchase quantities larger than they could sell in a reasonable amount of time, tying up money with unneeded inventory and decreasing profits. Only investigational drugs are still ordered from the manufacturer. Pharmacies that work with research institutions acquire investigational drugs from the lead investigator or manufacturer. In institutions, the materials management department may contract with manufacturers for small and large volume intravenous solutions, such as D_5W or normal saline, which are used throughout the entire facility.

In the past, patients were often responsible for the full cost of medications. That has changed. More recently, insurance providers, pharmacy benefit managers (PBM), and health maintenance organizations determine the cost of patient medications.

The average wholesale price (AWP) of a drug is the average price that wholesalers charge the pharmacy. Pharmacies and institutions negotiate for lower prices using the leverage of a buying group. Usually, third parties reimburse the pharmacy based on the APW less than an agreed-upon discount. The reimbursement price is calculated using the formula:

$$\text{APW} - \text{percentage} + \text{dispensing fee} = \text{reimbursement}$$

Example 9.1 shows how this formula can be applied to the purchase of the hypothetical drug Lipidbuster.

Example 9.1

The PBM for a patient's drug insurance plan has a contract to reimburse the pharmacy for brand name drugs on its formulary at AWP, minus 4% plus a $4.95 dispensing fee. The AWP for Lipidbuster is $100 per 30 tablets. The pharmacy's buying group negotiated a purchase price for Lipidbuster of AWP minus 5%.

How much will the pharmacy's gross profit be if it sells 30 tablets of Lipidbuster?

This is a three-part problem.

First, calculate how much the PBM will reimburse the pharmacy for the prescription.

$$\text{AWP} - \text{percentage} + \text{dispensing fee} = \text{reimbursement}$$

$$\$100 - (0.04 \times 100) + \$4.95 =$$

$$\$100 - \$4.00 + \$4.95 = \$100.95 \text{ (reimbursement)}$$

Second, determine how much the pharmacy paid for the drug.

$$\text{AWP} - \text{discount percentage} = \text{purchase price}$$

$$\$100 - (0.05 \times 100) =$$

$$\$100 - \$5.00 = \$95.00 \text{ purchase price}$$

Third, calculate the difference between the reimbursed price and the acquisition price. This is the gross profit.

$$\text{Reimbursement} - \text{purchase price} = \text{gross profit}$$

$$\$100.95 - \$95.00 = \$5.95 \text{ gross profit}$$

In this example, the pharmacy will make a gross profit of $5.95 for Lipidbuster for a patient on this insurance plan. For the pharmacy, it is important to try to find the best deal possible.

In addition to pharmaceuticals, the pharmacy technician is also responsible for ordering pharmacy supplies, prescription vials, bottles, labels, information sheets, measuring devices, and other items. In a hospital, the technician is responsible for ordering supplies from material management, the department in charge of ordering supplies for the entire institution, including syringes, needles, alcohol, personal protective equipment, and intravenous solutions used in compounding.

Ordering is the responsibility of all pharmacy employees. Some pharmacies have a perpetual inventory system on the computer programmed with minimum and maximum quantities the pharmacy should have on hand for each drug. The system automatically reorders needed stock at the end of the business day. Even with a perpetual inventory system, it is important to track and adjust the minimum and maximum quantities based on current trends.

Pharmacies that do not have a computerized perpetual inventory system track drug stocks by hand. Stickers on the shelves list the minimum and maximum quantities for each drug. When quantities get low, the technician notes it on an order sheet and calculates the quantity needed using the formula shown in Examples 9.2 and 9.3 on the next page.

Example 9.2

The pharmacy's maximum inventory of sertraline 100 mg tablets is 600 tablets and the minimum is 200 tablets. By the end of the day there are 100 tablets left on the shelf. How many bottles of sertraline 100 mg #100 per bottle should the pharmacy order?

maximum inventory − present inventory = amount needed to reach maximum

$$600 \text{ tablets} - 100 \text{ tablets} = 500 \text{ tablets}$$

The pharmacy needs to order 5 bottles of 100 tablets to bring the inventory up to the maximum level.

Example 9.3

The pharmacy buys sertraline in bottles of 30 tablets that only need to be labeled before dispensing, saving the pharmacy the cost of a prescription vial. Using the scenario in Example 9.2, How many bottles of 30 tablets need to be ordered to meet the pharmacy's maximum inventory?

maximum inventory − present inventory = amount needed to reach maximum

$$600 \text{ tablets} - 100 \text{ tablets} = 500 \text{ tablets}$$

500 tablets/30 tablets per bottle = 16.67 bottles. Round down to 16 bottles of 30 tablets so the order does not exceed the maximum inventory.

Pharmacies also use an order book to track inventory. When an item falls below the minimum, the technician places a sticker in the book. At the end of the day the technician keys in the order and transmits it to the wholesaler. This system works as long as everyone in the pharmacy remembers to reorder when stock is low. It also requires staff to know when to reorder bulk items that come in bottles of 500 to 1,000 tablets.

Discount Purchasing Value

Like consumers, pharmacies seek to benefit from sale prices. But before purchasing a large quantity of a product on sale, the pharmacy must consider how long it will take to sell the product and make a profit. Gross profit is the difference between the purchase price and the selling price. But before the pharmacy can make a profit on an item, it must factor in the cost of overhead. Overhead is the cost of wages, rent, utilities, equipment, and insurance required to operate the pharmacy. Net profit is the difference between the purchase price and the sale price once overhead costs are factored in. A negative profit (loss) occurs when the selling price is lower than the purchase price plus overhead.

When considering purchasing a large quantity of a drug or other item, the technician must calculate the additional time it will take to sell the additional quantity at a profit (see Example 9.4).

Example 9.4

The supplier offers a sale on calamine lotion: buy six cases, get the seventh case free. Each case sells for $6 and contains 12 bottles. All invoices must be paid in 30 days, or the pharmacy is charged interest. Last year, the pharmacy sold 76 bottles of calamine. If sales remain the same, how long will it take the pharmacy to sell all seven cases?

time to all sold = quantity to sell/sales history

time to all sold = (7 cases × 12 bottles)/76 bottles in 12 months

time to all sold = 14+ months

If it takes 14 months for the pharmacy to realize its return, is it a good idea to buy the product, even if it is on sale? Probably not. The gross profit from the discounted price is absorbed into the overhead costs, leaving little net profit. Calamine lotion is a low-dollar inventory item. What if this scenario involved an expensive pharmaceutical like Vytorin, which is used for treating hyperlipidemia? The pharmacy pays $100 or more for a bottle of Vytorin. In that case, the pharmacy would not want to wait 14 months to see a return on its investment. To avoid costly mistakes, pharmacies use an ABC classification system.

ABC Classification System

By classifying products into categories by sales volume, the pharmacy can more easily monitor the most expensive and high-use products and use just-in-time ordering to keep inventory costs down while ensuring there is sufficient quantity in stock to meet patient needs.

Table 9.1 shows how the classification system can be used to allocate pharmacy resources. Items in category A are more expensive and consume the largest amount of pharmacy resources. Category C accounts for the least amount of inventory resources, and category B for items in the middle. Loss of control of a few products in category A is more detrimental to the bottom line than the loss of control of a large number of items in category C.

TABLE 9.1 ABC Classifications

Category	% of Resource $
A	80%
B	15%
C	5%

Some classes of pharmaceuticals account for a large percentage of a pharmacy's inventory, including antiretrovirals, antipsychotics, antibiotics, and chemotherapeutic agents. The pharmacy wants these products to turn over quickly and not sit on the shelf longer than necessary. It is important to track the movement of these high-dollar items and order only when necessary, without making patients wait for medications. Many pharmacies dispense these drugs with auxiliary labels that read, "This item is special ordered for you, please call a few days prior to needing refills."

When ordering, it is important to know how soon the product will be available. This is called lead time. A compounding pharmacy must also consider the time it takes to compound or mix as part of the lead time.

To ensure the pharmacy does not run out of a drug, pharmacies keep a safety net supply on hand. This is known as safety stock. Safety stock provides a cushion so that if orders exceed the daily average, the pharmacy can still fill every prescription in a timely manner. To calculate safety stock, the technician must know the maximum potential daily usage, the average daily usage, and the lead time. Example 9.5 shows how to calculate the amount of safety stock needed for atenolol, a beta blocker used to treat high blood pressure and angina.

Example 9.5

The pharmacy dispenses an average of 400 tablets of atenolol 50 mg tablets daily, but it has sold as many as 750 tablets in one day. How many bottles of atenolol 50 mg 100 tablets should the pharmacy keep as safety stock if it takes 1 day to receive a new supply?

$$\text{safety stock} = (\text{maximum potential daily usage} - \text{average daily usage}) \times \text{lead time}$$

$$\text{safety stock} = (7.5 \text{ bottles} - 4 \text{ bottles}) \times 1 \text{ day}$$

$$\text{safety stock} = 3.5 \text{ bottles of 100 tablets of atenolol 50 mg}$$

Use the safety stock to calculate when the pharmacy should reorder. This is called the reorder point. Example 9.6 shows how to calculate the reorder point for atonolol.

Example 9.6

Reorder Point

$$\text{reorder point} = \text{average usage per unit} \times \text{lead time} + \text{safety stock}$$

$$\text{reorder point} = 4 \text{ bottles/day} \times 1 \text{ day} + 3.5 \text{ bottles}$$

$$\text{reorder point} = 7.5 \text{ bottles of atenolol 50 mg}$$

The pharmacy should have 7.5 bottles of atenolol available at the beginning of the day to make sure it can fill every prescription.

If the pharmacy runs out of a medication before more stock arrives and cannot fill prescriptions, the pharmacy experiences what is known as a shortage cost. Shortage cost is difficult to measure. The pharmacy may offer to have the medication delivered to the patient at home, incurring extra cost. If a medication is unavailable too often, the pharmacy may lose a customer.

As a purchasing agent, it is important to balance the expense of inventory against other operating costs. Knowing the pharmacy's inventory turnover rate—the number of times the inventory turns over per year—helps in evaluating the effectiveness of the pharmacy's inventory control system.

A high turnover rate is good. It means the pharmacy has closely estimated the inventory needed to meet patient needs, but not so closely that the pharmacy runs out of medications and loses business. A low turnover rate indicates the inventory is sitting on the shelves too long. Example 9.7 demonstrates how to calculate the inventory turnover rate by dividing the annual cost of purchases by the amount of inventory on hand.

Example 9.7

The pharmacy purchases $20,000 per month and has $93,000 in inventory in stock. What is the inventory turnover rate?

$$\text{inventory turnover rate} = \text{annual purchases/inventory on hand}$$

$$\text{inventory turnover rate} = (\$20{,}000 \text{ per month} \times 12 \text{ months per year}) \div \$93{,}000$$

$$\text{inventory turnover rate} = \$240{,}000 \div \$93{,}000$$

$$\text{inventory turnover rate} = 2.58$$

As Example 9.7 shows, this pharmacy is not controlling its inventory well. On average, a turnover rate of 5 or 6 is considered desirable. Inventory turnover rate does not usually exceed 10; 2.5 is extremely low. An increase in turnover would reduce the amount of inventory sitting on the shelf and save the pharmacy money.

Profit and Markup

The owner of the pharmacy has an objective for the year—to make a profit. How is profit calculated? Remember from Chapter 2 that markup is the difference between the selling price and the purchase price and is expressed in dollars and cents. To turn a profit, the pharmacy has to mark up products to cover the wholesale cost plus overhead. Overhead includes the cost of salaries, insurance, taxes, equipment, utilities, and other expenses. Although there is no hard percentage markup for every item, at the end of the year, income must exceed expenses. Review Chapter 2 to refresh your knowledge on markup, markup rate, discounts, and discount rate calculations.

Closed or Open Formulary

A formulary is a list of medications approved for use by an insurance company or hospital. Insurers sometimes have what are called closed formularies; drugs not on the formulary list are not covered by the insurer. Most insurance companies use a more lenient multi-tiered formulary. In Tier 1, the preferred drug (usually a generic) might require a minimal payment by the patient. Tier 2 requires a higher payment, and tier 3 (usually a brand name drug) has the highest patient cost. If a drug is not on the insurer's formulary but the physician feels it is medically necessary, the physician will have to seek prior approval before the insurance company will pay for the medication. Pharmacists and technicians can help patients find the most cost-effective medication option. Often, this involves contacting the prescribing physician to get approval for a therapeutic substitution (a pharmaceutically equivalent drug product). This can lengthen the time needed to fill a prescription. It is important for the technician to keep patients informed of any delay.

The community pharmacy does not use a formulary; it stocks pharmaceuticals to serve all of the patients in a community. If the pharmacy is owned by a health maintenance organization or private insurer, the Veterans Administration, for example, the pharmacy may have a formulary based on the larger organization's accepted standard of care.

In a hospital, a formulary is a tool to provide the patients with the appropriate therapy while controlling healthcare costs. Hospitals try to control expenses by reducing the number of pharmaceuticals in the formulary, based on purchasing groups and best practices established by the medical community. For example, the hospital may purchase one proton pump inhibitor (PPI) and make a therapeutic substitution for any PPI ordered. If omeprazole is the least expensive, then any medication order for lansoprazole, esomeprazole, or pantoprazole would be changed to omeprazole. Typically, any substitution has to be approved by the Pharmacy and Therapeutics (P&T) Committee, which includes members of the medical staff.

Receiving

Pharmaceuticals are delivered from the wholesaler, warehouse, or manufacturer, or through overnight mail in sealed storage units or totes. The technician receives the shipment, verifies the number of totes, and signs for the delivery.

If the delivery contains Schedule II drugs, the pharmacist may need to perform the inventory and sign the delivery order. If this is not the practice, the technician should make sure to verify the contents delivered (i.e., noncontrolled, controlled, Class II controls) before signing. If something is missing, the pharmacy will be charged after the delivery order is signed.

The technician then verifies the contents against the invoice and updates the computer inventory, acknowledging receipt of the items listed. This is called posting an order. Shortages, damaged items, and overages are reported immediately to the supplier for credit or pickup. Drugs not currently available from the supplier are reordered, if available soon, or ordered from an alternative supplier. Back orders have become common and technicians need to be savvy about finding other sources with competitive prices. It is important to keep the rest of the pharmacy staff alert to shortages, back orders, and recalls.

If the pharmacy has a computerized perpetual inventory system, the technician updates the perpetual inventory after the invoice is posted to ensure the computer reorders the appropriate quantities. In some systems, posting includes updating prices and expiration dates as well.

After posting, invoices should be sent to the accounts payable department in a timely manner. Many purchasing agreements stipulate that discounts are available only on invoices paid within 15 days. A delay in processing the invoice could cost the pharmacy money.

To review processes for ordering, receiving, and storing controlled substances, see Chapter 4.

Storage

After medications are received, they must be stocked or shelved according to proper labeling and storage requirements. Refrigerated and frozen pharmaceuticals are delivered in specially marked storage totes packed with ice or dry ice. These should be posted and stored as soon as possible. Do not touch dry ice. Place it in a well-ventilated area until it completely dissolves. Vaccines come in a tote with a color-coded device to indicate whether the vaccine has been exposed to temperatures outside the proper storage range. If stored improperly, the vaccine must be discarded and the supplier should be contacted for credit or replacement.

Medications and items stored at room temperature should have a designated space and shelf label. It is important to stock medications on the correct shelf and identify each by strength and dosage unit to minimize dispensing errors. For example, to avoid any sound-alike or look-alike errors, metformin 500 mg, a common diabetic drug, should not be placed on the shelf assigned to metformin ER 500 mg.

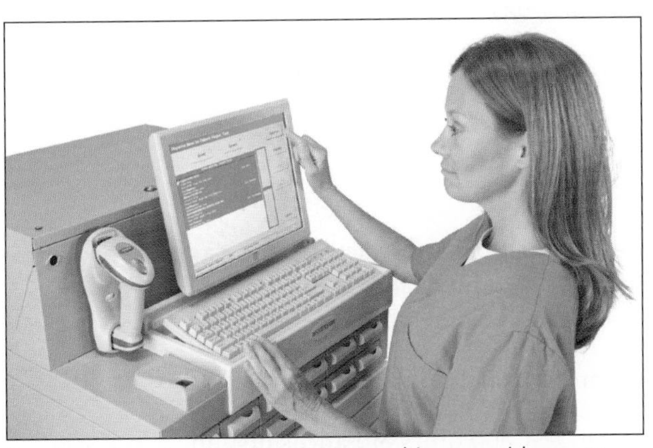

Automated medication dispensing machines provide secure storage and perpetual inventory control, and can charge the patient account at the point of administration.

In the hospital pharmacy, the technician is often responsible for restocking IV solutions used in sterile compounding and floor stock medications stored in automated dispensing units such as the Pyxis and Omnicell. These units provide a secure, locked storage area for frequently used drugs, including controlled substances, prescription drugs, and over-the-counter products. Floor stock units include a perpetual inventory system and automatically charge the appropriate patient account at the point of administration.

Zostavax and other vaccines and intravenous pharmaceuticals that need to be kept frozen should be stored at 5 °F or −15 °C. Zostavax must be used within 30 minutes after it is reconstituted with a diluent. Remember to check and log the freezer temperature daily. Where state law allows, many pharmacists are certified in administering vaccines, including flu vaccine clinics in the fall and early winter, and year-round vaccinations for Zostavax and other drugs.

Pharmacy refrigerator temperatures are kept in the range of 36 °F to 46 °F, or 2 °C to 8 °C. Refrigerated drugs include insulin, suppositories, NuvaRing™, and many injectable drugs. Chemotherapy agents that require refrigeration should be stored either in a separate refrigerator or isolated to avoid contamination if a leak or spill occurs. Any open refrigerated drug must be dated with its beyond-use date to ensure it is discarded at the appropriate time. Once opened, most insulins have a beyond-use date of 28 days. Patients need to be aware of this and instructed that insulin should be stored in the refrigerator until first use, and then discarded after 28 days. Patients do not need to refrigerate a vial or insulin pen after first use. Examples 9.8 and 9.9 show how to calculate how long an insulin vial or pen will last and how much medication, if any, will need to be discarded after the beyond-use date.

Example 9.8

If Mrs. Jones takes 20 units of Lantus insulin at bedtime daily, how long would a Lantus Solostar pen with 3 mL or 100 units/mL last? Will she need to throw out any of the drug after 28 days?

$$\text{volume} \times \text{concentration} = \text{total amount of drug available}$$

$$3 \text{ mL} \times 100 \text{ units/mL} = 300 \text{ units of Lantus insulin}$$

$$\text{total amount of drug/dose per day} = \text{number of days' supply}$$

$$300 \text{ units}/20 \text{ units/day} = 15 \text{ days' supply}$$

Mrs. Jones will not need to throw out any of the drug because each Lantus Solostar lasts 15 days.

Example 9.9

Instead of the insulin pen used in Example 9.8, calculate the days' supply if Mrs. Jones uses Lantus insulin in a 10 mL vial at a concentration of 100 units/mL. Will any of the insulin be wasted?

$$\text{volume} \times \text{concentration} = \text{total amount of drug available}$$

$$10 \text{ mL} \times 100 \text{ units/mL} = 1{,}000 \text{ units of Lantus insulin}$$

$$\text{Total amount of drug/dose per day} = \text{number of days' supply}$$

$$1{,}000 \text{ units}/20 \text{ units/day} = 50 \text{ days}$$

Because insulin should be discarded 28 days after first use, Mrs. Jones would have to dispose of more than 20 days' supply of insulin after its beyond-use date. It is important that diabetic patients understand that the strength of the insulin may decline after the beyond-use date, reducing its effectiveness.

Insulin must be stored under proper conditions. If a vial or syringe is frozen or left in the heat of a car or by a light, the medication should not be used and should be discarded. In warm climates or in summer, patients may be advised to transport their insulin home from the pharmacy in a cooler, especially if they are not returning home immediately.

Patients should be informed about how to properly store medication at home. For example, a reconstituted antibiotic suspension is stable for a limited time, about 10 days, and should be discarded once the treatment is complete. Antibiotics such as azithromycin, clarithromycin, and cefdinir are stored at room temperature; penicillin is stored in the refrigerator after it has been reconstituted.

NDC 0088-2220-33
℞ ONLY
Lantus®
insulin glargine (rDNA origin) injection
100 units/mL (U-100)
FOR SUBCUTANEOUS INJECTION ONLY
DO NOT MIX WITH OTHER INSULINS
STORE REFRIGERATED – DO NOT FREEZE
One 10mL Vial
sanofi-aventis U.S. LLC, Bridgewater, NJ 08807
Origin Germany 50085711
Lot
Exp

Some drugs, such as insulin, require refrigeration. The pharmacy technician is responsible for ensuring proper storage.

Room temperature is generally considered below 86°F or 30°C. Some temperature variation may occur during a short-term power outage, but any long-term storage above room temperature can affect medications, and patients should contact the manufacturer of the product for more information.

Nitroglycerin, used in lifesaving emergencies, has strict storage requirements. The sublingual tablets are unstable in the presence of air, moisture, and light, and must be stored in the original brown glass container from the manufacturer or a specially designed airtight container. Nitroglycerin should be stored at temperatures below 77°F or 25°C. Even body temperature will decrease its potency. To ensure potency, patients should purchase a new bottle of 25 tablets every three months. Intravenous nitroglycerin must be protected from light by covering the solution during administration.

Instructions for special storage and handling requirements for pharmaceuticals are included on package inserts. These requirements are in line with the United States Pharmacopeia and National Formulary (USP-NF) reference standards.

Technicians should also make sure to rotate drug stock, placing the oldest stock in front and the new stock behind—unless the new stock has an earlier expiration date than the stock on the shelf. Make sure that pharmaceuticals with the earliest expiration dates are used first.

Pharmaceutical Removal and Disposal

Removal of outdated or nearly outdated pharmaceuticals has been discussed in several chapters in this book. Nearly outdated pharmaceuticals may not be dispensed unless it is certain the patient will use the medication before the expiration date. It is wise to start removing nearly outdated pharmaceuticals as soon as it is clear they will not be used before the expiration date. Outdated drugs are nonsalable and should be stored in a location away from salable stock.

Outdated or nonsalable items may have some value, however, and should not be discarded in the trash. As discussed in Chapter 5, the Environmental Protection Agency (EPA) is concerned about the quantity of pharmaceuticals ending up in the water supply and in landfills that leach into the water supply. Some nonsalable products may be returned to the manufacturer for credit with the appropriate forms. Reverse distribution companies offer an efficient means for pharmacies to dispose of outdated nonsalable items. A company representative visits the pharmacy, conducts an inventory, boxes the nonsalable pharmaceuticals, and provides the pharmacy with a copy of the inventory. Once the product has been returned to the manufacturer, the pharmacy receives credit, replacement product, or a check. Companies do not accept unused patient medications. Some communities have drug disposal days or sites, or patients can dispose of unused medications in the garbage.

Pharmaceuticals also become nonsalable when the Food and Drug Administration (FDA) or a drug manufacturer issues a drug recall, withdrawing a drug or a batch of drugs from the market. There are three types, or classes, of recalls based on the potential for serious adverse health effects. Depending on the type of recall (see Table 9.2), patients who have purchased the recalled medication may also need to be notified.

TABLE 9.2 Recall Classifications

Class	Risk
Class I	A reasonable probability exists that use of the product will cause or lead to serious adverse health events or death. An example of a product that could fall into this category is a label mixup on a lifesaving drug.
Class II	The probability exists that use of the product will cause adverse health events that are temporary or medically reversible. One example is a drug that is under strength but that is not used to treat life-threatening situations.
Class III	The use of the product will probably not cause an adverse health event. Examples might be a container defect, a strange taste, or an odd color in a liquid.

Recall notification will be provided in writing and may come from the manufacturer or the wholesaler. The notification will include a letter describing the drug, dose, dosage form, manufacturer, package size, national drug code number (NDC), lot number, and expiration date along with a return postcard to document whether the pharmacy has any of the recalled product. The technician should isolate the product in question and wait for further instructions for return and credit. Only Class I recalls require the pharmacy to notify the patients who have received the drug. Additional information will be provided on the procedure for returning those drugs and receiving credit.

Some medications are still saleable but not needed by the pharmacy because prescribing trends have changed or too much was ordered. These medications can be returned to the wholesaler for credit if unopened and in salable condition. Most wholesalers charge a reshelving fee, so it is important to return only items the pharmacy cannot use. Returning items for credit is an important part of successful inventory management.

All pharmacies do a physical inventory of drug stocks annually for tax and accounting purposes. The physical inventory should be verified by documentation from purchases and sales. Although there can be some loss due to theft of over-the-counter medications, the prescription area should not have such problems. Discrepancies may be the result of improper receiving or poor management of nonsalable items.

Inventory management is an important part of a pharmacy technician's job. It affects the pharmacy's bottom line and profitability. Inventory management should not be done in a rush. It should receive the same attention to detail as filling a prescription.

Skills Quiz

Reflect on the information presented in the chapter by answering the following questions.

1. Before being dispensed, Humalog insulin should be stored
   a. at room temperature.
   b. in the freezer.
   c. between 68°F and 86°F.
   d. between 2°C and 8°C.

2. Which drug must be stored in the manufacturer's original brown glass vial or approved airtight container?
   a. NuvaRing
   b. nitroglycerin SL
   c. Lantus Solostar
   d. sertraline tablets

3. A recall for fentanyl patches is categorized as a Class II. If there is a recall, the technician should
   a. file the recall.
   b. isolate all the recalled lot number.
   c. remove all fentanyl patches from stock.
   d. return all fentanyl to the wholesaler.

4. A patient brings in a prescription for Zostavax and intends to pick up the following day to take to her physician for administration. Where should the prescription be stored once it is ready to dispense?
   a. in the refrigerator
   b. on the pickup shelf
   c. in the freezer
   d. in a cooler tote

5. Excessive inventory in the community pharmacy compromises
   a. profit levels.
   b. patient safety.
   c. medication storage.
   d. work space.

6. The wholesaler is offering a special buy on docusate sodium 100 mg. A case contains 12 bottles of 100 capsules. If the pharmacy buys six cases, it receives one free. Last month the pharmacy sold 48 bottles of docusate sodium at a gross profit of $2.18. How long will it take to sell all the bottles in this special offer?
   a. 1 month
   b. 2 months
   c. 3 months
   d. 4 months

7. Friendly Pharmacy does an annual inventory on June 30 every year. This year, the total inventory is $150,000 and the pharmacy averages $75,000 in monthly purchases. What is the inventory turnover rate?
   a. 2
   b. 4
   c. 6
   d. 8

8. Which of the following is not a reason to remove a pharmaceutical from the pharmacy stock?
   a. salability
   b. outdated
   c. recalled
   d. nonsalability

9. After posting invoices, what activity ensures the pharmacy will get all the discounts offered by a wholesaler?
   a. shelve items immediately
   b. submit invoices to accounts payable
   c. call wholesaler with any discrepancies
   d. store refrigerated items immediately

10. What relationship does the safety point have to inventory management?
    a. accounts for overhead expenses
    b. provides limits for discounts
    c. provides a cushion for increased sales
    d. guarantees that recalls are removed
11. Friendly Pharmacy has a minimum stock level of 100 tablets and a maximum of 750 tablets of simvastatin 20 mg tablets. At the end of business, there are only 50 tablets left in stock. The wholesaler has bottles of 90 tablets and 500 tablets. How many bottles of each should be ordered?
    a. one bottle of 500 tablets and two bottles of 90 tablets
    b. two bottles of 500 tablets
    c. six bottles of 90 tablets
    d. one bottle of 500 tablets and three bottles of 90 tablets
12. When must the pharmacy notify patients about a drug recall?
    a. never, that is the supplier's job
    b. if it is a Class I recall
    c. if it is a Class II recall
    d. if it is a Class III recall
13. A patient has a prescription for Avapro 150 mg and, according to her insurer's formulary, this is a tier 3 drug. What will be the cost to the patient?
    a. nothing, it is a preferred generic
    b. lowest copay
    c. highest copay
    d. middle copay
14. What technique can a technician use to decrease the amount of inventory that becomes outdated?
    a. reverse distribution
    b. perpetual inventory
    c. posting
    d. stock rotation
15. Good Care Hospital's formulary fills orders for any proton pump inhibitor with pantoprazole. Which drug would be substituted based on this policy?
    a. ranitidine
    b. omeprazole
    c. atorvastatin
    d. fluoxetine
16. Mr. Smith has a prescription for Advair 500/50. He gets a three-month supply at a time. Advair is expensive and you ask him to call when he is half done with his last inhaler so you can order more. What type of purchasing is this?
    a. just-in-time
    b. prime vendor purchasing
    c. discount purchasing
    d. buying-group purchasing
17. When posting an invoice for an order just received, you notice that you are short three items. Two items are back ordered and there is no charge from the wholesaler. There is a charge for one of the missing items. What should you do?
    a. Tell the pharmacist about the back ordered items and reorder all three items.
    b. Call the wholesaler about the one missing item, ask when the other two items are expected, and update the pharmacy staff.
    c. Put away the rest of the order and send the invoice to accounts payable.
    d. Reorder the two back ordered items and notify the pharmacist about the shortage.
18. What is the gross profit of a prescription for levothyroxine 100 mcg #90 tablets if a bottle of 1,000 tablets costs $9.88 and the prescription is sold for $10.95?
    a. $1.07
    b. $9.94
    c. $10.07
    d. $10.86

19. A physician prescribes Lipitor but the drug is not on the patient's insurance formulary. What process should the physician use to explain why the prescription should be filled as written?
    a. approved preferred product
    b. prior approval
    c. reverse distribution
    d. formulary review

20. Friendly Pharmacy has a computer program that maintains a perpetual inventory system with maximum and minimum stock levels for every drug. After receiving an order, what should the technician do to maintain the integrity of future orders?
    a. enter expiration dates
    b. update the purchase price
    c. enter the quantity received
    d. rotate the stock

Thinking Beyond the Exam

While filling in for the technician who usually does the ordering and receiving, you notice that you do not need to order as much of the controlled substance hydrocodone/APAP this week as is usually ordered. For the last three months the technician has ordered two bottles of 1,000 tablets per week. The shelf has the necessary supply. Prescription volume has not changed. What would you do? Consider the possibility that the technician is diverting drugs. What would you expect to happen next?

Pharmacy Billing and Reimbursement

10

Learning Objectives

- Determine eligibility for third-party reimbursement by identifying key components of a patient's prescription insurance card.
- Understand coordination of benefits for patients with more than one prescription drug plan.
- Identify rejected insurance claims and the process for notifying both patient and prescriber.
- Be familiar with the tiered copayment system used by insurers.
- Know how to handle prescription drug coupons presented for medication payment.
- Understand the difference between copayment and coinsurance payment.

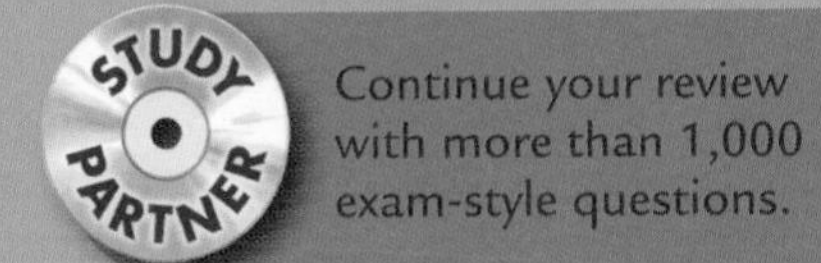

The pharmacy technician does not provide direct patient care, but having the knowledge and skill to properly enter insurance information into the pharmacy computer and correctly interpret insurance regulations and requirements provides a valuable service to patients. The eighth domain of the new PTCB exam tests knowledge of pharmacy billing and reimbursement processes and procedures.

Insurance Billing and Problem Solving

Most patients have some type of insurance coverage to help pay for prescription costs. Patients may have prescription insurance through their employer's insurance, through Medicaid or another state program, or through a federal program such as Medicare Part D. Some employers contract with a health maintenance organization (HMO), and others work with a preferred provider organization (PPO); both types of organizations use managed care to provide care and control costs. Verifying patient insurance information up front reduces unnecessary requests to insurers, which reduces the pharmacy's investment in terms of time and money and decreases customer wait time.

A working knowledge of the insurance card information is necessary to secure payment, including the prescription bank identification number (BIN), processing control number (PCN), group number, identification number, and person codes. The technician must be familiar with insurance providers' rejection codes and error messages, as well as be able to help troubleshoot payment. Sometimes, to get a claim paid, the pharmacy technician needs to call the pharmacy benefits manager (PBM) to resolve a billing issue.

A PBM is an entity that serves as a third-party administrator of prescription drug programs. Examples of PBMs include Merck-Medco, CVS Caremark, and Argus. Typically, the PBM is under contract with one or more insurance companies to perform certain aspects of claim administration, including processing and paying claims, developing and updating formularies, negotiating discounts with drug manufacturers, educating plan members about ways to lower prescription drug costs, performing utilization reviews for plan members, and claims adjusting to resolve prescription drug coverage disputes.

A pharmacy technician may also notify the prescriber of a rejected claim to allow the prescriber to seek prior authorization for a non-formulary medication. Prior authorization (PA) is the term for the process of getting insurance company approval for a medication not covered by the insurer's plan. For example, a prescriber might request prior authorization for Lipitor because the patient had an allergic reaction to the generic drug, atorvastatin, but has been able to take the brand name product successfully in the past. In this situation, the prescriber would contact the insurance plan either by phone, email, or in writing to request coverage of the more expensive brand name drug. The PBM has a staff of physician, nurse, and pharmacist consultants that reviews each case to determine the merits and approve or deny payment. The technician who understands the reason claims are rejected can initiate these calls.

A pharmacy technician must also be familiar with copayment and coinsurance requirements. Copayment requires the patient to pay a flat fee for every prescription, regardless of the actual cost of the medication. Coinsurance, another method of prescription drug reimbursement, requires that the patient pay a percentage of the retail cost of the drug. For example, if a patient has an 80-20 coinsurance benefit, the patient pays 20 percent of the medication cost and the insurer pays 80 percent. The patient's portion of a $50 medication would be $10, but the patient would pay $30 for a medication that costs $150.

Usually, the message from the PBM confirming payment of a claim, also known as claim capturing, includes information on preferred formulary products that will lower the copayment or the adjusted copayment for certain choices. This is also important for Medicare Part D patients who are required to pay the entire cost of their medications once they reach the "donut hole," which refers to a period of time when the insurer stops paying until the patient has contributed the necessary out-of-pocket payments.

Providing information on cost savings to the patient and prescriber can help curb rising out-of-pocket medication costs for patients and save insurers money, and perhaps help lower future premiums.

Insurance Reimbursement Eligibility

After reviewing a new prescription or refill order, the technician in a community pharmacy is responsible for updating any changes to the patient's demographic and insurance information. Each prescription is then automatically billed online (known as online adjudication) to an insurance provider before it is filled and dispensed to the patient. If a patient has more than one prescription insurance plan, or coupons or manufacturer discounts, the technician needs to enter all payment data before submitting the claim. Many patients have more than one type of insurance. Coordination of benefits (COB) is the online billing of primary and secondary insurance. The technician has to make sure that both types of insurance are entered in the proper sequence in the patient profile. Once the primary insurance acknowledges acceptance and payment, the secondary insurance will be automatically billed for further payment or to establish the patient's final copayment. Technicians need to remember that when a patient has two insurance policies and one is a state-funded Medicaid insurance program, Medicaid is the secondary insurance. Legally, Medicaid cannot be billed until the primary insurance carrier has paid. Providers will occasionally give patients coupon cards to help defray the cost of a medication. The technician must enter billing information from the coupon card into the patient insurance profile. Some coupon cards pay first and then bill the balance to the insurance company. Others pay the copayment after the insurer has been billed. Read the fine print. These cards often do not cover Medicaid copayments. Once the card has been billed, the technician needs to inactivate the card and billing information.

Information from the patient's insurance card (see Figure 10.1) or coupon information must be entered correctly for the prescription to be processed. The patient's name and birth date must match the information in the insurance database. If this information is not on file, the technician should request the insurance card. All new patients should be asked to provide a prescription insurance card to eliminate delays in filling a prescription. If no insurance coverage is on file, the patient is expected to pay for the prescription in full. The prescription insurance card includes:

- identification number (with or without person code)
- processor control number (PCN)
- six-digit bank identification number (BIN)
- group number/letters

Depending on the pharmacy's computer software, the person code is usually two or three digits for the primary card holder (000, 001), spouse (001, 002), and children (002, 003, 004, etc.). A group number may or may not be required for all plans.

An insurer may also place limits on the medications and quantity of medication covered by a plan. In many cases, the insurer will pay for only a 30 days' supply of medication each time the prescription is filled, regardless of the quantity on the prescription. Many insurers provide patients with an incentive to use mail order pharmacies authorizing a three-month supply for the equivalent of two copayments. If the prescription is filled at a local retail pharmacy, only a 30-day supply is allowed. Insurance may not cover any of the cost of some medications, such as diet pills, nerve pills, cough medicine, vitamins, or OTC drugs.

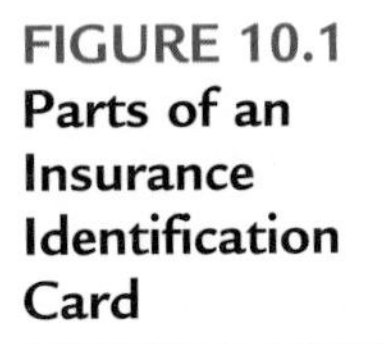

FIGURE 10.1 Parts of an Insurance Identification Card

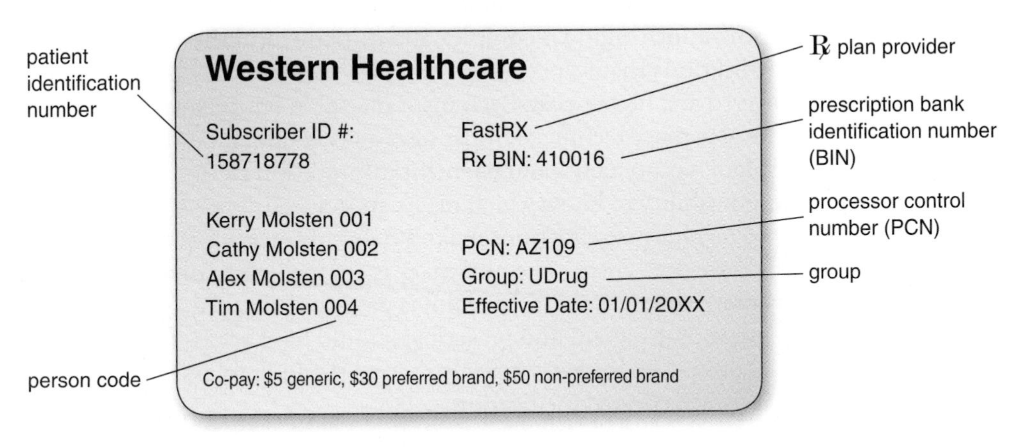

Insurers may also limit the quantity of certain types of medication during a 30-day period. For example, insurance may cover only nine tablets of the migraine drug sumatriptan (Imitrex) every 30 days because the drug is intended for use only during acute attacks. Erectile dysfunction drugs like Viagra, Levitra, and Cialis may have similar limitations, which vary with the insurance provider.

Brand name drugs generally require the patient to make a higher copayment than generic drugs. This is called a tiered copayment system. Tier 1 is the cheapest for the patient and usually is used for generic drugs. Tier 2 includes preferred brand name drugs that require a higher copayment. Tier 3 is for brand name drugs for which the insurer has determined cheaper alternatives are available. Some high-cost brand name medications require prior authorization and fall into the tier 3 category. If prior authorization is needed, the technician notifies the patient that the medical office must call the insurer to justify the prescribed medication. The technician will print the reason for the insurance company rejection and fax the information to the prescriber, including information needed to apply for a PA (prior authorization), and a web address where the prescriber can find the PA form and a list of alternative drug choices covered by the insurer. If the patient has not had success with other, lower-cost drugs or cannot tolerate other drugs, insurance will generally authorize payment. If the insurer refuses the PA request, the prescriber is encouraged to use a generic or alternate therapy.

A patient may request a three-month (or 90-day) supply of medication to save money; most pharmacies try to fill such prescriptions for non-controlled medications as long as the prescriber approves the request, there are sufficient refills available, and the insurer approves the request. For example, a prescription for verapamil 240 mg PO b.i.d. #60 with two refills could be filled for verapamil 240 mg PO b.i.d. #180 with no refills. However, the technician or pharmacist will need to call the prescriber for a new order with the larger quantity.

If the insurance information entered is correct and the prescription drug is covered, the technician can print a label and a receipt with copayment information. At the beginning of the calendar year, patient medication costs may be higher because many insurance plans require patients to pay a deductible before covering prescription costs. A deductible is the amount of money paid directly by the insured person each year before the insurance coverage is available. An insurance plan with a low annual deductible generally costs more than a high-deductible plan. In Medicare Part D prescription plans (mostly for those over age 65), the plan pays first up to a certain amount. Once that cap has been reached, the patient must pay a certain amount out of pocket before the Medicare plan D starts to pay again. This is often referred to as the Medicare donut hole. Patients on many medications may find themselves in the donut hole later in the calendar year.

Insurance billing is complex and difficult, and there are frequent changes. Medications that were covered by a plan last year may no longer be covered, or may be covered at a higher cost. Each insurance plan has its own preferred drug list (PDL). The pharmacy technician must have a good understanding of insurance to be able to explain requirements and payment information to the patient. It is the patient's responsibility to know which drugs are covered.

The pharmacy does not make a habit of tracking or sending test prescriptions to the insurer to check. The pharmacy is charged every time a claim is submitted to an insurer, whether or not the claim is paid, and charged again if it has to reverse the request. The patient and prescriber should have access to the PDL at work, at home, and online. Pharmacies may also access the PDL to assist a patient and prescriber in selecting a covered medication.

Skills Quiz

Reflect on the information presented in the chapter by answering the following questions.

1. An insurance card BIN and PCN provide information for
   a. updating a patient's demographics.
   b. filling a prescription.
   c. locating a complete medical record.
   d. billing prescriptions online.

2. A prescription for the migraine drug Imitrex reads 100 mg #9 with the instructions "take at onset of headache; may repeat in 2 hours." How often will insurance cover the cost of the drug?
   a. every 5 days
   b. every 9 days
   c. every 30 days
   d. every 90 days

3. The patient requests a 90-day supply of "amlodipine 5 mg 1 tab PO daily #30 with 1 refill." How can the pharmacy technician process this request?
   a. fill the prescription for amlodipine 5 mg #90 with 1 refill
   b. fill the prescription for amlodipine 5 mg #90 with no refills
   c. fill the prescription for amlodipine 10 mg #45 using ½ tab PO daily with no refills
   d. call the prescriber to request a change in the prescription

4. Which term describes the process used when an insurer requires that a medical office justify a prescription for a brand name drug?
   a. prior authorization
   b. coordination of benefits
   c. donut hole
   d. preferred drug list

5. A patient with a coinsurance of 25 percent will pay how much of the price of a prescription with a retail cost of $179.00? (Assume that the deductible has been met.)
   a. $179.00
   b. $139.25
   c. $44.75
   d. $25.00

6. When entering patient insurance information, you identify the patient has two prescription plans: CVS Caremark and the state Medicaid prescription plan. Which should be billed first?
   a. CVS Caremark
   b. state Medicaid
   c. neither, the patient cannot legally have two prescriptions plans
   d. bill both at the same time and collect the maximum from both

7. In a tiered copayment plan, the tiers are based on
   a. generic versus brand name.
   b. abuse and cost.
   c. prescription and OTC.
   d. chronic use and acute use.

8. Where can a patient or prescriber find an up-to-date list of preferred drugs paid for by a patient's insurance plan?
   a. the Physician's Desk Reference
   b. the patient's original insurance contract
   c. the patient's employer human resource department
   d. on the insurer's website

9. If a patient wants a three-month supply of medication to take to Florida for the winter, what must the technician do?
   a. make sure the patient has enough refills to cover three months all at once
   b. check to make sure the insurer will allow payment for a three-month supply
   c. contact the prescriber if the prescription is written for a month supply per fill
   d. all of the above

10. You receive a prescription for Lexapro 20 mg and the patient wants the brand name drug. What should you tell the patient?
    a. insurance will not cover brand name
    b. the generic equivalent costs less
    c. the brand name costs less
    d. that you do not have a choice, the pharmacy fills it with the cheapest product

11. Mrs. Jones' insurer rejects her prescription claim and she is waiting in the pharmacy. What should you do?
    a. give her the prescription back and tell her to talk to her doctor
    b. tell her to keep waiting; it will not take too much longer
    c. tell her the claim was rejected and ask if she wants to wait or come back later
    d. fill the prescription and tell her that she has to pay in cash

Thinking Beyond the Exam

In the retail pharmacy, the pharmacy technician needs to become an expert in insurance billing. Look at your own insurance card and identify the necessary information to bill a prescription.

Have everyone in the class bring their prescription insurance cards and discuss how many different companies there are for pharmacies to bill.

Find the website that describes Medicare Plan D and discuss how this system works.

Pharmacy Information System Usage and Application

11

Learning Objectives

- Discuss computer data storage techniques.
- Understand the importance of the login and password.
- Know which drugs should never be put in a pill counting machine.
- Know the difference between hardware and software.
- Discuss the advantages of newer technologies, such as e-prescribing, medication dispensing machines, and online adjudication.
- List uses for barcode technology in health care.

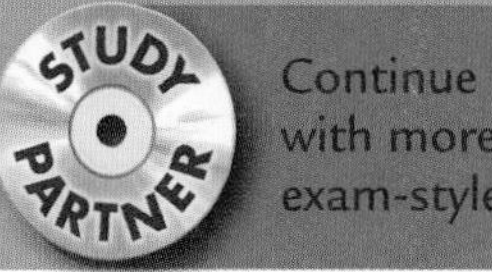

Continue your review with more than 1,000 exam-style questions.

The days of using paper and a typewriter in pharmacy are long past. Technology is the present and future of pharmacy. The computerization of health care provides better data management, greater cost savings, and new error prevention strategies. Ten percent of the pharmacy technician certification exam is related to the technological advances in pharmacy, including electronic medical records, drug interaction monitoring, inventory management, and drug diversion prevention.

Computer Basics

The pharmacy technician needs to have a working knowledge of computers, adequate typing skills, and the ability to learn how to use pharmacy-specific software programs on the job. The computer is an essential tool in every pharmacy for processing prescriptions, filing insurance claims, tracking inventory, and many other uses. A variety of software programs is available for pharmacy use, and the type of program used varies from pharmacy to pharmacy.

Every pharmacy employee is given an individual login and password that provides access to the computer system. It is essential to keep this information confidential. It will be used to track and monitor a technician's activities on the computer and evaluate competency and job performance. Computer tracking can also be used to identify the source of medical errors and identify individuals who need additional training to prevent future errors. A technician is responsible for all activity on the computer that occurs under his or her login.

Pharmacies use two basic types of data storage. Smaller or independent pharmacies may use a smart terminal with its own processing capacity and storage, much like a personal computer. When using this system, it is important to back up the computer regularly to prevent data loss in the event of a computer system or software failure. Most larger pharmacies and hospital pharmacies use a dumb terminal system. There is a computer monitor and keyboard for data entry, but the terminal has no storage or processing capabilities. The terminal is connected to a remote computer or mainframe at a headquarters, home office, or central location in an institution. Data is stored and backed up on the mainframe or offsite.

Most pharmacies use a database management system that allows staff to quickly enter, retrieve, and query patient records. Most of these are Windows-based, menu-driven programs that require minimal keystrokes. The patient profile, physician database, and drug inventory are examples of database management systems.

The patient profile database includes fields for demographic, insurance, and prescription information. Changes can be easily made to any of these fields, new prescriptions entered, and medication labels printed.

Modern pharmacy computer systems offer a wide range of functions, including drug utilization review (DUR), which can automatically alert pharmacy staff to any potential patient allergies, adverse drug reactions, or drug interactions. For example, if a patient has an existing prescription for the blood thinner warfarin and brings in a new prescription from an emergency room visit for Bactrim DS, an antibiotic used for urinary tract and other infections, the computerized drug utilization review will alert the technician to a potential drug interaction. Bactrim is also used as a blood thinner and, if combined with warfarin, it could produce a potentially life-threatening interaction. Because the ER doctor might not have known the patient was taking warfarin, it is the pharmacist's responsibility to alert the physician to prevent the problem.

Pharmacies are also using computers to process prescription claims quickly and efficiently. The process, called online adjudication, allows the pharmacy's computer to submit a prescription claim directly to the insurer's prescription benefits manager (PBM) and receive a rapid response, often in less than 30 seconds. The response includes the amount the pharmacy should charge the patient for a medication and the amount the pharmacy will be reimbursed. It alerts the pharmacy if the medication is not covered by the insurer or if the patient needs to meet a deductible before payment is available. The PBM can also notify the pharmacy if the patient has filled the prescription at another pharmacy or has a prescription at another pharmacy that may cause an adverse drug interaction.

For patients who have more than one type of prescription coverage, online adjudication also makes it possible for the pharmacy to bill the primary insurer first and then bill the unpaid balance to the secondary insurer. This is referred to as coordination of benefits.

Increasingly, the electronic prescription, also known as e-prescribing, is becoming more common in health care. It allows a prescriber to submit a patient's prescription directly to the pharmacy computer. It is important for pharmacy technicians to know the state and federal laws and regulations that pertain to electronic prescribing. The federal Drug Enforcement Administration regulates e-prescriptions for controlled substances (discussed in Chapter 4), and individual states may have additional rules. E-prescriptions reduce prescription forgery and medication errors stemming from a physician's hard-to-read handwriting.

Physicians can submit an e-prescription to the pharmacy while documenting the information in the patient's chart. This is a time saver for physicians. It also saves time for the pharmacy by reducing time spent talking on the phone and entering information from written prescriptions, and reduces wait time for patients. In many cases, a prescription can be ready before the patient arrives at the pharmacy.

Institutional Pharmacy

Technology is changing the practice of health care in the institutional setting. Hospitals, clinics, and physicians are transitioning from paper records to electronic records. Patient charts are typed directly into a computerized form called an electronic health record (EHR) or electronic medical record (EMR). Hospitals are moving to fully computerized systems from admission to discharge. Computerized physician order entry (CPOE) will be the norm in the future, as electronic orders replace written orders. Nurses will administer medications to patients based on data from an electronic medication administration record (eMAR).

Computers are changing medication distribution as well. Hospitals have long used medication carts to organize patient medications on the floor, but this manual system contributes to medication errors and medication diversion. New automated systems, such as Omnicell and Pyxis, dispense medications based on an eMAR. These automated medication storage units placed throughout the hospital provide a secure, accurate, and efficient means of dispensing and tracking patient medications. Medication storage units also provide diversion prevention, improve inventory control, reduce costs, increase compliance protocols, monitor for violations, and eliminate mistakes.

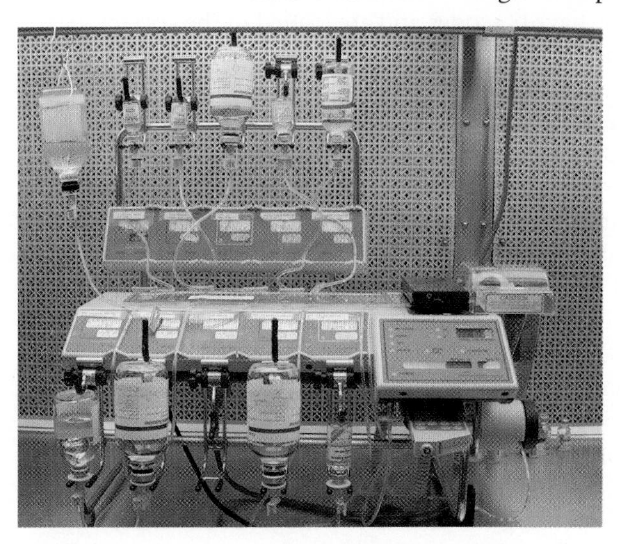

This automated compounding device (ACD) adds micronutrients to TPN solutions. This procedure is done within a laminar airflow workbench.

Technology is helping to prepare compounded products in the hospital pharmacy. Automatic compound devices (ACD) are used to compound injectable pharmaceuticals, especially in large medical centers that produce a high volume of parenterals. ACDs improve efficiency and reduce labor costs. The machines are programmed to reliably add electrolytes or additives to total parenteral nutrition, reducing the potential for medication errors and contamination. USP Chapter <797> guidelines must be followed to ensure the accuracy and maintenance records of ACDs.

Community Practice

Computer software allows pharmacy technicians to prepare prescriptions, freeing up time for the pharmacist who need only to perform a final check. All of the information the pharmacist needs for final verification of a prescription is available on the computer, including an image of the tablet or capsule, the national drug code number, an image of the hard copy prescription, and drug utilization review information. This leaves the pharmacist more time for patient counseling, medication therapy management (MTM), vaccinations, and other patient care services.

Community and institutional pharmacies use computer barcode scanning programs to select and verify dispensed medications and for inventory management. In hospitals, patients receive wristbands with barcodes that provide identification information. Nursing staff use a barcode reader to scan the patient's wristband and match it against the medication barcode and the eMAR information. This ensures that the 5Rs of medication administration are followed and helps to prevent medication errors.

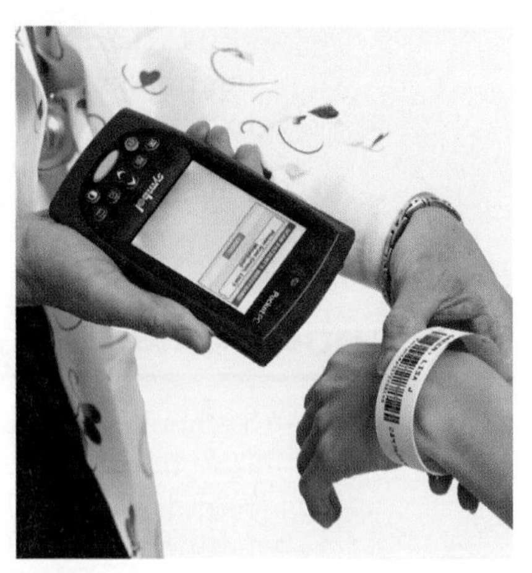

Barcode scanning helps to reduce medication errors.

Pharmacy Robots

Computerized robots select medication used to fill medication carts, automatic dispensing cabinets, prescriptions, and other repetitive tasks. The robot uses barcode scanning to identify and select drug products. The pharmacy technician is responsible for making sure all pharmaceuticals have barcodes and are loaded in the correct location in the robot. Attention to detail is important to ensure accuracy.

Medication dispensing machines count and fill prescriptions in busy pharmacies. Pill counting machines count tablets or capsules as they fall through a beam of light. The technician should make sure the machine is cleaned regularly. Automated pill counting machines should never be used to count penicillin, sulfonamides, or codeine products because cross-contamination with other products could be life threatening for a patient who has medication allergies.

In institutional pharmacies, all medications are now dispensed in unit-dose packs. If the manufacturer does not supply the product in a unit-dose pack, the technician repackages the medication and labels it with the drug name, strength, lot number, expiration date, beyond-use date, and barcode. Software programs, such as the Wasp labeler, print sheet labels for unit-dose pods after they are filled.

Medication delivery to a floor or hospital unit is a big part of a technician's job in many institutions. Delivering medication to patient care units and refilling medication storage areas and automatic dispensing cabinets uses a mix of old and new technology. The technician is instrumental in reloading the medication cabinets and filling individual medication drawers. Some larger hospitals also use a pneumatic system to deliver medication to the floor, usually for "stat" doses. Some companies are developing motorized robots to deliver medication to patient care units.

Automation technology in the pharmacy provides a variety of tools that allows staff to work smarter. Technology is helping pharmacies cope with rising demand for prescriptions while controlling costs, and computers are increasing efficiency and reducing medication errors.

Skills Quiz

Reflect on the information presented in this chapter by answering the following questions.

1. Who should have access to your login and password?
   a. director of pharmacy
   b. staff pharmacist
   c. only you
   d. human resources

2. What type of computer terminal in the pharmacy does not store its own data or have its own processing capacity?
   a. smart terminal
   b. dumb terminal
   c. off-site storage
   d. desktop

3. A prescription sent electronically from the doctor's office to the pharmacy is called
   a. keyboarding.
   b. CPOE.
   c. e-prescribing.
   d. eMAR.

4. A nurse will scan a _______________ on the patient, on the drug, and on the medication administration record before giving medication to a patient.
   a. computer disc
   b. insurance card
   c. written code
   d. barcode

5. Who is responsible for entering orders in the process of CPOE?
   a. physician
   b. nurse
   c. pharmacist
   d. pharmacy technician

6. What USP chapter must be followed if you are using an ACD?
   a. Chapter <797>
   b. Chapter <595>
   c. Chapter <795>
   d. Chapter <597>

7. Electronic health records will eliminate ________ in the hospital.
   a. parenteral admixtures
   b. pharmacy technicians
   c. paper charts
   d. unit-dose packs

8. How do medications get delivered to the patient care unit?
   a. hand delivery by pharmacy technicians
   b. pneumatic tube system
   c. automatic dispensing cabinets
   d. all of the above

9. Which piece of information is not needed on a unit-dose label created by a pharmacy technician?
   a. chemical name
   b. generic name
   c. lot number
   d. barcode

10. A prescription entered by a pharmacy technician will be checked by the pharmacist. A computer software program that displays _______ will help the pharmacist verify that the correct drug is dispensed.
    a. barcode
    b. image of tablet
    c. adjudication results
    d. DUR information

Thinking Beyond the Exam

Search online to find examples of medication errors that could have been prevented with modern technology. Compare the cost of computer technology with its potential for decreasing medication errors. What kinds of errors may be created by reliance on technology and how can they be prevented?

Appendix A

Most Commonly Prescribed Drugs

This table presents the most commonly prescribed drugs in the United States. The drugs are listed by their generic names.

Generic Name	Pronunciation	Classification	Brand Name
acetaminophen/ codeine	a-seat-a-MIN-oh-fen/ KOE-deen	opioid analgesic	Tylenol/ codeine
acyclovir	ay-SYE-kloe-veer	antiviral	Zovirax
albuterol	al-BYOO-ter-ole	beta-2 agonist	Ventolin HFA
albuterol (nebulizer solution)	al-BYOO-ter-ole	beta-2 agonist	AccuNeb
albuterol HFA	al-BYOO-ter-ole	beta-2 agonist	Pro-Air HFA
alendronate	a-LEN-droe-nate	bisphosphonate	Fosamax
allopurinol	al-o-PURE-i-nole	antigout agent xanthine oxidase inhibitor	Zyloprim
alprazolam	al-PRAY-zoe-lam	benzodiazepine	Xanax
amitriptyline	a-mee-TRIP-ti-leen	antidepressant tricyclic	Elavil
amlodipine	am-LOE-di-peen	antianginal calcium channel blocker	Norvasc
amoxicillin	a-moks-i-SIL-in	antibiotic penicillin	Amoxil
amoxicillin ER	a-moks-i-SIL-in	antibiotic penicillin	Moxatag
aripiprazole	ay-ri-PIP-ra-zole	antipsychotic	Abilify
aspirin (EC)	AS-pir-in	antiplatelet	Bayer Aspirin EC
atenolol	a-TEN-oh-lole	beta blocker	Tenormin
atorvastatin	a-TORE-va-sta-tin	antilipemic	Lipitor
azithromycin	az-ith-ro-MYE-sin	antibiotic macrolide	Zithromax, Z-Pak
baclofen	BAK-loe-fen	skeletal muscle relaxant	Lioresal
benazepril	ben-AY-ze-pril	ACE inhibitor	Lotensin
benzonatate	ben-ZO-na-tate	antitussive	Tessalon

Generic Name	Pronunciation	Classification	Brand Name
bisoprolol-hydrochlorothiazide	bis-OH-proe-lol hye-droe-klor-oh-THYE-a-side	beta blocker/diuretic	Ziac
budesonide/formoterol	byoo-DES-oh-nide/ for-MOH-te-rol	beta-2 agonist/ corticosteroid	Symbicort
buprenorphine/ naloxone	byoo-pre-NOR-feen/ nal-OKS-own	opioid analgesic	Suboxone
bupropion	byoo-PROE-pee-on	antidepressant	Budeprion, Wellbutrin, Zyban
bupropion SR	byoo-PROE-pee-on	antidepressant	Budeprion SR, Wellbutrin SR
bupropion XL	byoo-PROE-pee-on	antidepressant	Budeprion XL, Wellbutrin XL
butalbital acetamino-phen-caffeine	byoo-TAL-bi-tal a-seat-a-MIN-oh-fen KAF-een	barbiturate	Fioricet, Esgic Plus
carisoprodol	kar-eye-so-PROE-dole	skeletal muscle relaxant	Soma
carvedilol	kar-ve-DI-lole	beta blocker	Coreg
cefdinir	SEF-di-ner	antibiotic cephalosporin	Omnicef
celecoxib	sele-KOKS-ib	NSAID	Celebrex
cephalexin	sef-a-LEKS-in	antibiotic cephalosporin	Keflex
chlorhexidine gluconate	klor-HEKS-i-deen GLOO-ko-nate	antiseptic	Peridex
ciprofloxacin	sip-roe-FLOX-a-sin	antibiotic quinolone	Cipro
citalopram	sye-TAL-oh-pram	antidepressant SSRI	Celexa
clarithromycin	kla-RITH-roh-my-sin	antibiotic macrolide	Biaxin
clobetasol	kloe-BAY-ta-sol	corticosteroid	Temovate, Olux
clonazepam	kloe-NAZ-e-pam	benzodiazepine	Klonopin
clonidine	KLON-i-dine	alpha-2 adrenergic agonist	Catapres
clopidogrel	kloe-PID-oh-grel	antiplatelet agent	Plavix
clotrimazole-betamethasone	kloe-TRIM-a-zole bay-ta-METH-a-sone	antifungal/corticosteroid	Lotrisone
colchicine	KOL-chi-seen	antigout	Colcrys
cyclobenzaprine	sye-kloe-BEN-za-preen	skeletal muscle relaxant	Flexeril
dextroamphetamine-amphetamine	deks-troe-am-FET-a-min am-FET-a-meen	stimulant	Adderall

Generic Name	Pronunciation	Classification	Brand Name
dextroamphetamine-amphetamine XR	deks-troe-am-FET-a-meen am-FET-a-meen	stimulant	Adderall XR
diazepam	dye-AZ-e-pam	benzodiazepine	Valium
diclofenac	dye-KLOE-fen-ak	NSAID	Cataflam
dicyclomine	dye-SYE-kloe-meen	anticholinergic	Bentyl
digoxin	di-JOKS-in	antiarrhythmic	Lanoxin
diltiazem CD	dil-TYE-a-zem	antianginal calcium channel blocker	Cardizem CD
divalproex	dye-VAL-pro-ex	anticonvulsant	Depakote
donepezil	doh-NEP-e-zil	acetylcholinesterase inhibitor	Aricept
doxazosin	doks-AY-zoe-sin	alpha-1 blocker	Cardura
doxycycline	doks-i-SYE-kleen	antibiotic tetracycline	Vibramycin
duloxetine	doo-LOKS-e-teen	antidepressant SSRI	Cymbalta
dutasteride	do-TAS-teer-ide	5-alpha-reductase inhibitor	Avodart
enalapril	e-NAL-a-pril	ACE inhibitor	Vasotec
escitalopram	es-sye-TAL-oh-pram	antidepressant SSRI	Lexapro
esomeprazole	es-oh-MEP-rah-zole	proton pump inhibitor	Nexium
estradiol	es-tra-DYE-ole	estrogen	Estrace, Climara, Femring
estrogens (conjugated)	ES-troe-jenz	estrogen	Premarin
eszopiclone	es-zoe-PIK-lone	hypnotic	Lunesta
ethinyl estradiol-drospirenone	ETH-in-yl es-tra-DYE-ole droh-SPYE-re-none	contraceptive	Ocella, Yaz
ethinyl estradiol-etonogestrel	ETH-in-yl es-tra-DYE-ole et-noe-JES-trel	contraceptive	NuvaRing
ethinyl estradiol-levonorgestrel	ETH-in-yl es-tra-DYE-ole LE-voe-nor-jes-trel	contraceptive	Aviane
ethinyl estradiol-norethindrone and ferrous fumerate	ETH-in-yl es-tra-DYE-ole nor-eth-IN-drone	contraceptive	Loestrin 24 FE
ethinyl estradiol-norgestimate	ETH-in-yl es-tra-DYE-ole nor-JES-ti-mate	contraceptive	Tri-Sprintec, Ortho Tri-cyclen Lo, Sprintec, TriNessa

Generic Name	Pronunciation	Classification	Brand Name
ezetimibe	ez-ET-i-mibe	antilipemic	Zetia
ezetimibe-simvastatin	ez-ET-i-mibe SIM-va-stat-in	antilipemic	Vytorin
famotidine	fa-MOE-ti-dine	H_2 antagonist	Pepcid
fenofibrate	fen-oh-FYE-brate	antilipemic	TriCor
fenofibric acid	fen-oh-FYE-brik AS-id	antilipemic	Trilipix
fentanyl (transdermal)	FEN-ta-nil	opioid analgesic	Duragesic
ferrous sulfate	FER-us SUL-fate	iron supplement	Feosol, Slow FE
fexofenadine	feks-oh-FEN-a-deen	antihistamine H_1 antagonist	Allegra
finasteride	fi-NAS-teer-ide	5-alpha-reductase inhibitor	Proscar
fluconazole	floo-KOE-na-zole	antifungal	Diflucan
fluoxetine	floo-OKS-e-teen	antidepressant SSRI	Prozac
fluticasone (HFA)	floo-TIK-a-sone	corticosteroid	Flovent
fluticasone (nasal spray)	floo-TIK-a-sone	corticosteroid	Flonase
fluticasone/salmeterol	floo-TIK-a-sone/sal-ME-ter-ole	beta-2 agonist/ corticosteroid	Advair
folic acid	FOE-lik AS-id	vitamin	Folate
furosemide	fyoor-OH-se-mide	diuretic	Lasix
gabapentin	GA-ba-pen-tin	anticonvulsant	Neurontin
glimepiride	GLYE-me-pye-ride	antidiabetic sulfonylurea	Amaryl
glipizide	GLIP-i-zide	antidiabetic sulfonylurea	Glucotrol
glipizide ER	GLIP-i-zide	antidiabetic sulfonylurea	Glucotrol XL
glipizide XL	GLIP-i-zide	antidiabetic sulfonylurea	Glucotrol XL
glyburide	GLYE-byoor-ide	antidiabetic sulfonylurea	DiaBeta, Glynase
glyburide/metformin	GLYE-byoor-ride/met-FOR-man	antidiabetic biguanide/sulfonylurea	Glucovance
guaifenesin/codeine	gwy-a-FEN-e-sin/KOE-deen	antitussive	Cheratussin AC
hydralazine	hye-DRAL-a-zen	vasodilator	Apresoline
hydrochlorothiazide	hye-droe-klor-oh-THYE-a-side	diuretic	Microzide

Generic Name	Pronunciation	Classification	Brand Name
hydrocodone/ acetaminophen	hye-droe-KOE-done/ a-seat-a-MIN-oh-fen	opioid analgesic	Lortab, Vicodin, Norco
hydroxyzine	hy-DROKS-i-zeen	H_1 antagonist	Vistaril, Atarax
ibandronate	eye-BAN-droh-nate	bisphosphonate derivative	Boniva
ibuprofen	eye-byoo-PROE-fen	NSAID	Advil, Motrin
insulin aspart	IN-soo-lin AS-part	antidiabetic	NovoLog
insulin glargine	IN-soo-lin GLAR-jeen	antidiabetic	Lantus
insulin lispro	IN-soo-lin LYE-sproe	antidiabetic	Humalog
ipratropium-albuterol	i-pra-TROE-pee-um al-BYOO-ter-ole	anticholinergic beta-2 agonist	Combivent
irbesartan	ir-be-SAR-tan	angiotensin II receptor blocker	Avapro
isosorbide	eye-soe-SOR-bide	antianginal vasodilator	Imdur
lamotrigine	la-MOE-tri-jeen	anticonvulsant	Lamictal
latanoprost	la-TA-noe-prost	antiglaucoma prostaglandin	Xalatan
levetiracetam	lee-va-tyre-RA-se-tam	anticonvulsant	Keppra
levothyroxine	lee-voe-thye-ROKS-een	thyroid hormone replacement	Synthroid, Levoxyl
lisdexamfetamine	les-dex-am-FET-a-meen	stimulant	Vyvanse
lisinopril	lyse-IN-oh-pril	ACE inhibitor	Prinivil, Zestril
lisinopril-hydrochlorothiazide	lyse-IN-o-pril hye-droe-klor-oh-THYE-a-side	ACE inhibitor/diuretic	Prinzide, Zestoretic
lorazepam	lor-AZE-pam	benzodiazepine	Ativan
losartan	loe-SAR-tan	angiotensin II receptor blocker	Cozaar
losartan-hydrochlorothiazide	loe-SAR-tan hye-droe-klor-oh-THYE-a-side	angiotensin II receptor blocker	Hyzaar
lovastatin	LOE-va-sta-tin	antilipemic agent	Mevacor
meclizine	MEK-li-zeen	antiemetic H_1 antagonist	Antivert
meloxicam	mel-OKS-a-kam	NSAID	Mobic
memantine	me-MAN-tine	N-Methyl-D-Aspartate receptor agonist	Namenda
metformin	met-FOR-min	antidiabetic biguanide	Glucophage
methocarbamol	meth-oh-KAR-ba-mole	skeletal muscle relaxant	Robaxin
methotrexate	meth-oh-TREKS-ate	antineoplastic	Rheumatrex
methylphenidate	meth-il-FEN-i-date	stimulant	Concerta
methylprednisolone	meth-il-pred-NIS-o-lone	corticosteroid	Medrol

Generic Name	Pronunciation	Classification	Brand Name
metoclopramide	met-oh-KLOE-pra-mide	antiemetic	Reglan
metoprolol (succinate)	me-toe-PROE-lole	beta blocker	Toprol XL
metoprolol (tartrate)	me-toe-PROE-lole	antianginal	Lopressor
metronidazole	met-roe-NYE-da-zole	antibiotic and amebicide	Flagyl
mirtazapine	mir-TAZ-a-peen	antidepressant	Remeron
mometasone	moe-MET-a-sone	corticosteroid	Nasonex
montelukast	mon-te-LOO-kast	leukotriene receptor agonist	Singulair
moxifloxacin	moks-i-FLOKS-a-sin	antibiotic quinolone	Vigamox
nabumetone	na-BYOO-me-tone	NSAID	Relafen
naproxen	na-PROKS-en	NSAID	Aleve, Anaprox
nebivolol	ne-BIV-oh-lole	beta blocker	Bystolic
niacin	NYE-a-sin	antilipemic	Niaspan
nifedipine ER	nye-FED-i-peen	antianginal calcium channel blocker	Adalat, Procardia
nitroglycerin	nye-tro-GLIS-er-in	antianginal vasodilator	Minitran, Nitro-Dur
nortriptyline	nor-TRIP-ti-leen	tricyclic antidepressant	Pamelor
nystatin (topical)	nye-STAT-in	antifungal	Nystop
olanzapine	oh-LANZ-a-peen	antipsychotic	Zyprexa
olmesartan	ole-me-SAR-tan	angiotensin II receptor blocker	Benicar
omega-3 acid	oh-MEG-a three AS-id	antilipemic	Lovaza
omeprazole	oh-MEP-ra-zole	proton pump inhibitor	Prilosec
oxycodone ER	oks-i-KOE-done	opioid analgesic	OxyContin
oxycodone-acetaminophen	oks-i-KOE-done a-seat-a-MIN-oh-fen	opioid analgesic	Percocet, Tylox
pantoprazole	pan-TOE-pra-zole	proton pump inhibitor	Protonix
paroxetine	pa-ROKS-e-teen	antidepressant SSRI	Paxil
phenazopyridine	fen-az-oh-PEER-i-deen	urinary analgesic	Pyridium, Azo-Standard
phentermine	FEN-ter-meen	anorexiant	Adipex-P
pioglitazone	pye-oh-GLI-ta-zone	antidiabetic thiazolidine	Actos
polyethylene glycol	pol-i-ETH-i-leen GLY-col	laxative	MiraLAX
potassium chloride	poe-TASS-e-um KLOR-ide	electrolyte supplement	Klor-Con

Generic Name	Pronunciation	Classification	Brand Name
potassium chloride ER	poe-TASS-e-um-KLOR-ide	electrolyte supplement	K-Dur, Klor-Con M
pravastatin	prav-a-STAT-in	antilipemic agent	Pravachol
prednisolone	pred-NISS-oh-lone	corticosteroid	Orapred, Pediapred
pregabalin	pre-GAB-a-lin	analgesic anticonvulsant	Lyrica
promethazine	pro-METH-a-zeen	antiemetic	Phenergan
promethazine-codeine	pro-METH-a-zeen KOE-deen	opioid analgesic	Phenergan/codeine
propranolol	proe-PRAN-oh-lol	beta blocker	Inderal
quetiapine	kwe-TYE-a-peen	antipsychotic	Seroquel
quinapril	KWIN-a-pril	ACE inhibitor	Accupril
rabeprazole	ra-BEP-ra-zole	proton pump inhibitor	AcipHex
raloxifene	ral-OKS-i-feen	estrogen receptor modulator	Evista
ramipril	RA-mi-pril	ACE inhibitor	Altace
ranitidine	ra-NI-ti-deen	H_2 antagonist	Zantac
risperidone	ris-PER-i-done	antipsychotic	Risperdal
rosuvastatin	roe-soo-va-STAT-in	antilipemic	Crestor
sertraline	SER-tra-leen	antidepressant SSRI	Zoloft
sildenafil	sil-DEN-a-fil	phosphodiesterase-5-enzyme inhibitor	Viagra
simvastatin	sim-va-STAT-in	antilipemic	Zocor
sitagliptin	sit-a-GLIP-tin	antidiabetic DPP-4 inhibitor	Januvia
spironolactone	speer-on-oh-LAK-tone	diuretic	Aldactone
sumatriptan	soo-ma-TRIP-tan	serotonin 5-HT 1 receptor agonist	Imitrex
tadalafil	tah-DA-la-fil	phosphodiesterase-5 enzyme inhibitor	Cialis
tamsulosin	tam-SOO-loe-sin	alpha-1 blocker	Flomax
temazepam	te-MAZ-e-pam	benzodiazepine	Restoril
terazosin	ter-AY-zoe-sin	alpha-1 blocker	Hytrin
tiotropium	ty-oh-TRO-pee-um	anticholinergic	Spiriva
tizanidine	tye-ZAN-i-deen	alpha-2 adrenergic agonist	Zanaflex
tolterodine LA	tole-TER-oh-deen	anticholinergic	Detrol LA
topiramate	toe-PIE-ruh-mate	anticonvulsant	Topamax

Generic Name	Pronunciation	Classification	Brand Name
tramadol	TRA-ma-dole	opioid analgesic	Ultram
trazodone	TRAZ-oh-done	antidepressant SSRI	Desyrel
triamcinolone	try-am-SIN-oh-lone	corticosteroid	Kenalog
triamterene-hydrochlorothiazide	try-AM-ter-en hye-droe-klor-oh-THYE-a-side	diuretic	Dyazide, Maxzide
trimethoprim-sulfamethoxazole	try-METH-oh-prim sul-fa-meth-OKS-a-zole	antibiotic sulfa	Bactrim
valacyclovir	val-ay-SYE-kloe-veer	antiviral	Valtrex
valsartan	val-SAR-tan	angiotensin II receptor blocker	Diovan
valsartan-hydrochlorothiazide	val-SAR-tan hye-droe-klor-oh-THYE-a-side	angiotensin II blocker/diuretic	Diovan/HCT
venlafaxine XR	ven-la-FAX-een	antidepressant SSRI	Effexor XR
warfarin	WAR-far-in	anticoagulant	Coumadin
zolpidem	zole-PI-dem	hypnotic	Ambien
zolpidem CR	zole-PI-dem	hypnotic	Ambien CR

Appendix B

Practice Exams

The two practice exams in Appendix B are made up of 90 multiple-choice questions. Read the questions and select the best answer. Check your answers against the answer key in Appendix C. The answer keys include additional information about the answer choices and the chapters in which the information is located.

The companion Study Partner CD for this text offers extensive opportunities for additional exam practice, including a bank of more than 1,000 exam-style questions that can be used to randomly generate an unlimited number of unique practice exams. Students have the option of receiving immediate, question-by-question feedback, or taking the exam in Reported mode, a timed test that more closely resembles the high-stakes testing environment with performance graded at the end of the exam.

Practice Exam 1

1. Which of the following drugs may cause photosensitivity?
   a. azithromycin
   b. omeprazole
   c. doxycycline
   d. levothyroxine

2. The cost of 1,000 capsules of amoxicillin is $27.95. How much will the pharmacy charge for 30 capsules to yield a 34 percent profit margin with a $9.50 dispensing fee?
   a. $10.63
   b. $1.13
   c. $10.34
   d. $9.79

3. How many grams of 5% hydrocortisone ointment can be made with 10 g of hydrocortisone powder?
   a. 200 g
   b. 2,000 g
   c. 0.5 g
   d. 50 g

4. How many 500 mg metronidazole tablets are needed to make a two-week supply of metronidazole oral solution for a patient who must take 500 mg per nasogastric (NG) tube b.i.d.?
   a. 14 tablets
   b. 28 tablets
   c. 30 tablets
   d. 14,000 tablets

5. Which medication should be dispensed in its original brown glass container?
   a. oxycodone 5 mg tablets
   b. levofloxacin 500 mg tablets
   c. digoxin 0.125 mg tablets
   d. nitroglycerin 0.4 mg tablets

6. The pharmacy dispensing fee for prescriptions is $6.50. How much should you charge for 50 capsules of fluoxetine 20 mg if 100 capsules cost the pharmacy $12.43?
   a. $12.72
   b. $9.47
   c. $7.12
   d. $6.22

7. Mrs. Jones is refilling her heart medication. Which medication should the technician refill?
   a. Nexium
   b. Diovan
   c. Premarin
   d. Zoloft
8. How many grams of dextrose are needed to compound 250 mL of a 45% dextrose solution?
   a. 45 g
   b. 112.5 g
   c. 11.25 g
   d. 11,250 g
9. Aseptic technique is the process of manipulating sterile products to prevent the introduction of
   a. an active ingredient.
   b. pathogens.
   c. water.
   d. inactive ingredient.
10. What document does every employee of a community or institutional pharmacy sign that guarantees the privacy of patient health information?
    a. DUR warning
    b. OBRA-90 guarantee
    c. OSHA requirements
    d. HIPAA notice
11. Which of the following drugs is a Schedule II controlled substance?
    a. oxycodone
    b. acetaminophen with codeine
    c. buprenorphine
    d. lorazepam
12. Which drug would be considered a high-alert/ high-risk medication that requires special attention when administered to prevent a serious adverse event?
    a. heparin
    b. cephalexin
    c. citalopram
    d. buspirone
13. Documentation of a patient's adverse drug reaction should be made to the FDA online using the _________ form.
    a. MedWatch
    b. MSDS
    c. PharmAlert
    d. Drug Watch
14. What is the name of the official list of medications approved for use in a hospital by the Pharmacy and Therapeutics Committee?
    a. United States Pharmacopeia
    b. DESI list
    c. *Orange Book*
    d. formulary
15. An azithromycin prescription with the directions "2 tablets stat 1 PO daily × 4 for URI" would be dispensed with what patient instruction?
    a. Take two tablets now, then one tablet by mouth daily for 4 days for urinary tract infection.
    b. Take two tablets now, then one tablet by mouth daily for 4 days for upper respiratory infection.
    c. Take two tablets by mouth daily for 4 days for upper respiratory infection.
    d. Take two tablets as soon as possible, then one tablet four times daily for upper respiratory infection.
16. Where should the pharmacy store doxorubicin, a hazardous substance that needs to be refrigerated?
    a. next to other refrigerated products on wire racks
    b. separate from other drugs in the drug refrigerator in bins that prevent breakage and control leakage
    c. in the hood where chemotherapy is admixed
    d. at room temperature, as long as the room is air conditioned
17. For a generic drug to be considered bioequivalent, it must contain the same active ingredient as the original and be identical in strength, route of administration, and
    a. color.
    b. inactive ingredients.
    c. price.
    d. dosage form.

18. The pharmacy technician receives a prescription for amlodipine. A review of the patient profile shows that a prescription for verapamil was filled a week ago. What should the pharmacy technician do?
    a. Fill the prescription because it is not for the same drug.
    b. Notify the pharmacist of a potential duplication of therapy.
    c. Call the physician to discuss the duplication of therapy.
    d. Discontinue the verapamil prescription and fill the amlodipine.

19. Which of the following concepts does the federal law referred to as OBRA-90 require?
    a. confidentiality
    b. compliance
    c. medication errors
    d. counseling

20. Retail pharmacies receive electronic prescriptions and hospitals use computer technology called______ to transmit medication orders to the pharmacy.
    a. CPOE
    b. online adjudication
    c. Micromedex
    d. file maintenance

21. A Pyxis machine is an example of
    a. a pneumatic delivery system.
    b. a class-100 environment.
    c. automatic dispensing technology.
    d. a sterile compounding machine.

22. You need to measure out 6 mL of sterile water to mix azithromycin suspension. Where is the volume of fluid measured in a conical graduate?
    a. top of the meniscus
    b. center of the meniscus
    c. bottom of the meniscus
    d. one mark above the bottom of the meniscus

23. A medication order for ampicillin 1 g IVPB q4h is started at 6:00 a.m. When will the next two doses be given?
    a. 1200, 1800
    b. 1000, 1400
    c. 0900, 1300
    d. 0800, 1200

24. How many milligrams are in a ¼-grain thyroid USP tablet?
    a. 15 mg
    b. 25 mg
    c. 30 mg
    d. 60 mg

25. The reason a drug utilization evaluation (DUE) might pop up on the computer screen for Coumadin is because the medication has a high
    a. rate of side effects and drug interactions.
    b. cost index and a low margin.
    c. incidence of patients sharing prescriptions.
    d. incidence of addiction and potential for abuse.

26. Which of the following IV antibiotics is an antineoplastic that a nurse should never mix on the patient unit?
    a. erythromycin
    b. gentamicin
    c. azithromycin
    d. bleomycin

27. You are asked to compound a pediatric suspension of spironolactone that is 1 mg/5 mL. The prescription is for a 30-day supply, and the patient takes 1.5 tsp PO b.i.d. All you have in stock are 25 mg tablets. How many tablets will you need to crush to fill the order?
    a. four tablets
    b. three tablets
    c. two tablets
    d. one tablet

28. A patient who is allergic to penicillin may also be sensitive to
    a. cephalexin.
    b. erythromycin.
    c. sulfisoxazole.
    d. levofloxacin.

29. The FDA requires pharmacies to include a patient information insert every time a prescription is filled for which drug class?
    a. antihypertensives
    b. birth control tablets
    c. dietary supplements
    d. antibiotics

30. A pharmacy technician is filling a prescription for eye drops that reads "2 gtt OD t.i.d." How many drops will the patient use a day?
    a. 12 gtt
    b. 8 gtt
    c. 6 gtt
    d. 3 gtt

31. A shipment of vaccine arrives at the pharmacy. When it is opened, the temperature monitoring strip shows the vaccine container temperature was above the acceptable temperature. What should you do?
    a. Place the vaccine in the refrigerator for use.
    b. Throw out the vaccine.
    c. Notify the supplier so a new shipment can be sent.
    d. Place the vaccine in the freezer for storage.

32. The patient requests a refill for her little pink water pills. Which drug from her patient profile will you select?
    a. Synthroid 200 mcg
    b. hydrochlorothiazide 25 mg
    c. propranolol 10 mg
    d. allopurinol 300 mg

33. What computer function in the pharmacy helps identify drug interactions or therapeutic duplication?
    a. drug utilization review
    b. prior authorization notification
    c. medication assistance program
    d. incompatibility notification

34. Amoxicillin is available as 200 mg/tsp and 400 mg/tsp suspension, and 250 mg and 500 mg capsules. Which dosage form and strength would you dispense for a 13-month-old child who weighs 18 lbs if the prescribed dose is 25 mg/kg/day?
    a. 200 mg/tsp suspension
    b. 400 mg/tsp suspension
    c. 250 mg capsule
    d. 500 mg capsule

35. A patient presents a prescription for alendronate 70 mg, with directions "1 tab PO q Wk." How many tablets must be dispensed for a 3-month supply?
    a. 4 tablets
    b. 12 tablets
    c. 30 tablets
    d. 90 tablets

36. Which abbreviation(s) should not be used on a medication order because of the potential for error?
    a. U, IU
    b. QID
    c. qHS
    d. BID

37. What is inventory?
    a. a record of drugs purchased
    b. a record of drugs sold
    c. a list of all items available for sale
    d. the value of merchandise in stock

38. Gloves, gowns, respirators, face masks, and needle guards are all examples of
    a. compounding equipment.
    b. personal protective equipment.
    c. medical disposable material.
    d. ISO class 5 equipment.

39. A 70 kg adult requires aminophylline IV at 0.7 mg/kg/hr. The premixed solution is 500 mg/500 mL. What is the correct rate?
    a. 0.7 mL/hr
    b. 24.5 mL/hr
    c. 49 mL/hr
    d. 490 mL/hr

40. All chemicals used in a pharmacy or institution must have accompanying documentation that details the characteristics of the chemical and explains what measures should be taken in the event of a spill or human exposure. What is this document called?
    a. policy and procedure
    b. formulary
    c. PPI
    d. MSDS

41. One reason to extemporaneously compound a product is to
    a. increase the pharmacy's profit margin by making patented products.
    b. make a dose form not manufactured by a pharmaceutical company.
    c. make a supply to sell to physicians who may then sell it from their offices.
    d. make an otherwise unknown drug you think will work in humans.

42. Serum potassium levels should be checked on a patient taking which drug?
 a. erythromycin
 b. sertraline
 c. valproic acid
 d. furosemide

43. What is the trade name for fluoxetine?
 a. Cymbalta
 b. Strattera
 c. Prozac
 d. Celexa

44. To prevent a data entry error when selecting a patient profile, always get the correct spelling of the patient's name, address, and
 a. allegies.
 b. past medical history.
 c. date of birth.
 d. weight.

45. What two drugs are found in the combination product Vicodin?
 a. propoxyphene, acetaminophen
 b. propoxyphene, aspirin
 c. hydrocodone, acetaminophen
 d. acetaminophen, codeine

46. A child can take ¾ tsp t.i.d. of Tylenol. How many milliliters will the child take in a day?
 a. 15 mL
 b. 3.75 mL
 c. 2.25 mL
 d. 11.25 mL

47. Which of the following drugs should be stored in a refrigerator even after it is dispensed to the patient?
 a. Nitrostat
 b. NuvaRing
 c. Combivir
 d. Patanol

48. The interface between the pharmacy and the automatic dispensing machine on the patient care unit prevents medication errors by
 a. limiting drug selection for administration to the patient.
 b. eliminating the need to interpret a physician's hand writing.
 c. dispensing the correct drug at the correct time.
 d. preventing drug diversion by drug seeking staff.

49. A pharmacy offers a 10% discount to elderly patients who pay cash for prescriptions. If a prescription regularly costs $56.75, what is the senior discount price?
 a. $56.75
 b. $5.68
 c. $51.07
 d. $62.43

50. Which of the following drugs is an inhaled treatment for COPD?
 a. Ventolin
 b. Flonase
 c. Relenza
 d. NebuPent

51. A company that administers prescription drug benefits for individuals covered by multiple different insurance companies is called a
 a. comprehensive insurance company.
 b. health maintenance organization (HMO).
 c. pharmacy benefit manager (PBM).
 d. preferred provider organization (PPO).

52. To ensure the safety of employees, hazardous drugs, such as those used for chemotherapy, must be mixed
 a. in a vertical airflow hood.
 b. in a horizontal airflow hood.
 c. only by the pharmacist.
 d. only by the oncology nurse.

53. Which of the following drugs is a proton pump inhibitor?
 a. cimetidine
 b. dexlansoprazole
 c. sucralfate
 d. metoclopramide

54. A patient is to receive 2 L of D_5 0.45 NS with 40 mEq of KCl over 12 hr. What is the flow rate?
 a. 83 mL/hr
 b. 166 mL/hr
 c. 42 mL/hr
 d. 50 mL/hr

55. What technique could be used to prevent look-alike/sound-alike medication selection errors?
 a. avoid trailing zeros
 b. locate similar names together on the shelf
 c. limit purchasing of similar named drugs
 d. tall man lettering

56. The pharmacy technician should contact the pharmacist for any interaction with a patient involving
  a. location of an item in the store.
  b. adverse drug reaction.
  c. dispensing of prepared refill of a prescription.
  d. ordering a refill of a prescription.

57. The generic name for Seroquel is
  a. fluoxetine.
  b. omeprazole.
  c. alprazolam.
  d. quetiapine.

58. What vitamin is administered during a Coumadin overdose?
  a. vitamin A
  b. vitamin E
  c. vitamin C
  d. vitamin K

59. What is an advantage of using technology in the pharmacy?
  a. less need for technical help
  b. increased efficiency
  c. decreased need for pharmacist double-check
  d. increased expense

60. Which of the following items is necessary to clean up a chemotherapy leak in the hospital?
  a. emergency box
  b. latex gloves
  c. spill kit
  d. isopropyl alcohol

61. A patient with a history of peptic ulcer disease (PUD) should purchase _____ for pain.
  a. acetaminophen
  b. aspirin
  c. ibuprofen
  d. naproxen

62. What is the approved temperature range for refrigerated storage?
  a. 35°F to 45°F
  b. 15°C to 30°C
  c. 25°C to 2°C
  d. 15°F to 30°F

63. A physical inventory of Schedule II controlled substances must be done
  a. daily.
  b. monthly.
  c. yearly.
  d. every two years.

64. A DEA 222 form must be filled out to purchase a supply of
  a. heroin.
  b. oxycodone.
  c. tramadol.
  d. diazepam.

65. Which drug recall is issued as a result of a patient's death and requires the immediate removal of the drug from the market and from any patient who received it?
  a. Class I
  b. Class II
  c. Class III
  d. Class IV

66. What part of the computer connects the computer to a remote network via telephone lines?
  a. central processing unit
  b. operating system
  c. random access memory
  d. modem

67. How often should a patient's allergy information be updated?
  a. only at the patient's first visit
  b. once a year
  c. never
  d. at every visit with a new prescription

68. When is the last day that a drug with an expiration date of 1/1/2018 can be dispensed from a retail pharmacy?
  a. 1/1/2018
  b. six months after the original bottle is opened
  c. 1/31/2018
  d. up to 1/1/2018 as long as the patient uses it up before 1/1/2018.

69. What report is used to identify employees who currently have access to the pharmacy database?
   a. override report
   b. interface report
   c. user access report
   d. diversion report

70. Melatonin is a(n)
   a. antidiarrheal.
   b. laxative.
   c. dietary supplement.
   d. fiber supplement.

71. If the selling price of a product is AWP minus 10% plus a dispensing fee of $9, what will 90 Lipitor 10 mg cost if the AWP is $112.25 per 100 tablets?
   a. $90.90
   b. $101.02
   c. $110
   d. $99.72

72. How much haloperidol is in 0.75 mL of a 5 mg/mL injectable solution?
   a. 4.5 mg
   b. 3.75 mg
   c. 2.25 mg
   d. 3.5 mg

73. What new technology is used in pharmacies to help the technician verify the correct drug has been selected for a prescription refill?
   a. barcode scanning
   b. electronic patient profile
   c. online claim processing
   d. automatic dispensing machines

74. The prescription reads:
   Phenobarbital ½ grain po b.i.d.
   Disp: 1 month supply

   If the tablets are 65 mg each, how many will you dispense?
   a. 15 tablets
   b. 30 tablets
   c. 45 tablets
   d. 60 tablets

75. Which auxiliary label should be included on a prescription for metformin?
   a. Take with food.
   b. Avoid calcium-containing foods and vitamins.
   c. Take on an empty stomach.
   d. This medication may cause drowsiness.

76. Which of the following tasks is a pharmacy technician *not* allowed to do?
   a. counsel a patient about a prescription
   b. offer counseling to a patient about his or her prescription
   c. receive a written prescription from a patient
   d. update a patient profile on the computer

77. If an insurer rejects a patient's prescription, the pharmacy technician may be required to call the physician to request what?
   a. prior authorization
   b. a refill
   c. clarification of the prescription
   d. a written prescription

78. Which federal agency regulates drug manufacturers researching new drugs?
   a. Drug Enforcement Administration (DEA)
   b. Food and Drug Administration (FDA)
   c. Department of Health and Human Services (DHHS)
   d. Consumer Product Safety Commission (CPSC)

79. A patient may have more than one prescription insurance plan or a coupon to help cover the cost of a prescription. The process to ensure the correct claims payment is called
   a. coordination of benefits.
   b. medication assistance programming.
   c. health maintenance organization.
   d. pharmacy benefit management.

80. Purchasing done frequently in quantities to meet current demand is called
   a. direct purchasing.
   b. prime vendor purchasing.
   c. JIT.
   d. ASAP.

81. A patient's prescription coverage does not allow a retail pharmacy to fill more than a 30-day supply of medications, but a mail-order pharmacy may fill a 90-day supply. This is called a
    a. rejected claim.
    b. prior authorization.
    c. par level.
    d. plan limitation.

82. What is the brand name for simvastatin?
    a. Zocor
    b. Zetia
    c. Xanax
    d. Mevacor

83. What federal standards regulate the extemporaneous compounding of nonsterile preparations?
    a. USP Chapter <795>
    b. USP Chapter <797>
    c. the Food, Drug, and Cosmetic Act
    d. the Orphan Drug Act

84. Which of the following DEA numbers is falsified?
    a. AB1234549
    b. AB3261930
    c. AB2347627
    d. AB1928374

85. The most common source of contamination when preparing sterile products is
    a. air.
    b. water.
    c. alcohol.
    d. touch.

86. Customer service is demonstrated by
    a. smiling and making eye contact when communicating.
    b. pointing to the location of items in the aisle.
    c. not putting the caller on hold while they wait for the pharmacist.
    d. waiting on as many customers as possible at one time.

87. Which computer report is used to manage inventory?
    a. diversion report.
    b. override report.
    c. patient adherence report.
    d. usage report.

88. When breaking the top of an ampule, break it
    a. away from you.
    b. toward the high-efficiency particulate air (HEPA) filter.
    c. toward you.
    d. outside the hood.

89. What is the first thing a pharmacy technician should do when exposed to a hazardous substance?
    a. Notify the pharmacy director.
    b. Flood any exposed skin with water and thoroughly clean with soap and water.
    c. Call environment service for help with clean up.
    d. Go to the emergency department.

90. What advantage is there to monitoring inventory?
    a. increase in expired products
    b. decrease in capital that is tied up
    c. increased risk of diversion
    d. need for increased storage space

Practice Exam 2

1. What federal law protects the confidentiality of a patient's medical information?
   a. Prescription Drug Marketing Act of 1987
   b. Health Insurance Portability and Accountability Act of 1996
   c. Omnibus Budget Reconciliation Act of 1990
   d. FDA Modernization Act

2. Prescription transfer between pharmacies
   a. is never allowed.
   b. is under the control of each individual state.
   c. may only be done by a registered pharmacist.
   d. is under the control of each pharmacy's owner.

3. What is the generic name for Plavix?
   a. celecoxib
   b. clopidogrel
   c. clonidine
   d. citalopram

4. Which drug is in the same therapeutic class as Effexor?
   a. Cymbalta
   b. Clozaril
   c. Cordarone
   d. Cardizem

5. Who is responsible for publishing the *Orange Book* of approved drug products and bioequivalent generics?
   a. DEA
   b. ISMP
   c. CMS
   d. FDA

6. Which statement regarding policy and procedure manuals is correct?
   a. Technicians should always check their employer's policy and procedure manual when unsure of safe operation of the pharmacy.
   b. State pharmacy boards write the policy and procedure manuals that will be used in pharmacies in each state.
   c. Federal law dictates what topics will be included in a policy and procedure manual.
   d. Technicians should always do what the pharmacist tells them, even when the policy and procedure manual disagrees.

7. A high level of cholesterol in the bloodstream is a risk factor for
   a. diabetes.
   b. atherosclerosis.
   c. deep vein thrombosis.
   d. cancer.

8. A patient refilling his prescription for his albuterol inhaler states that he is having more shortness of breath than usual and has been using his inhaler more than usual. The technician notices on his profile that he takes medication for congestive heart failure and asthma. What should the technician do?
   a. Fill the prescription for the inhaler.
   b. Call the patient's physician to report an early refill of the inhaler.
   c. Suggest that the patient take more of his diuretic, and that might help his breathing.
   d. Suggest the patient talk to the pharmacist while you get the inhaler ready.

9. The pharmacy receives a prescription for Zithromax 250 mg tablets
   Disp: 5
   Sig. ii stat then i PO daily × 4D

   What is wrong with the prescription?
   a. The drug should be taken for 10 days total and needs to be written for 11 tablets.
   b. The drug is only available intravenously (IV) and given in a hospital.
   c. The quantity should be six tablets to complete the five days of therapy.
   d. The drug is only available as a capsule and must be ordered that way.

10. What ordering technique requires the pharmacy staff to write down items that need to be reordered?
    a. minimum and maximum product levels
    b. order book
    c. inventory cards
    d. computerized inventory system

11. Which of the following nicotine replacement products delivers nicotine over a continuous 24-hour period?
   a. nicotine lozenge
   b. nicotine gum
   c. nicotine inhalation
   d. nicotine patch

12. Which of the following is an error of omission?
   a. patient only takes seven days of a 10-day antibiotic regimen
   b. an intravenous antibiotic to be given at 8 a.m. is given at 8 p.m.
   c. a nurse administers only half the bag of intravenous antibiotic
   d. the automatic compounding machine releases too much antibiotic into the IV bag

13. Which numbers in the national drug code 0002-8215-01 for Humulin R, manufactured by Lilly and Company, identify the manufacturer?
   a. 0002
   b. 8215
   c. 01
   d. none of the above

14. Ondansetron (Zofran) is an IV therapy to
   a. prevent nausea and vomiting.
   b. prevent organ transplant rejection.
   c. treat breast cancer.
   d. dissolve blood clots.

15. A drug order from a wholesaler should be checked against what document?
   a. invoice
   b. want book
   c. purchase order
   d. last 24-hour usage

16. What alternative medicine might be used in place of a prescription sedative or hypnotic?
   a. ginger
   b. ginkgo
   c. saw palmetto
   d. melatonin

17. Which of the following is a near homonym or homograph, or both, of each other?
   a. clonidine, Klonopin
   b. clonidine, Catapres
   c. clonazepam, Klonopin
   d. clonazepam, clonidine

18. A patient buys Lantus U-100 insulin and syringes at your pharmacy. If she uses 52 units of insulin at bedtime, how many vials or pens will she need for 30 days?
   a. 2 vials of 10 mL
   b. 1 vial of 10 mL
   c. 5 pens of 3 mL
   d. 3 pens of 3 mL

19. A patient presents a prescription for Lyrica. What is the maximum number of refills allowed?
   a. none
   b. one
   c. five
   d. six

20. What special auxiliary label should be on a prescription label for ziprasidone (Geodon) when it is dispensed to a patient?
   a. keep refrigerated
   b. drowsiness warning
   c. avoid sunlight warning
   d. take with food

21. Which of the following medications requires special handling, preparation, and waste disposal?
   a. fluorouracil
   b. fluoxetine
   c. fluticasone
   d. fenofibrate

22. The prescription reads:

   Bactrim DS
   Disp: XIV
   Sig. 1 tab po BID

   How many tablets will be dispensed?
   a. 14
   b. 56
   c. 16
   d. 30

23. If cefazolin vial contains 1 g of drug, how many doses of 200 mg can be made from one vial?
   a. 1
   b. 3
   c. 5
   d. 7

24. The stock 10 mL vial of folic acid is 5 mg/mL. How much will need to be drawn up in a syringe to equal 2 mg?
   a. 0.2 mL
   b. 0.25 mL
   c. 0.4 mL
   d. 0.6 mL

25. A patient weighs 154 lbs. and is prescribed Levaquin at 7 mg/kg/dose. What is the dose in milligrams?
   a. 250 mg
   b. 500 mg
   c. 750 mg
   d. 1,000 mg

26. Which of the following pieces of data would be found in the drug database?
   a. special handling
   b. drug utilization review
   c. storage information
   d. national drug code

27. A category of drugs on the ISMP high-alert medication list is
   a. antithrombotic.
   b. antibiotics.
   c. corticosteroids.
   d. contraceptives.

28. Which abbreviation is considered dangerous by the Institute for Safe Medication Practices (ISMP) and should not be used according to Joint Commission standards?
   a. t.i.d.
   b. q.d.
   c. mg
   d. PO

29. What type of software program is commonly used in a pharmacy computer system?
   a. DBMS
   b. DUR
   c. smart terminal
   d. dumb terminal

30. The instrument used to pick up and transfer weights to and from the balance to avoid transferring moisture and oils to the weights is called a
   a. spatula.
   b. pestle.
   c. forceps.
   d. pipette.

31. The area in which the computer software backup should be stored is
   a. the sterile product room.
   b. a high-traffic area.
   c. an area of high humidity.
   d. secure and fire proof.

32. When preparing the nonsterile compound 10% hydrocortisone ointment, the compounding record
   a. is not necessary.
   b. only requires the name of the product compounded and the preparer of the compound.
   c. includes a record of the compounding, including ingredients, amounts of ingredients, preparer's name, and name of supervising pharmacist.
   d. is the recipe for how to make a compounded product.

33. The laminar airflow hood should be given a thorough cleaning with isopropyl alcohol
   a. every six months.
   b. at the end of the day.
   c. every 30 days.
   d. several times a day.

34. What is the name of the procedure used to prevent infection caused by exposure to blood or other bodily fluids?
   a. blood precautions
   b. universal precautions
   c. sterile precautions
   d. aseptic technique

35. Inventory control is important to prevent overstocking. As a pharmacy technician, what computer report would be useful to decide the par levels of medications?
   a. override report
   b. work total report
   c. usage report
   d. diversion report

36. Prozac Liquid is available as 20 mg/5 mL. How many milliliters will you draw up if the patient is to receive 1 mg of Prozac?
   a. 5 mL
   b. 2.5 mL
   c. 1 mL
   d. 0.25 mL

37. Compounded prescriptions are priced at cost plus 30% plus a $10 compounding fee. If the cost of the compounded ingredients is $8.76, how much should you charge the patient?
   a. $8.76
   b. $11.39
   c. $18.76
   d. $21.39

38. The minimum inventory level for Cytoxan is 10 vials of 500 mg and the maximum inventory level is 20 vials. You use all but two vials compounding chemotherapy medication orders. Cytoxan is available from your wholesaler in packages of 10 vials of 500 mg and 10 vials of 200 mg. How many vials should you order?
   a. 8 vials of 500 mg
   b. 10 vials of 500 mg
   c. 20 vials of 500 mg
   d. 10 vials of 200 mg

39. A special REMS program, iPLEDGE, is mandated by the FDA to promote patient safety for what drug?
   a. thalidamide
   b. clozapine
   c. isotretinoin
   d. olanzapine

40. Which diuretic is potassium sparing?
   a. hydrochlorothiazide
   b. triamterene
   c. metolazone
   d. furosemide

41. Which of the following drugs is indicated to treat Alzheimer's disease?
   a. AcipHex
   b. Accutane
   c. Accupril
   d. Aricept

42. A patient comes to the pharmacy counter and complains that the pharmacy incorrectly filled her prescription. She was supposed to get medicine to treat her high blood pressure and instead was given the same medicine her friend takes for migraine headaches. What do you tell her?
   a. "Your friend has the wrong medicine, not you, and your friend should contact her pharmacy."
   b. "We never make mistakes, you are wrong."
   c. "Many medications have more than one use, this may be one, let me get the pharmacist."
   d. "Call your physician. He made the mistake."

43. At what age may a female purchase the morning after pill without a prescription?
   a. 15
   b. 16
   c. 17
   d. 14

44. When preparing capsules, which part is used to *punch* the powder?
   a. top
   b. bottom
   c. body
   d. cap

45. What size hard-shell capsule is the smallest?
   a. 000
   b. 0
   c. 1
   d. 5

46. What does a the FDA's black box warning indicate about a drug?
   a. it should not be used in pregnancy
   b. the drug is not approved for human use
   c. extra information should be given to pharmacists and physicians
   d. the product must be recalled from the market

47. Which drug must be dispensed for the treatment of narcotic detoxification and maintenance at specially licensed hospitals or clinics?
   a. buprenorphine
   b. naloxone
   c. butorphanol
   d. methadone

48. Augmentin belongs to which family of antibiotics?
   a. penicillins
   b. tetracyclines
   c. aminoglycosides
   d. cephalosporins

49. If a patient is allergic to erythromycin and says that she stopped breathing once when she had it, what drug is she is also allergic to?
    a. gentamicin
    b. clarithromycin
    c. penicillin
    d. doxycycline

50. When compounding sterile products, you work at least _____ inches from the edge of the hood.
    a. 6
    b. 10
    c. 12
    d. 4

51. Which is an example of reverse distribution?
    a. returning overstock to the wholesaler
    b. patient returning an unused prescription for credit
    c. returning outdated drugs for credit
    d. selling prescription drugs to a physician's office

52. What identifies you as a user of the pharmacy computer system and should not be shared?
    a. identification badge
    b. BIN and PCN
    c. login and password
    d. override code

53. Which of the following duties may be done by a pharmacy technician?
    a. checking and verifying finished prescriptions
    b. receiving verbal prescriptions in person or by telephone
    c. receiving written prescriptions
    d. verifying that weighing and measuring is done properly

54. When should a pharmacy technician inquire about a patient's insurance prescription coverage?
    a. never
    b. if the patient is new to the pharmacy
    c. if the online claim is rejected for non-formulary reasons
    d. every time the patient requests a refill

55. Which of the following pieces of information is legally required on a prescription?
    a. indication for use
    b. date written
    c. responsible party for payment
    d. refill information

56. What is required on a controlled substance prescription for MS Contin that is *not* needed for a prescription written for metoprolol?
    a. DEA number
    b. physician's signature
    c. address of physician
    d. date written

57. There is a drug recall on albuterol HFA inhalers, which are Class I. How will you identify all the patients who received an albuterol inhaler from your pharmacy?
    a. Class I does not require you to contact the patient
    b. run a usage report for albuterol HFA inhalers
    c. from memory, think of all of the asthma patients and contact them to see if they have one
    d. go through all of the written prescriptions looking for albuterol HFA inhalers

58. Checking the temperature of the refrigerators that store medications is an example of
    a. a method to ensure proper storage of medications and avoid waste.
    b. a mechanism to control inventory.
    c. repackaging requirements.
    d. one of the five rights of filling a prescription.

59. Which choice is an example of a quality control measure used when mixing a sterile product?
    a. turning the hood on right before starting to mix
    b. cleaning all interior working surfaces of the hood with isopropyl alcohol
    c. turning on the air conditioner to keep the area cool while compounding
    d. placing all the necessary materials on a shelf behind the hood

60. Zolpidem would most likely be ordered
    a. every morning.
    b. twice daily.
    c. four times daily.
    d. at bedtime.

61. Duplicate therapy, allergy, food-drug interaction and drug-drug interactions are all examples of what function done by the pharmacy computer program?
    a. drug utilization review
    b insurance plan limitations
    c. medication adherence program
    d. override reports

62. What is the proper way to write Coumadin *five milligrams* to prevent a medication error?
    a. 5.0 mg
    b. 5 mg
    c. 0.5 mg
    d. 0.005 g

63. What is the advantage of e-prescribing for patient safety?
    a. fewer phone calls to the pharmacy
    b. prescription is ready when the patient arrives at the pharmacy
    c. decreases the risk of handwritten prescription misinterpretation
    d. saves time for the physician

64. Which of the following pregnancy risk levels means that isotretinoin is an absolute contraindication?
    a. A
    b. C
    c. D
    d. X

65. What role does the National Drug Code (NDC) play in medication safety?
    a. selection of the accurate drug
    b. inventory management
    c. storage requirement
    d. claim reconciliation

66. A patient taking the pain reliever tramadol should be told to avoid
    a. dairy products.
    b. driving.
    c. sunlight.
    d. food.

67. The name for an infection acquired while in the hospital is
    a. nosocomial.
    b. empirical.
    c. aerobic.
    d. superinfection.

68. If the biennial inventory is not up-to-date, which agency is charged with enforcement?
    a. FDA
    b. Consumer Product Safety Commission
    c. DEA
    d. U.S. Department of Health and Human Services

69. Which medication is used to treat gout?
    a. acetaminophen
    b. amlodipine
    c. atenolol
    d. allopurinol

70. The term used to describe having more receipts than expenses is
    a. turnover.
    b. profit.
    c. markup.
    d. dispensing fee.

71. Tylenol Arthritis Strength is a Class II recall. What should happen to the store's inventory of the affected lots?
    a. nothing
    b. mark down to sell
    c. remove from stock
    d. throw out in trash

72. When stocking pharmaceuticals received from the wholesaler, always place products with the closest expiration dates
    a. behind the other stock.
    b. on the counter.
    c. in front of the other stock.
    d. next to the other stock.

73. Which of these numbers would you find on the patient's prescription insurance card?
    a. social security number
    b. date of birth
    c. bank identification number
    d. employer's phone number

74. If a product on the formulary is not available from the manufacturer in unit-dose packaging, the technician should
    a. recommend it be taken off the formulary.
    b. order bulk and repackage in unit-dose packaging.
    c. order bulk and send bulk package to the floor for patient use.
    d. interchange with a therapeutic equivalent drug available in unit-dose packaging.

75. Which of the following medications must be refrigerated after dispensing?
    a. cephalexin pediatric suspension
    b. sulfamethoxazole and trimethoprim pediatric suspension
    c. Dilantin pediatric suspension
    d. fluoxetine oral solution

76. Information on how to handle hazardous substances at your facility might be found in a
    a. compounding logbook.
    b. repackaging logbook.
    c. policy and procedure manual.
    d. human resources manual.

77. What is the name of the rigorous voluntary inspection process conducted by the Joint Commission?
    a. registration
    b. licensure
    c. certification
    d. accreditation

78. In the following prescription, how many tablets should be dispensed?

    Prednisone 10 mg
    1 tab q.i.d. × 4 days
    1 tab t.i.d. × 4 days
    1 tab b.i.d. × 2 days
    1 tab daily × 2 days
    ½ tab daily × 2 days

    a. 14
    b. 42
    c. 35
    d. 40

79. A prescription for Patanol reads *OU*. What do you type on the label?
    a. both ears
    b. both eyes
    c. right eye
    d. right ear

80. Which of the following is exempt from the Poison Prevention Act?
    a. hormone replacement therapy
    b. oral contraceptives in the manufacturer's dispensing package
    c. isosorbide mononitrate
    d. potassium chloride tablets

81. NuvaRing should be stored before dispensing
    a. at room temperature.
    b. in the freezer.
    c. in the controlled-substance cabinet.
    d. in the refrigerator.

82. Your computer in the retail pharmacy automatically fills prescriptions for chronic medications if a patient requests. If a patient calls and says he will not need a refill this month, what might be the problem outside of your control?
    a. your computer filled the prescription too often
    b. the patient is not being compliant with the medication
    c. a duplicate label was printed and filled by mistake
    d. the counting machine is not accurate

83. What is a pharmacy benefits manager (PBM)?
    a. the pharmacy's human resource person
    b. third party administrator of prescription drug plans
    c. the employer's human resource department
    d. pharmacy personnel who help patients find health insurance

84. Who is responsible for contacting the insurance provider for prior authorization (PA) for a prescription?
    a. pharmacist
    b. patient
    c. pharmacy technician
    d. prescriber

85. The federal government restricts the sale of ___________ because of its use in making methamphetamine.
    a. pseudoephedrine
    b. syringes
    c. Plan B
    d. dextromethorphan

86. What might indicate that a prescription for Vicodin has been forged?
    a. there is no date on the written prescription
    b. there is no DEA number on the written prescription
    c. the quantity has been changed
    d. the patient is very nervous

87. If a technician notices that the tablets in a vial do not appear to be the right color, what should he or she do?
    a. dispense to the patient because it was already checked by the pharmacist
    b. return to the filling area for review and documentation
    c. throw out and reprint the label for another filling
    d. dispense to the patient but warn the patient that the tablets look different

88. Barcoding a prescription unit-dose drug container
    a. facilitates choosing the right drug for the prescription or medication order.
    b. supplements inventory management required by the DEA.
    c. allows the patient to be assured that the product is FDA-approved.
    d. supports the prevention of theft from the pharmacy.

89. An elderly patient does not understand why you are asking her to pay for her prescription when all year long, her medicine has been free. She has a Medicare Part D plan. What is the most likely problem?
    a. she is in the donut hole
    b. she did not pay her premiums
    c. she is mistaken and has always paid
    d. her plan stopped paying for the drug

90. Which medication might an insurance company limit the number of tablets dispensed per 30 days because it is not recommended for use daily?
    a. atenolol
    b. sumatriptan
    c. gemfibrozil
    d. metformin

Appendix C

Answer Keys

Pretest

1. a Chapter 4
2. c Chapter 6
3. a Chapter 4
4. b Chapter 11
5. b Chapter 4
6. d Chapter 10
7. c Chapter 11
8. c Chapter 8
9. b Chapter 11
10. a Chapter 8
11. c Chapter 8
12. a Chapter 3
13. b Chapter 10
14. a Chapter 11
15. c Chapter 5
16. a Chapter 7
17. b Chapter 9
18. b Chapter 9
19. c Chapter 8
20. b Chapter 10
21. b Chapter 6
22. d Chapter 10
23. a Chapter 9
24. d Chapter 8
25. c Chapter 8
26. d Chapter 5
27. a Chapter 10
28. a Chapter 6
29. a Chapter 7
30. b Chapter 7
31. b Chapter 5
32. a Chapter 5
33. c Chapter 7
34. d Chapter 5
35. b Chapter 7
36. c Chapter 8
37. c Chapter 8
38. a Chapter 8
39. a Chapter 9
40. c Chapter 4
41. a Chapter 6
42. d Chapter 6
43. c Chapter 6
44. d Chapter 11
45. b Chapter 5
46. a Chapter 5
47. d Chapter 9
48. b Chapter 9
49. c Chapter 9
50. c Chapter 4
51. a Chapter 11
52. a Chapter 4
53. d Chapter 4
54. b Chapter 4
55. b Chapter 4
56. b Chapter 4
57. a Chapter 10
58. d Chapter 5
59. c Chapter 4
60. d Chapter 11
61. c Chapter 4
62. d Chapter 10
63. c Chapter 10
64. b Chapter 10
65. a Chapter 11
66. a Chapter 8
67. b Chapter 6
68. b Chapter 6
69. b Chapter 6
70. c Chapter 7
71. b Chapter 8
72. c Chapter 8
73. c Chapter 8
74. a Chapter 5
75. b Chapter 8
76. c Chapter 8
77. c Chapter 9
78. b Chapter 7
79. a Chapter 8
80. b Chapter 3
81. d Chapter 3
82. a Chapter 3
83. b Chapter 3
84. a Chapter 3
85. c Chapter 3
86. d Chapter 3
87. a Chapter 3
88. b Chapter 3
89. d Chapter 3
90. c Chapter 3

Calculations Practice Exam

1. **a.** Set up a proportion between the concentration of the available product and the dose required.

$$25 \text{ mg}/1 \text{ mL} = 6.25 \text{ mg}/x \text{ mL}$$

Cross-multiply $25x = 1 \times 6.25$

Divide by 25 $x = 1 \times 6.25/25$

$$x = 0.25 \text{ mL}$$

2. **b.** The diphenhydramine is available as 25 mg/mL. The prescription calls for a 50 mg dose. Set up a proportion to solve.

$$25 \text{ mg}/1 \text{ mL} \times 50 \text{ mg}/x \text{ mL}$$

$$25x = 1 \times 50$$

$$x = 2 \text{ mL}$$

3. **c.** The dose of ceftriazone is 125 mg and the diluted vial is 250 mg/mL. Set up the proportion.

$$250 \text{ mg/mL} = 125 \text{ mg}/x \text{ mL}$$

$$250x = 125 \text{ mg} \times 1$$

$$x = 0.5 \text{ mL}$$

The dose of azithromycin is 2 grams, which is 2000 mg. Set up the proportion.

$$250 \text{ mg}/1 \text{ tablet} = 2000 \text{ mg}/x \text{ tablets}$$

$$250x = 2000 \times 1$$

$$x = 8 \text{ tablets}$$

4. **c.** Each dose is ½ tablet. "TID" means three times a day. The patient will need 1.5 tablets per day. Multiply by 30 days or set up proportion:

$$1.5 \text{ tablets}/1 \text{ day} = x \text{ tablets}/30 \text{ days}$$

$$1.5 \times 30 = 1x$$

$$x = 45 \text{ tablets}$$

5. **d.** The Vicodin has 500 mg of acetaminophen per tablet and the patient takes 2 tablets per day or 1000 mg. The Advil is acetaminophen free. The Tylenol tablets have 325 mg of acetaminophen per tablet and the patient takes 2 per day, or 650 mg.

$$1000 \text{ mg} + 650 \text{ mg} = 1650 \text{ mg per day of acetaminophen}$$

6. **b.** The vial is 200 mg vial and the patient needs 100 mg per dose. Set up a proportion.

$$100 \text{ mg}/1 \text{ dose} = 200 \text{ mg}/x \text{ doses}$$

$$x = 2 \text{ doses}$$

7. **c.** Two different strengths could be dispensed in combination; it is easier for the patient to take one strength and have only one copayment. The dose 62.5 mcg is half of 125 mcg. Therefore, the best option is to dispense 125 mcg tablets with instructions to cut the tablet in half. A 90 days' supply would require 45 tablets.

8. **a.** Calculate the total amount of ointment that will be contained in the 24 jars.

$$1 \text{ oz} = 30 \text{ grams}$$

$$4\text{oz} = 120 \text{ grams}$$

$$120 \text{ grams} \times 24 \text{ jars} = 2880 \text{ grams}$$

10% hydrocortisone means 10 grams hydrocortisone per 100 grams of total ointment

$$\frac{10 \text{ grams HC}/}{100 \text{ grams Oint.}} = \frac{x \text{ gram}/}{2880 \text{ grams Oint.}}$$

$$x = 288 \text{ grams of hydrocortisone powder}$$

9. **d.** The final ointment is to be 0.5% menthol. From question 8 you know there will be 2880 grams total ointment, and 0.5% means 0.5 grams menthol per 100 grams of ointment. Set up a proportion.

$$\frac{0.5 \text{ gram menthol}/}{100 \text{ grams Oint.}} = \frac{x \text{ grams menthol}/}{2880 \text{ grams Oint.}}$$

$$x = 14.4 \text{ grams}$$

10. **c.** Use a proportion to calculate the milligram dose.

$$20 \text{ mg}/5 \text{ mL} = x \text{ mg}/ 1.25 \text{ mL}$$

$$x = 5 \text{ mg of fluoxetine}$$

11. **c.** Every 15 minutes for 4 hours would be 16 doses of 17 grams each.

$$16 \text{ doses} \times 17 \text{ gram/dose} = 272 \text{ grams.}$$

The patient will need to purchase the 357 gram bottle to have enough for the bowel prep.

12. **c.** This is a basic calculation of quantity used in retail pharmacy. The first 14 days will require 14 tablets, the second 14 days require 28 tablets, and the final 2 weeks require 42 tablets.

$$14 + 28 + 42 = 84 \text{ tablets.}$$

13. **b.** Because the manufacturer's expiration date is greater than 1 year from the date of repackaging, you may use the 1-year beyond-use date.

14. **d.** The patient will use 8 puffs per day. Figure out the number of puffs for 90 days and then divide by the size of the inhaler.

$$8 \text{ puffs/day} \times 90 \text{ days} = 720 \text{ puffs}$$

$$720 \text{ puffs} \times 1 \text{ inhaler}/120 \text{ puffs} = 6 \text{ inhalers}$$

15. **c.** First, calculate the total daily dose:

$$50 \text{ mg/kg/day} \times 20 \text{ kg} = 1000 \text{ mg/day}$$

Divide by 3 to get the dose to be given every 8 hours.

$$1000 \text{ mg/day} \times 1 \text{ day}/3 \text{ doses} = 333 \text{ mg}$$

16. **d.** First, calculate the dose per day (1 teaspoon = 5 mL)

$$5 \text{ mL/dose} \times 4 \text{ doses/day} = 20 \text{ mL /day}$$

Then calculate total number of doses for 14 days.

$$20 \text{ mL/day} \times 14 \text{ days} = 280 \text{ mL}$$

The 300 mL bottle comes closest to the size needed for the 14 day therapy.

17. **d.** The patient will need to check blood sugar 4 times a day for 3 months (90 days), requiring at least 360 glucometer strips. Dispense 4 containers of 100 strips.

18. **c.** Calculate the total number of units needed for 30 days.

$$70 \text{ units/day} \times 30 \text{ days} = 2100 \text{ units for 30 days}$$

Each pen has 3 mL of 100 units/mL for a total of 300 units/pen

$$2100 \text{ units}/30 \text{ days} \times 1 \text{ pen}/300 \text{ units} = 7 \text{ pens}$$

19. **d.** U-500 insulin has a concentration of 500 units per 1 mL. The patient needs 125 units per dose. Use a simple proportion to calculate.

$$500 \text{ units}/1 \text{ mL} = 125 \text{ units}/x \text{ mL}$$

$$x = 125/500$$

$$x = 0.25 \text{ mL of U-500 insulin is equal to 125 units}$$

20. **b.** A varying dose schedule for warfarin is not uncommon. The easiest way to calculate this is to look at the total milligrams needed for the cycle, then figure out how many cycles in the month and calculate total milligrams needed, and then divide by strength of the tablets.

$$1 \text{ cycle} = 3 \text{ days}$$

$$2.5 \text{ mg} + 2.5 \text{ mg} + 3.75 \text{ mg} = 8.75 \text{ mg}$$

$$30 \text{ days} = 10 \text{ cycles}$$

$$8.75 \text{ mg/cycle} \times 10 \text{ cycle} = 87.5 \text{ mg}$$

$$87.5 \text{ mg/month} \times 1 \text{ tablet}/2.5 \text{ mg} = 35 \text{ tablets}$$

21. **b.** Change your information to similar units. Instead of 250 mL/1hr, write 250mL/60 min. The drop set is a 15 gtt/mL set.

$$250 \text{ mL}/60 \text{ min} \times 15 \text{ gtt/mL} = 62.5 \text{ gtt/min}$$

22. **c.** Add the first, third, and fifth digits together: $5 + 9 + 2 = 16$. Add the second, fourth, and sixth digits and multiply by 2: $4 + 7 + 1 = 12 \times 2 = 24$. Add the first and second answers together and the last digit will be the last digit of the DEA number: $16 + 24 = 40$

23. **a.** The concentration 0.5% is also written a 0.5 grams/100 mL.

    Calculate how many grams of clindamycin will be needed for 30 mL.

    $$0.5 \text{ gram}/100 \text{ ml} = x \text{ gram}/30 \text{ mL}$$

    $$x = 0.15 \text{ gram}$$

    Convert grams to milligrams.

    $$1000 \text{ mg}/1 \text{ gram} = x \text{ mg}/0.15 \text{ gram}$$

$x = 150$ mg, which is the content of 1 capsule of clindamycin

24. **d.** The patient still has $7 to pay toward the deductible. The insurer will pay all but $10 of the cost of the prescription. The patient must pay $7 + $10 = $17; the insurer will pay $12.65.

25. **d.** Convert 3 liters to milliliters.

    $$1000 \text{ mL}/1 \text{ L} \times 3 \text{ L} = 3000 \text{ mL}$$

    There are 24 hours in a day, so divide total volume by time.

    $$3000 \text{ mL}/24 \text{ hours} = 125 \text{ mL/hr}$$

26. **a.** To calculate the final concentration, divide the amount in the bottle by the final volume. This will take into account the powder volume. 1200 mg/15mL = 80 mg/mL.

27. **d.** Add how many were used today: $30 + 30 + 60 + 8 + 45 = 173$

    Subtract starting inventory from amount used: $420 - 173 = 247$ capsules left in stock

    Order enough to reach the maximum: $750 - 247 = 503$ capsules

    Order 5 bottles of 100 capsules to bring inventory to 747, near the maximum allowed.

28. **b.** A proportion will be used to figure out the percentage.

    $$x/100 = 97/120$$

    $$x = 80.8 \text{ or } 80.8\%$$

29. **a.** Calculate the AWP for 30 tablets.

    $$x/30 \text{ tablets} = \$26.59/100 \text{ tablets}$$

    $$x = \$7.98$$

    Subtract the 5%.

    $$\$7.98 \times 0.05 = \$0.40$$

    $$\$7.98 - \$0.40 = \$7.58$$

    Subtract the amount paid by the cost for the dispensing fee.

    $$\$13.16 - 7.58 = \$5.58 \text{ dispensing fee}$$

30. **c.** The previous WBC was 7.6. If a WBC reading below 5.6 requires retesting, a WBC 5.6 or above does not require retesting.

31. **c.** Calculate the total dose allowed in a lifetime.

    $$550 \text{ mg}/1 \text{ m2} = x \text{ mg}/ 2.1 \text{ m2}$$

    $$x = 1155 \text{ mg}$$

    Subtract the amount already received.

$1155 \text{ mg} - 400 \text{ mg} = 755$ mg left before the lifetime limit is reached.

32. **c.** The least amount sold is 2700 films. Divide 2700 by 30 days to get the minimum of 90 films.

    The largest amount sold in a month was 3500 films; divide by 30 for 120 films as a maximum to prevent over stock.

33. **c.** The 0.9% solution could be used in the correct answer provided the correct amount of sterile water is used. Answer "d" does not provide the correct amounts of either so answer "c" is correct. If you use 0.45% and sterile water the correct volume will be calculated using alligation:

Use alligation:

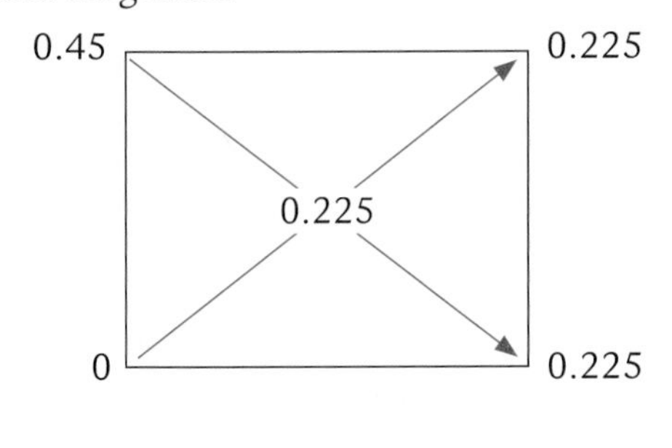

0.45

Then, set up the proportions and solve to calculate the quantity of each solution needed to make the final product.

0.225/0.45 × 1000 mL = 500 mL of 0.45% NaCl

0.225/0.45 × 1000 mL = 500 mL of sterile water

34. **d.** Calculate how many milliliters are in 8 ounces.

1 ounce/30 mL = 8 ounces/x mL

x = 240 mL

Because the ratio is equal amounts of all 3 ingredients, then 240 mL/3 = 80 mL of each ingredient.

35. **b.** This is a multiple-step problem.

Calculate the dose for the 50 kg patient.

50 kg × 20 mcg/kg/min = 1000 mcg/min

Calculate the amount per hour.

1000 mcg/min × 60 min/hr = 60,000 mcg/hr

Or, change to mg/hr by moving the decibel point 3 places to the left to get 60 mg/hr.

Based on the concentration of the dopamine as 400 mg/500 ml

60mg/x mL = 400 mg/500 mL

x = 75 mL

75 mL is 60 mg so, based on the proportion of 60 mg per hour, the solution will be administered at 75 mL/hr.

36. **b.** Set up a proportion.

1 mg/5 mL = x mg/150 mL

x = 30 mg

Each tablet is 10 mg, so it will take 3 tablets to compound the solution.

37. **c.** Calculate how many milligrams are in 200 mL of a 20 mg/5 mL solution.

x mg/200 mL = 20 mg/5 mL

x = 800 mg of fluoxetine

38. **b.** Concentration is in grams per 100 mL. Set up the proportion

10 gram/200 mL = x/100 mL

x = 5 grams/100 mL or 5%

39. **c.** Calculate the number of grams of hydrocortisone powder in 120 grams of 10% cream.

10 gram HC/100 gram = x gram HC/120 gram

x = 12 gram of HC powder

How many grams of a 5% cream can be made with 12 grams of HC powder?

5 gram HC/100 gram = 12 gram HC/x gram

x = 240 gram of cream

There are already 120 grams of Eucerin in the 10% ointment; adding 120 grams will produce 240 grams of a 5% cream.

40. **a.** Divide the case price by 12 to determine the unit price cost, then multiply by 0.3 and add that amount to the acquisition cost.

$$\$71.52/12 = \$5.96$$

$$\$5.96 \times 0.3 = \$1.79$$

$$\$5.96 + \$1.79 = \$7.75$$

41. **b.** Convert time to hours because the answer is in mL/hr.

$$15 \text{ gtt/min} \times 60 \text{ min/1 hr} = 900 \text{ gtt/hr}$$

If the set is 60 gtt/mL, determine how many mL there are in 900 gtts. This is the rate per hour.

$$900 \text{ gtt/hr} \times 1 \text{ mL/60 gtt} = 15 \text{ mL/hr}$$

42. **d.** Each vial has 10 doses, and there are 10 vials, so there are 100 doses in 10 vials.

$$1 \text{ dose/0.5 mL} = x \text{ doses/5 mL}$$

$$x = 10 \text{ doses}$$

43. **a.** A 5 mL vial has 10 doses on 0.5 mL.

Calculate the cost of each dose.
$125/10 = $12.50

Calculate the profit.
$25.00 per dose - $12.50 cost = $12.50

The profit per dose is $12.50. There are 10 doses per vial. Therefore, the profit per vial is $125.00

44. **d.** A liter of fluid is 1000 mL. It takes 4 hours to infuse the 1000 mL bag of D_5W.

Calculate the infusion rate.

$$1000 \text{ mL/4 hr} = 250 \text{ mL/hr}$$

45. **c.** Using the formula $(9/5 \times °C) + 32 = °F$, then $(9/5 \times 5) + 32 = 41°F$

46. **a.** First, convert the weight to kilograms using the conversion factor 1 kg = 2.2 lbs.

$$1 \text{ kg/2.2 lbs} = x \text{ kg/120 lbs}$$

$$x = 54.5 \text{ kg}$$

Multiply.

$$54.5 \text{ kg} \times 60 \text{ mg/kg/day} = 3270 \text{ mg}$$

3250 mg is the closest answer.

47. **b.** Ratio strength is used for weak solutions of drugs. It is expressed as *x* gram : *x* mL. Convert the 10 mg to grams or 0.01 gram in 10 mL and then reduce the ratio to whole numbers in a proportion.

$$0.01 \text{ g/10 mL} = 1 \text{ g/} x \text{ mL}$$

$$x = 1000$$

The ratio would be 1:1000 of Atropine.

48. **d.** Set up a proportion to solve.

$$1 \text{ g/50 mL} = x \text{ g/100 mL}$$

$x = 2$ grams, so the answer is a 2% solution.

49. **c.** Convert 2 grams to milligrams.

$$2 \text{ g} \times 1000 \text{ mg/1 g} = 2000 \text{ mg.}$$

$$250 \text{ mg/1 cap} = 2000 \text{ mg/}x \text{ cap}$$

$$x = 8 \text{ capsules}$$

The dentist wants 3 doses:
$3 \times 8 = 24$ capsules

50. **c.** "qid" means 4 times a day. The patient uses 2 puffs per dose, 8 puffs a day. $200/8 = 25$ days' supply.

Pharmacology Practice Exam

1. b
2. c
3. a
4. d
5. b
6. b
7. d
8. a
9. c
10. c
11. a
12. b
13. b
14. c
15. a
16. d
17. a
18. c
19. b
20. c
21. b
22. c
23. a
24. d
25. b

Practice Exam 1

When checking your answers, review the correct answer, but be aware that understanding why the other answers are wrong may also help. Be sure to review the feedback for each incorrect answer, as well as the information about the correct answer. Each question's feedback includes a reference to the chapter in this text where you can review information related to the question.

1. Chapter 3
   a. Incorrect. Azithromycin (Zithromax) does not cause photosensitivity.
   b. Incorrect. Famotidine (Pepcid) does not cause photosensitivity.
   c. Correct. Tetracycline and drugs in the tetracycline family (e.g., doxycycline, minocycline) can cause photosensitivity.
   d. Incorrect. Levothyroxine does not cause photosensitivity.

2. Chapter 9
   a. Correct. First calculate the cost of 30 capsules: $x/30 caps = $27.95/1000 caps, $x = $0.84. Calculate markup: $0.84 × 0.34 = $0.29. Next add all the prices together: $0.84 + $0.29 + $9.50 = $10.63.
   b. Incorrect. Only the cost and markup
   c. Incorrect. Only the dispensing fee and cost
   d. Incorrect. Only the dispensing fee and markup

3. Chapter 2
   a. Correct. Since 5% means 5 g is in 100 g of ointment, solve by setting up a proportion: x g/10 g = 100 g/5 g, x g = 200 g of ointment.
   b. Incorrect. Assuming that the percentage means 5 g in 1000 g, for 5%, you would make this error.
   c. Incorrect. Multiplying 10 g by 0.05 would give you this number, which is the value of 5% of 10 g.
   d. Incorrect. Multiplying 5 by 10 will produce this number, and it has no meaning to this calculation.

4. Chapter 2
   a. Incorrect. The quantity would only last 1 week because the directions are to use it twice a day.
   b. Correct. Since *b.i.d.* means *two times a day,* the patient needs 500 mg/dose × 2 doses/day. Each tablet is 500 mg; therefore, this amount is equivalent to two tablets per day: 2 capsules/day × 14 days = 28 capsules.
   c. Incorrect. This will give more than a 2-week supply and would lead to incorrect filling of the quantity that the physician prescribed.
   d. Incorrect. Multiplying 500 mg × 28 capsules = 14,000 mg, which is the actual number of milligrams the patient will take in the 2-week period.

5. Chapter 8
   a. Incorrect. All narcotics require child-resistant packaging.
   b. Incorrect. Antibiotics should be in child-resistant containers.
   c. Incorrect. Digoxin is highly toxic if accidentally taken by children and should be in a child-resistant container unless the patient requests otherwise.
   d. Correct. Nitroglycerin sublingual tablets must be dispensed in the original brown glass bottle from the manufacturer to prevent drug loss when exposed to light.

6. Chapter 2
   a. Correct. First, solve for the cost of the 50 tablets, which is \$12.43 divided by 2, or \$6.22. Then, add the dispensing fee of \$6.50.
   b. Incorrect. By adding the dispensing fee to the cost for 100 tablets then dividing by 2, you obtained this number, which does not include the full dispensing fee.
   c. Incorrect. The decimal point is misplaced on the cost per tablet during the calculation process.
   d. Incorrect. This is the cost of the drug without any dispensing fee.

7. Chapter 3
   a. Incorrect. Nexium is a proton pump inhibitor used for stomach and intestinal ulcers.
   b. Correct. Diovan (valsartan) is a cardiovascular agent used to treat hypertension.
   c. Incorrect. Premarin is part of estrogen replacement therapy.
   d. Incorrect. Zoloft is a selective serotonin reuptake inhibitor used to treat depression.

8. Chapter 2
   a. Incorrect. This is the weight of dextrose in 100 mL, as the 45% represents.
   b. Correct. 45% means 45 g of dextrose in 100 mL of solution. Set up a proportion to determine the amount of dextrose needed for 250 mL: x g/250 mL = 45 g/100 mL, x g = 112.5 g.
   c. Incorrect. The percentage is mistaken as meaning 45 g of dextrose in 1000 mL.
   d. Incorrect. Multiplying 250 mL by 45 does not take into consideration the meaning of percentage.

9. Chapter 5
   a. Incorrect. During the aseptic technique process, you are introducing some active drug, electrolyte, or nutrient to treat the patient.
   b. Correct. By practicing aseptic technique you are preventing the contamination of a sterile product by a pathogen.
   c. Incorrect. You may have to add water to a preparation as long as it is water for injection if it is an injectable preparation.
   d. Incorrect. Inactive as well as active ingredients may be added to a compounded product.

10. Chapter 4
    a. Incorrect. A DUR warning occurs when information on a patient's profile is flagged as a problem with a prescription drug being filled.
    b. Incorrect. OBRA-90 guarantees a patient the right to counseling by a pharmacist.
    c. Incorrect. OSHA monitors the work environment for safety.
    d. Correct. HIPAA notice is signed by employees to ensure patient's confidentiality.

11. Chapter 4
    a. Correct. Oxycodone is a Schedule II drug.
    b. Incorrect. Plain codeine is a Schedule II drug; in combination with acetaminophen, aspirin, or ibuprofen, codeine is a Schedule III drug.
    c. Incorrect. Buprenorphine is a Schedule III drug.
    d. Incorrect. Lorazepam is a Schedule IV.

12. Chapter 6
    a. Correct. Heparin is an anticoagulant and if not monitored closely and dosed correctly, the patient could hemorrhage.
    b. Incorrect. Cephalexin is an antibiotic that is not considered a high-risk, high-alert drug.

c. Incorrect. Citalopram is an SSRI and is not on the high-risk/high-alert med list.
d. Incorrect. Buspirone is an antianxiety medication that is not high risk/high alert.

13. Chapter 6
a. Correct. MedWatch is the document to fill out if a patient has an adverse reaction to a drug.
b. Incorrect. MSDS are information sheets with information on chemicals.
c. Incorrect. PharmAlert is a marketing tool to update pharmacists about pharmaceuticals.
d. Incorrect. Drug Watch is a made-up name.

14. Chapter 9
a. Incorrect. This is the official United States compendium of drug monographs.
b. Incorrect. DESI lists are lists of drugs that the FDA has determined do not have enough data to prove efficacy.
c. Incorrect. This is the list of bioequivalent drug products established by the FDA.
d. Correct. A formulary is a list of drugs selected by a committee of healthcare professionals to supply the medication needs of an institution.

15. Chapter 8
a. Incorrect. URI is not the abbreviation for urinary tract infection.
b. Correct. These are the correct directions for the Sig, with the abbreviation URI meaning upper respiratory tract infection. A drug such as Zithromax would have this Sig.
c. Incorrect. This is not specific enough; you have excluded the terms *tablet* and *by mouth*.
d. Incorrect. The duration is missing and the directions are not 4 times a day.

16. Chapter 7
a. Incorrect. They may be stored next to other refrigerated products but should be placed in bins for containment in case of leaks.
b. Correct. Although having a separate refrigerator for hazardous substances is ideal, if they are to be stored with other medications in the refrigerator, then they need to be separated and stored in a bin or container that prevents a spill if an item leaks or is damaged.
c. Incorrect. The drug product is placed in the hood only at the time of mixing.
d. Incorrect. A drug requiring refrigeration may not be stable at room temperature.

17. Chapter 4
a. Incorrect. The color of the final product is not a requirement.
b. Incorrect. The inactive ingredients may vary as long as the pharmacokinetics of the final product are similar to those of the brand name product.
c. Incorrect. To substitute a generic for a brand name, it must be cheaper for the patient.
d. Correct. Besides the same active ingredient, strength, and route of administration, it must be the same dosage form to be considered bioequivalent.

18. Chapter 4
a. Incorrect. Amlodipine and verapamil are both calcium channel blockers, and a duplication-of-therapy warning should have appeared when the computer system scanned the patient profile.
b. Correct. As a technician, a duplication of therapy such as verapamil and amlodipine would produce a warning flag on the computer, and the technician should notify the pharmacist about the problem.
c. Incorrect. The pharmacist should call the physician.
d. Incorrect. Never discontinue a prescription without instruction from the pharmacist.

19. Chapter 3
a. Incorrect. The Health Insurance Portability and Accountability Act of 1996 (HIPAA) is the federal law guaranteeing confidentiality.
b. Incorrect. Compliance is a patient adhering to a medication regimen.
c. Incorrect. Medication error reporting is voluntary.
d. Correct. OBRA-90 is a federal law that requires patients to be counseled by a pharmacist when picking up a new prescription.

20. Chapter 11
    a. Correct. Computerized Physician Order Entry is the process in which prescribers enter orders into the electronic health record, which is transmitted to the pharmacy.
    b. Incorrect. Online adjudication is the transmission of prescription information to a PBM for payment.
    c. Incorrect. Micromedex is a drug information program that interfaces with computer systems for DUE.
    d. Incorrect. File maintenance is the keeping of the computer data.

21. Chapter 11
    a. Incorrect. A pneumatic delivery system allows medications to be delivered from the pharmacy to the patient floor via a tube system under pressure.
    b. Incorrect. A Class 100 environment is used for sterile compounding.
    c. Correct. This is a machine that dispenses patient medications when requested by the nurse and verified via an interface with the pharmacy computer system.
    d. Incorrect. This is used in a Class 100 environment to mix IV products with multiple additions.

22. Chapter 5
    a. Incorrect. The top of the meniscus is the slightly higher edge of the concaved edge of the liquid and will give you a measurement that is too high.
    b. Incorrect. Measuring accurately to the center is impossible.
    c. Correct. When reading the amount of liquid in a conical graduate, the reading is taken at the bottom of the meniscus.
    d. Incorrect. This will give you a measurement that is too high.

23. Chapter 8
    a. Incorrect. This represents a q6h regimen.
    b. Correct. In hospitals, military time is routinely used to schedule medications. If the first dose is given at 0600, add 4 hours to that time for 1000 (equivalent to 10:00 A.M.) and another 4 hours to that for 1400 (equivalent to 2:00 P.M.).
    c. Incorrect. The second dose is given 3 hours after the first dose.
    d. Incorrect. The second dose is given 2 hours after the first dose.

24. Chapter 2
    a. Correct. If 1 grain = 60 mg, then ¼ grain = 15 mg.
    b. Incorrect. This amount is too high if you use the conversion 1 grain = 60 mg.
    c. Incorrect. This is a ½ grain measurement.
    d. Incorrect. This is a 1 grain measurement.

25. Chapter 3
    a. Correct. A DUE is a review of a medication or therapy to ensure appropriate dosing and monitoring and is usually done on medication with a high incidence of side effects and toxicity.
    b. Incorrect. Although the cost may be a reason to initiate a DUE, it is not the reason in this case.
    c. Incorrect. This is not a common occurrence with blood thinners.
    d. Incorrect. Narcotics are addictive and have abuse potential.

26. Chapter 6
    a. Incorrect. A macrolide antibiotic, which may be difficult to dissolve, may be mixed on a nursing unit.
    b. Incorrect. An aminoglycoside antibiotic, which is nephrotoxic and ototoxic, is not difficult to mix.
    c. Incorrect. An azalide antibiotic is similar to macrolides.
    d. Correct. This is classified as an antibiotic but is an antineoplastic used to treat some cancers and should be mixed using necessary precautions.

27. Chapter 2
    a. Correct. Since 1 tsp = 5 mL, then 1.5 tsp = 7.5 mL. Determine the amount of milligrams in a dose using the ratio-proportion method: x mg/7.5 mL = 1 mg/5 mL, x mg = 1.5 mg. Since the patient is to take this dose b.i.d., 1.5 mg/dose × 2 doses/day = 3 mg/day. Use this to determine the amount needed in 30 days: 3 mg/day × 30 days = 90 mg. Given that the drug comes in multiples of 25 mg, you

will need 90 mg/treatment ÷ 25 mg/tablet = 3.6 tablets, rounded to 4 tablets.
b. Incorrect. This amount will not make a 1-month supply.
c. Incorrect. This amount will not make a 1-month supply.
d. Incorrect. This amount will not make a 1-month supply.

28. Chapter 3
a. Correct. Cephalexin is a cephalosporin that is similar to penicillin (a beta-lactam) in structure, and patients who are allergic to penicillin may be allergic to cephalosporins.
b. Incorrect. In many instances, a macrolide antibiotic is used when patients are allergic to penicillin.
c. Incorrect. This is a sulfonamide antibiotic.
d. Incorrect. This is a fluoroquinolone antibiotic.

29. Chapter 6
a. Incorrect. Antihypertensives do not need a patient package insert dispensed every time a prescription is filled.
b. Correct. Every time an oral contraceptive or hormone replacement therapy is dispensed, a patient package insert is to be dispensed.
c. Incorrect. Dietary supplements do not require patient package inserts to be dispensed; they are usually over-the-counter products.
d. Incorrect. Antibiotics do not require a patient package insert to be dispensed every time they are filled.

30. Chapter 8
a. Incorrect. This is the number of drops if both eyes are involved.
b. Incorrect. This is the number of drops if used q.i.d.
c. Correct. 2 gtt × 3 times/day = 6 gtt/day
d. Incorrect. This is correct only if you use one drop three times a day.

31. Chapter 9
a. Incorrect. A vaccine that is not stored properly may not be effective and should not be dispensed.
b. Incorrect. Do not throw it out until you have replacement stock from the supplier or the pharmacy will be out a lot of money.
c. Correct. The supplier should be notified so the vaccine can be replaced.
d. Incorrect. Most vaccines only need be refrigerated, except Zostavax, and if the vaccine is not stored correctly it will be ineffective.

32. Chapter 11
a. Incorrect. Synthroid is for thyroid hormone replacement.
b. Correct. Hydrochlorothiazide is a diuretic and is a peach- or pink-colored tablet.
c. Incorrect. Propranolol is a heart medicine to control heart rate and blood pressure.
d. Incorrect. Allopurinol is used to prevent gout.

33. Chapter 4
a. Correct. The DUE alerts the pharmacist or technician that there is a problem with the new prescription listed and a drug or allergy on the patient's profile.
b. Incorrect. Prior authorization is given for a medication not covered by an insurer.
c. Incorrect. Medication assistance programs help patients pay for their medications.
d. Incorrect. Incompatibility refers to mixing two or more pharmaceuticals that will interfere with each other, such as precipitation or inactivation.

34. Chapter 8
a. Correct. A suspension is a good choice for a 13-month-old child.
b. Incorrect. While this a suspension, it would not be the most appropriate choice because of its higher concentration.
c. Incorrect. A capsule is not a good dosage form for a 13-month-old child.
d. Incorrect. A capsule is not a good dosage form for a 13-month-old child.

35. Chapter 8
a. Incorrect. This is a 30 days' supply.
b. Correct. Only 1 tablet per week and because 3 months is 12 weeks, it would require 12 tablets for the 3-month supply.
c. Incorrect. Thirty tablets would last 30 weeks.
d. Incorrect. Ninety tablets would last 90 weeks or almost 2 years.

36. Chapter 6
  a. Correct. Any drug dosed in units should have "units" written out.
  b. Incorrect. QID, four times a day is not as error prone as "QD."
  c. Incorrect. QHS is allowed for "at bedtime."
  d. Incorrect. BID is allowed for "twice a day."

37. Chapter 9
  a. Incorrect. Although you may have purchased an item once, it may not still be in stock; therefore it is not part of the inventory.
  b. Incorrect. This is important to know so you can restock supply that is sold.
  c. Correct. Inventory is the term to describe all the items available for sale.
  d. Incorrect. This is inventory value.

38. Chapter 7
  a. Incorrect. Compounding equipment includes the items used to compound such as scale, spatula, etc.
  b. Correct. These are all examples of personal protective equipment.
  c. Incorrect. While they may be disposable, this is not the correct terminology.
  d. Incorrect. ISO class 5 equipment, such as a vertical or horizontal hood, is the sterile environment equipment.

39. Chapter 2
  a. Incorrect. The patient's weight has not been figured into the answer.
  b. Incorrect. Miscalculating the concentration of the stock solution as 2 mg/mL gives this answer. Be careful when reducing fractions to the smallest denominator.
  c. Correct. First, calculate the amount needed per hour: 0.7 mg/kg/hr $\times$ 70 kg = 49 mg/hr. Second, solve using a proportion: x mL/49 mg = 500 mL/500 mg, x mL = 49 mL. Therefore, the rate will be 49 mL/hr.
  d. Incorrect. Decimal placement errors will produce this answer.

40. Chapter 3
  a. Incorrect. Policy and procedures give institutional ways to do a given job.
  b. Incorrect. Formulary is the list of drugs accepted for use by a hospital or insurer.
  c. Incorrect. PPI's are information sheets about a drug.
  d. Correct. Material Safety Data Sheets must be on file for any chemical, from house cleaning products to chemotherapy agents, used in an institution.

41. Chapter 5
  a. Incorrect. Even in compounding, you cannot infringe on patent rights.
  b. Correct. Many times, a product may be needed for a pediatric patient that only comes in tablet form, therefore compounding allows a pharmacist to make a liquid or suppository.
  c. Incorrect. This constitutes manufacturing and requires a manufacturer's license, not a pharmacy license.
  d. Incorrect. This constitutes an investigational drug study and must first be approved by the FDA for further study.

42. Chapter 3
  a. Incorrect. Erythromycin is an antibiotic and does not affect potassium levels.
  b. Incorrect. Sertraline is an antidepressant and does not affect potassium levels.
  c. Incorrect. Valproic acid has many uses but does not affect potassium levels. Patients on valproic acid who are of pregnancy age should receive folic acid to prevent spina bifida in the newborn if they become pregnant.
  d. Correct. Furosemide is a diuretic, and all except the potassium-sparing diuretics may cause patients to lose potassium and require supplementation, requiring periodic serum potassium levels to be assessed.

43. Chapter 3
  a. Incorrect. Duloxetine is the generic for Cymbalta and is used to treat depression or neuropathic pain.
  b. Incorrect. Atomoxetine is the generic for Strattera and is used to treat ADHD.
  c. Correct. Prozac was the first selective serotonin reuptake inhibitor (SSRI) manufactured and is the brand name for fluoxetine.
  d. Incorrect. Citalopram is the generic name for Celexa, which is an SSRI.

44. Chapter 6
   a. Incorrect. While a patient's allergy information is important, it is not used to select a patient profile.
   b. Incorrect. Past medical information usually is not useful to select the correct patient.
   c. Correct. The date of birth is useful to select the correct patient profile particular with same name patient
   d. Incorrect. A patient's weight is useful for dosing a drug.

45. Chapter 8
   a. Incorrect. Propoxyphene and acetaminophen are the active ingredients in Darvocet N-100.
   b. Incorrect. This is the old Darvon compound formula.
   c. Correct. This is the Vicodin or Lortab combination.
   d. Incorrect. This is the Tylenol with codeine combination.

46. Chapter 2
   a. Incorrect. If the dose was 1 tsp, which is 5 mL, and was taken three times a day, you produce this answer.
   b. Incorrect. If you use 1 tsp = 15 mL, you produce this answer.
   c. Incorrect. This is actually the number of teaspoons a day. Be careful of the units when doing calculations.
   d. Correct. Since 1 tsp = 5 mL, and ¾ tsp = 0.75 tsp, determine the amount of drug in a dose using the ratio-proportion method: x mL/0.75 tsp = 5 mL/1 tsp, x mL = 3.75 mL. Since the child takes the drug t.i.d, 3.75 mL/dose × 3 doses/day = 11.25 mL/day.

47. Chapter 9
   a. Incorrect. Nitrostat should not be refrigerated.
   b. Correct. NuvaRing is refrigerated until inserted vaginally.
   c. Incorrect. Combivir is not stored in the refrigerator
   d. Incorrect. Patanol is not stored in the refrigerator.

48. Chapter 11
   a. Correct. The automatic dispensing machines will open a specific drug storage location with the medication selected for administration.
   b. Incorrect. CPOE is the technology to eliminate handwriting.
   c. Incorrect. Administering the correct drug at the correct time requires the nurse to use the electronic medication administration record.
   d. Incorrect. Drug diversion is controlled by limited access and medication unit counts.

49. Chapter 2
   a. Incorrect. A discount has not been subtracted.
   b. Incorrect. This is the amount of the discount.
   c. Correct. First, calculate the discount on the regular price: \$56.75 × 0.1 = \$5.68. Second, subtract the discount from the original price: \$56.75 − \$5.68 = \$51.07.
   d. Incorrect. The discount was added to the regular price.

50. Chapter 3
   a. Correct. Ventolin is the brand name for albuterol and is a bronchodilator used to treat asthma.
   b. Incorrect. Fluticasone (Flonase) is a nasal spray for allergic rhinitis. A fluticasone dose form (Flovent) is used to treat asthma.
   c. Incorrect. Rimantadine (Relenza) is an inhaled treatment for influenza A and B.
   d. Incorrect. Pentamidine (NebuPent) is an inhaled treatment for *Pneumocystic carinii* pneumonia.

51. Chapter 10
   a. Incorrect. This is another name for an insurance company that does not have member or provider restrictions.
   b. Incorrect. This is an organization that provides health insurance to members with contracted restrictions on use.
   c. Correct. Pharmacy benefit managers administer prescription drug plans for numerous insurance companies in an attempt to provide the best service for the lowest price.
   d. Incorrect. This is an insurance entity that has a defined group of physicians providing service for its members.

52. Chapter 5
   a. Correct. Vertical airflow hoods protect the employee, who is mixing the antineoplastic, from contamination with the product; they also provide a sterile environment to compound the parenteral product.
   b. Incorrect. Nonhazardous sterile products may be compounded using effective aseptic technique in the horizontal airflow hood.
   c. Incorrect. Pharmacy technicians can be adequately trained to mix chemotherapy drugs.
   d. Incorrect. Although the oncology nurse is an expert on chemotherapy, the mixing of chemotherapy drugs is performed by the pharmacy staff members who have been appropriately trained in aseptic technique and handling of hazardous products.

53. Chapter 3
   a. Incorrect. Cimetidine (Tagamet) is an H_2 receptor blocker used to decrease stomach acid.
   b. Correct. Dexlansoprazole, which is the generic name for Dexilanta, is a proton pump inhibitor used to decrease acid production.
   c. Incorrect. Sucralfate (Carafate) is a coating agent used to treat ulcers.
   d. Incorrect. Metoclopramide (Reglan) is an antiemetic that promotes gastrointestinal motility.

54. Chapter 9
   a. Incorrect. This is the rate if it is to run over 24 hours.
   b. Correct. Since 2 L = 2000 mL, use the proportion: x mL/1 hr = 2000 mL/12 hr, x mL = 166.666 mL, or 166 mL/hr.
   c. Incorrect. If the volume was 1 L and ran over 24 hours, you produce this answer.
   d. Incorrect. This would deliver 600 mL in the 12-hour period.

55. Chapter 6
   a. Incorrect. Trailing zeros will prevent a tenfold overdose of a drug.
   b. Incorrect. Similar named products should not be stored close together.
   c. Incorrect. Limiting purchasing will not help in retail in which you must be able to fill prescriptions for all the patient's needs.
   d. Correct. Tall man lettering helps to highlight the different names of sound-alike/look-alike drugs.

56. Chapter 6
   a. Incorrect. Technicians should help customers locate products in the store.
   b. Correct. A patient's concern about any adverse drug reaction should be referred to the pharmacist.
   c. Incorrect. A prepared refill that has already been checked by the pharmacist can be dispensed by the technician.
   d. Incorrect. Technicians may take a request for a prescription refill.

57. Chapter 3
   a. Incorrect. The brand name is Prozac.
   b. Incorrect. The brand name is Prilosec.
   c. Incorrect. The brand name is Xanax.
   d. Correct. Quetiapine is the generic name of Seroquel.

58. Chapter 3
   a. Incorrect. This will not help treat a Coumadin overdose.
   b. Incorrect. This will not help treat a Coumadin overdose.
   c. Incorrect. This will treat scurvy but does not help treat a Coumadin overdose.
   d. Correct. The mechanism of action for Coumadin is to inhibit the vitamin K clotting factors; therefore, in an overdose, you would give vitamin K to overcome the inhibition.

59. Chapter 11
   a. Incorrect. The pharmacy technician spends a considerable amount of time maintaining the automation technology.
   b. Correct. Technology in pharmacy increases the efficiency of the staff in the pharmacy, which should increase the amount of time spent on clinical and direct patient care.
   c. Incorrect. All work done by a pharmacy technician, even if automation is involved, should be double-checked by the pharmacist.
   d. Incorrect. Although expense for automation may be considerable, it should save money in the long term.

60. Chapter 6
    a. Incorrect. An emergency box usually refers to a code blue box for cardiac or respiratory arrest.
    b. Incorrect. Gloves may be necessary but not the most important.
    c. Correct. The spill kit is a specialty kit that contains absorbent material, protective gear, and cleaning supplies for chemotherapy drug spills.
    d. Incorrect. Although used to clean the hoods, this is not the best chemical for cleaning up a chemotherapy drug spill.

61. Chapter 3
    a. Correct. Acetaminophen does not cause gastric mucosal irritation or peptic ulcer disease.
    b. Incorrect. Aspirin is contraindicated in PUD.
    c. Incorrect. This is a nonsteroidal anti-inflammatory drug (NSAID) that may aggravate PUD.
    d. Incorrect. This is an NSAID that may aggravate PUD.

62. Chapter 9
    a. Correct. Refrigeration temperature needs to be maintained between 35°F and 45°F and checked daily.
    b. Incorrect. This is room temperature.
    c. Incorrect. This is colder than refrigeration.
    d. Incorrect. This is colder than refrigeration.

63. Chapter 4
    a. Incorrect. Although your employer may require this, federal law does not.
    b. Incorrect. This is not required.
    c. Incorrect. Although your employer may do this at the yearly inventory, law does not require it.
    d. Correct. A physical inventory must be done biennially, or every two years.

64. Chapter 4
    a. Incorrect. Heroin may never be purchased because it is a C-I drug and has no medical use.
    b. Correct. This is a C-II drug that must be purchased with a DEA 222 form.
    c. Incorrect. Tramadol is not a controlled substance.
    d. Incorrect. Diazepam (Valium) is a C-IV drug and does not require a special order form.

65. Chapter 4
    a. Correct. Class I drug recalls are sent when the risk of a serious event, such as death, is possible.
    b. Incorrect. This does not involve death as the reason for the recall.
    c. Incorrect. This does not involve death as the reason for the recall.
    d. Incorrect. No such class of recall exists.

66. Chapter 11
    a. Incorrect. This is for processing data that is input before output or storage.
    b. Incorrect. This is the software that allows the computer to perform certain functions.
    c. Incorrect. This is the temporary, nonpermanent memory.
    d. Correct. A modem is connected through a telephone line; the pharmacy computer is connected with a remote computer or network via the modem.

67. Chapter 8
    a. Incorrect. Although this is important to assess initially, it should be updated at every visit.
    b. Incorrect. This is too long, and an allergy that occurred during the year may be missed.
    c. Incorrect. Allergy information is not static and needs to be updated regularly.
    d. Correct. Every time a patient visits the pharmacy with a new prescription, the inquiry about allergies should be made.

68. Chapter 9
    a. Incorrect. This is the date it expires and the patient would not be able to use it before expiration.
    b. Incorrect. Medications in the original bottle in the pharmacy are good until the expiration date on the bottle.
    c. Incorrect. The drug is 30 days outdated at this point.
    d. Correct. The patient must have enough time to use the medication before it expires.

69. Chapter 11
   a. Incorrect. Override reports document who has overridden a DUE.
   b. Incorrect. Not a real report in pharmacy.
   c. Correct. User access report documents all who have access to the system.
   d. Incorrect. Diversion report documents who fills/dispenses prescriptions for controlled substances.

70. Chapter 3
   a. Incorrect. Loperamide is an antidiarrheal.
   b. Incorrect. Senokot is a laxative.
   c. Correct. Melatonin is a supplement for insomnia found in the vitamin aisle.
   d. Incorrect. Metamucil is a source of fiber.

71. Chapter 2
   a. Incorrect. The dispensing fee was not added to the AWP minus 10%.
   b. Incorrect. The price for 100 tablets was used, and the dispensing fee was not added.
   c. Incorrect. The price for 100 was used.
   d. Correct. First, calculate the price per tablet: $112.25 ÷ 100 tablets = $1.12. Second, calculate the cost for 90 tablets: 90 tablets × $1.12/tablet = $100.80. Third, calculate the 10% discount: $100.80 × 0.1 = $10.08. Fourth, determine the final price: $100.80 − $10.08 discount + $9.00 dispensing fee = $99.72.

72. Chapter 2
   a. Incorrect. 0.9 mL is equal to 4.5 mg.
   b. Correct. Set up a proportion: x mg/0.75 mL = 5 mg/1 mL, x mg = 3.75 mg.
   c. Incorrect. 0.45 mL is equal to 4.5 mg.
   d. Incorrect. 0.7 mL is equal to 3.5 mg.

73. Chapter 7
   a. Correct. Barcode scanning helps select the correct drug for filling a prescription or medication order.
   b. Incorrect. The patient profile is filled with information about the patient.
   c. Incorrect. Online claim processing helps with payment of prescriptions.
   d. Incorrect. Automatic dispensing machines help nurses administer medication to patients.

74. Chapter 8
   a. Incorrect. This is a 15 days' supply.
   b. Correct. Because 1 grain is 65 mg, the patient will take ½ tablet twice a day (b.i.d.); the patient will need 30 tablets for 1-month supply.
   c. Incorrect. This is a 45 days' supply.
   d. Incorrect. This is a 60 days' supply.

75. Chapter 3
   a. Correct. Metformin should be taken with food.
   b. Incorrect. Calcium does not affect absorption of this drug.
   c. Incorrect. Metformin should not be taken on an empty stomach.
   d. Incorrect. Metformin does not cause drowsiness.

76. Chapter 10
   a. Correct. The pharmacist is the individual who is allowed to counsel a patient about a drug.
   b. Incorrect. Any time you give a patient a new prescription, you should offer to have the pharmacist counsel the patient about the medication.
   c. Incorrect. Although each state varies on taking telephone orders, all technicians may receive a written prescription.
   d. Incorrect. Any time a patient gives you updated information, it should be added to the patient profile.

77. Chapter 4
   a. Correct. A reject for a prescription claim may require the physician to call the insurer for prior authorization.
   b. Incorrect. A refill must be authorized before a claim can be transmitted.
   c. Incorrect. Clarification should be done before transmission.
   d. Incorrect. A written prescription is only needed for C-II prescriptions and not a notification given for online adjudication.

78. Chapter 4
   a. Incorrect. The DEA is responsible for controlled substances only.
   b. Correct. The FDA approves all new drug entities and studies being done on a drug.
   c. Incorrect. The U.S. Department of Health and Human Services is responsible for HIPAA, among other things.
   d. Incorrect. This group regulates the Poison Prevention Act.

79. Chapter 10
   a. Correct. Coordination of benefits occurs when patients have more than one insurance.
   b. Incorrect. Medication assistance programs help patients pay for prescriptions.
   c. Incorrect. HMOs are insurers.
   d. Incorrect. PBMs are the companies that pay prescription benefits for insurers.

80. Chapter 9
   a. Incorrect. This is purchasing direct from the manufacturer in larger quantities at less frequent intervals.
   b. Incorrect. This is a contractual situation in which a buyer purchase a certain percentage of pharmaceuticals from a wholesaler for a special price.
   c. Correct. JIT means *just in time,* which is the type of ordering done to keep inventory at a minimum but have sufficient stock available for immediate needs.
   d. Incorrect. ASAP is the abbreviation for *as soon as possible.*

81. Chapter 10
   a. Incorrect. A rejected claim is not paid by the insurer.
   b. Incorrect. Prior authorization is required for non-formulary drugs.
   c. Incorrect. Par levels are used to monitor inventory for reordering.
   d. Correct. Plan limitations are set by the insurer to control costs.

82. Chapter 3
   a. Correct. Simvastatin is an antihyperlipidemic agent that decreases the body's production of cholesterol and is sold under the brand name Zocor.
   b. Incorrect. This is the brand name for ezetimibe, an antihyperlipidemic drug.
   c. Incorrect. This is the brand name for alprazolam, a benzodiazepine.
   d. Incorrect. This is the brand name for lovastatin, an antihyperlipidemic drug.

83. Chapter 4
   a. Correct. Chapter <795> of the USP states the regulations concerning the compounding of nonsterile products.
   b. Incorrect. Chapter <797> of the USP states the regulations concerning the compounding of sterile products.
   c. Incorrect. The Food, Drug, and Cosmetic Act granted the FDA the authority to such products in 1938.
   d. Incorrect. The Orphan Drug Act provides incentives and programs for pharmaceutical companies to investigate and develop treatments for rare diseases.

84. Chapter 2
   a. Incorrect. This is a legitimate DEA number.
   b. Incorrect. This is a legitimate DEA number.
   c. Correct. Add the first, third, and fifth digits (2 + 4 + 6 = 12). Add the second, fourth, and sixth digits, and multiply by 2 (3 + 7 + 2) = 12 × 2 = 24). Add 12 + 24 = 36. The last digit of the DEA number *should* match the last digit of the total. In this case, it does not; therefore the number is not a valid DEA number.
   d. Incorrect. This is a legitimate DEA number.

85. Chapter 5
   a. Incorrect. Although this is a factor in contamination, it is not the most common source.
   b. Incorrect. Although this is a factor in contamination, it is not the most common source.
   c. Incorrect. Alcohol is used to clean the sterile field.
   d. Correct. Human touch is the most common source of contamination when mixing sterile products.

86. Chapter 7
   a. **Correct.** Good customer service techniques always start with a smile and direct eye contact with the individual you are helping.
   b. Incorrect. Escort the customer when possible to the location.
   c. Incorrect. Telephone etiquette is important.
   d. Incorrect. Although this might be considered multitasking, each customer deserves your undivided attention.

87. Chapter 11
   a. Incorrect. Diversion reports document controlled substance usage.
   b. Incorrect. Override reports document who overrides DUE.
   c. Incorrect. Patient adherence reports will help identify patients not compliant to drug usage.
   d. **Correct.** Usage reports help identify which drugs have been dispensed.

88. Chapter 7
   a. **Correct.** Always break an ampule away from your body and the HEPA filter but still inside the hood.
   b. Incorrect. Small glass pieces can be deposited in the filter.
   c. Incorrect. Small glass pieces may land on you.
   d. Incorrect. This will not maintain sterility.

89. Chapter 7
   a. Incorrect. Wait until you are cleaned up.
   b. **Correct.** Always wash the contaminant off yourself first, then seek help and medical attention.
   c. Incorrect. Clean yourself first.
   d. Incorrect. Clean yourself first.

90. Chapter 9
   a. Incorrect. Appropriate inventory control decreases expired products.
   b. **Correct.** Inventory control is a major way to contain costs and keep healthcare expenses down.
   c. Incorrect. Keeping stock at appropriate levels should decrease theft.
   d. Incorrect. Inventory control should help limit the space needed for stock.

Practice Exam 2

When checking your answers, review the correct answer, but be aware that understanding why the other answers are wrong may also help. Be sure to review the feedback for each incorrect answer, as well as the information about the correct answer. Each question's feedback includes a reference to the chapter in this text where you can review information related to the question.

1. Chapter 4
   a. Incorrect. This law is under scrutiny in recent years because senior citizens trying to save money on prescriptions are traveling to Canada and Mexico to purchase prescription drugs.
   b. **Correct.** HIPAA is the law that protects patients' private medical information.
   c. Incorrect. This act requires states that participate in Medicaid to establish standards of practice for pharmacists, including counseling patients and reviewing drug use.
   d. Incorrect. This act updates the labeling currently on prescription medications to *Rx only*.

2. Chapter 4
   a. Incorrect. Although this may be the law in some states, it is not in every state.
   b. **Correct.** Each state board of pharmacy determines whether transferring prescriptions between pharmacies is allowed and the manner in which this process will take place.
   c. Incorrect. Although this may be the law in some states, others allow pharmacy technicians to transfer prescriptions.
   d. Incorrect. An owner may choose not to participate in the transfer of prescriptions, but state rules and regulations establish the legality of this activity.

3. Chapter 3
   a. Incorrect. Celebrex is the brand name of celecoxib, a nonsteroidal anti-inflammatory agent.
   b. Correct. Plavix is the brand name for clopidogrel, an antiplatelet drug.
   c. Incorrect. Catapres is the brand name of clonidine, an antihypertensive.
   d. Incorrect. Celexa is the brand name of citalopram, an antidepressant.

4. Chapter 3
   a. Correct. Cymbalta is an antidepressant, like Effexor.
   b. Incorrect. Clozaril (clozapine) is an antipsychotic, which requires white blood cell counts because of the risk of agranulocytosis.
   c. Incorrect. Cordarone (amiodarone) is an antiarrhythmic.
   d. Incorrect. Cardizem (diltiazem) are both calcium channel blockers, for hypertension or arrhythmias.

5. Chapter 6
   a. Incorrect. The DEA is responsible for controlled substances.
   b. Incorrect. ISMP is a watch group that looks for ways to decrease medical errors.
   c. Incorrect. CMS has oversight for Medicare and Medicaid plans.
   d. Correct. The FDA is responsible for the *Orange Book* of bioequivalent products.

6. Chapter 4
   a. Correct. As an employee, any time you are not sure of the appropriate procedure to follow, the policy and procedure manual should be checked for directions.
   b. Incorrect. Relevant state and federal laws are taken into consideration when writing policy and procedures, but each employer writes his or her own manual.
   c. Incorrect. Few federal laws exist dictating anything about a policy and procedure manual.
   d. Incorrect. Technicians should be aware of the policy and procedure manual and follow the guidelines established in it.

7. Chapter 3
   a. Incorrect. Although high cholesterol may be secondary to diabetes, it does not cause diabetes.
   b. Correct. Atherosclerosis is the accumulation of fats in the arteries, clogging the vessels and limiting blood flow.
   c. Incorrect. Blood pooling from inactivity causes most cases of deep-vein thrombosis, blood clotting in veins.
   d. Incorrect. Cholesterol has not been linked to cancer, though a diet high in fat has been.

8. Chapters 4 and 10
   a. Incorrect. The patient may have symptoms of worsening congestive heart failure, not asthma. The patient needs to talk to his physician or pharmacist.
   b. Incorrect. Although this would notify the physician that something of importance is going on, the pharmacist should handle this situation.
   c. Incorrect. Although this may be what the physician may order, it is not up to the technician to use professional judgment and prescribe.
   d. Correct. The pharmacist should be notified and may be able to direct the patient to a more appropriate approach for dealing with the shortness of breath and encourage a dialogue with the physician.

9. Chapter 8
   a. Incorrect. The Zithromax Z-PAK is a five-day therapy.
   b. Incorrect. The drug is available in IV and dosage forms.
   c. Correct. The patient will need 6 tablets to complete the course of therapy.
   d. Incorrect. It is a tablet dosage form.

10. Chapter 9
   a. Incorrect. This system's predetermined levels decide if the item will be reordered.
   b. Correct. An order book is a system used to reorder drugs used during the day and requires anyone who fills a prescription or sells an item to write down the information.

c. Incorrect. Inventory cards establish an ongoing history of drug use and purchase.
d. Incorrect. The computer is programmed to order stock when a prescription is filled and when the predetermined minimum is reached.

11. Chapter 3
a. Incorrect. Lozenges have an immediate effect but are short acting.
b. Incorrect. Gum has an immediate effect but is short acting.
c. Incorrect. Inhalers have an immediate effect but are short acting.
d. Correct. The nicotine patch releases medication for up to 24 hours while wearing.

12. Chapter 6
a. Correct. Noncompliance by a patient is an error of omission.
b. Incorrect. This is a wrong time error.
c. Incorrect. This is a wrong dose error.
d. Incorrect. This is a technical error.

13. Chapter 6
a. Correct. The first 4 or 5 digits identify the manufacturer.
b. Incorrect. 8215 identifies the drug.
c. Incorrect. 01 identifies the package size.
d. Incorrect.

14. Chapter 3
a. Correct. This is one of the agents used before and after chemotherapy to prevent nausea and vomiting, which the antineoplastic may cause.
b. Incorrect. This use is not indicated, and an agent like cyclosporine is used to prevent rejection.
c. Incorrect. This drug is given before starting therapy to treat cancer, such as cyclophosphamide.
d. Incorrect. This drug is not indicated as a fibrinolytic, like streptokinase.

15. Chapter 9
a. Incorrect. This document helps identify if the pharmacy was charged inappropriately for items in the order but may differ from items actually ordered if they are out of stock.
b. Incorrect. This is not an effective document.
c. Correct. By checking the order that came in against the purchase order, you will make sure all the items you ordered are received, preventing a shortage later on.
d. Incorrect. The volume of pharmaceuticals used in a pharmacy each day does not make this an option.

16. Chapter 3
a. Incorrect. This may be effective as an antiflatulent.
b. Incorrect. This may be an effective circulatory stimulant.
c. Incorrect. This may be useful for prostate health.
d. Correct. Melatonin is a dietary supplement that has sedating qualities similar to eating a large meal.

17. Chapter 6
a. Correct. Sound-alike/look-alike drugs (SALADs) are responsible for medication errors resulting from the similarity in the names.
b. Incorrect. These two names are not commonly confused; Catapres is the brand name of clonidine.
c. Incorrect. These two names are not commonly confused.
d. Incorrect. These two names are not commonly confused.

18. Chapter 2
a. Correct. The patient uses 52 units/day × 30 days = 1560 units. Each vial is 10 mL of 100 units/mL = 1000 units per vials. So she would need 2 vials for 30 days.
b. Incorrect. This would only last 19 days.
c. Incorrect. Each pen is 3 ml × 100 units/mL × 5 pens = 1500 units, which is short 60 units for 30 days.
d. Incorrect. Only 900 units are available in 3 pens.

19. Chapter 4
a. Incorrect. Only C-II drugs do not allow refills by the CSA.
b. Incorrect. CSA allows up to 5 refills on C-V drugs
c. Correct. The CSA allows up to 5 refills in 6 months for C-III through C-V drugs.
d. Incorrect. This is not allowed for any controlled substance.

20. Chapter 8
    a. Incorrect. Ziprasidone is stored at room temperature.
    b. Incorrect. Drowsiness is not a side effect of ziprasidone.
    c. Incorrect. Sunlight does not have to be avoided with ziprasidone.
    d. Correct. The absorption of ziprasidone is dependent on food being eaten at the time the dose is taken.

21. Chapter 5
    a. Correct. Fluorouracil is an antineoplastic and needs to be handled as a hazardous substance, with strict adherence to handling and preparation precautions.
    b. Incorrect. This is the generic name for Prozac, a selective serotonin reuptake inhibitor.
    c. Incorrect. This is the generic name for Flovent and Flonase, corticosteroids.
    d. Incorrect. This is the generic name for Proscar, an agent for BPH that should not be handled by pregnant women because of its antitestosterone effects.

22. Chapter 8
    a. Correct. This is #14 in roman numerals. X=10, IV=4
    b. Incorrect. L = 50, V = 5, and I = 1, LVI tablets = 50 + 5 + 1 = 56 tablets.
    c. Incorrect. 16 is written XVI.
    d. Incorrect. 30 is written XXX.

23. Chapter 2
    a. Incorrect. You would waste 800 mg of drug if you made only one dose.
    b. Incorrect. Three doses of 200 mg is only 600 mg.
    c. Correct. Five doses of 200 mg is 1,000 mg or 1 gram.
    d. Incorrect. This is more than the original vial contains.

24. Chapter 2
    a. Incorrect. This would be 1 mg of folic acid.
    b. Incorrect. This would be 1.25 mg of folic acid.
    c. Correct. Solve a proportion: 2 mg/x mL = 5 mg/1 mL x = 0.4 mL
    d. Incorrect. This would be 3 mg of folic acid.

25. Chapter 2
    a. Incorrect. This is the lowest available strength of levofloxacin but not the correct answer.
    b. Correct. Convert the patient's weight to kilograms: 154 lb × 1 kg/2.2 lb = 70 kg. Calculate the dose: 70 kg × 7 mg/kg/dose = 490 mg/dose. Levaquin is available only in 250 mg, 500 mg, and 750 mg tablets.
    c. Incorrect. Using the incorrect conversion of pounds to kilograms might produce this answer.
    d. Incorrect. Not converting pounds to kilograms will give this answer.

26. Chapter 11
    a. Incorrect. Special handling would be found in the drug package insert and MSDS.
    b. Incorrect. DUE is a process the computer uses to review for problems when filling new prescriptions.
    c. Incorrect. Storage information would be found on the product or in the drug package insert.
    d. Correct. The NDC is on the drug database and used for billing and identification of drug selection.

27. Chapter 6
    a. Correct. Because of the risk of bleeding from thrombolytics, it is a high-risk/high-alert drug.
    b. Incorrect. Antibiotics are not considered high-risk/high-alert, though overuse can lead to resistance.
    c. Incorrect. Corticosteroids, like prednisone, have many side effects but are not considered high risk.
    d. Incorrect. Contraceptives are not high-risk drugs, even though they need to have a patient package insert dispensed with every fill.

28. Chapter 6
    a. Incorrect. *t.i.d.* is not considered a dangerous abbreviation. It is the abbreviation for "three times daily."
    b. Correct. *q.d.* is on the unacceptable list of abbreviations because it may be confused with *q.i.d.* when written in haste.

c. Incorrect. *mg* is not considered a dangerous abbreviation. It is the abbreviation for milligrams.
d. Incorrect. *PO* is not considered a dangerous abbreviation. It is the abbreviation for "by mouth."

29. Chapter 11
  a. Correct. Database management system is the type of software used in most pharmacy systems.
  b. Incorrect. DUR is a function of a pharmacy system.
  c. Incorrect. Smart terminals have their own processing system.
  d. Incorrect. Dumb terminals do not have their own processing system.

30. Chapter 5
  a. Incorrect. Spatulas are used to transfer solid materials to the weighing pans.
  b. Incorrect. The pestle is used to grind or mix ingredients in a mortar.
  c. Correct. Forceps or tweezers is the name for the tool used to transfer weights.
  d. Incorrect. A pipette is a long, thin, calibrated glass tube used for measuring liquid volumes less than 1.5 mL.

31. Chapter 11
  a. Incorrect. Only items necessary to sterile compounding should be in the sterile compounding room.
  b. Incorrect. High traffic areas are not safe and secure for computer back-up.
  c. Incorrect. Humidity may harm the back-up system.
  d. Correct. Secure and fireproof protects the data in case of a computer system failure.

32. Chapter 5
  a. Incorrect. Some sort of record-keeping is required for compounding.
  b. Incorrect. The ingredients and supervising pharmacist's name are also required.
  c. Correct. A compounding record should provide all the information someone would need to re-create the compounded product plus information on the products used in case of a recall.
  d. Incorrect. Although it may contain this information, it must also have the information listed in the correct answer.

33. Chapter 5
  a. Incorrect. The hood should be cleaned at least daily; an outside firm should inspect the hood every six months to make sure it is working properly.
  b. Incorrect. This does not help decrease contamination risk during the workday.
  c. Incorrect. LAFH should be cleaned at least daily.
  d. Correct. USP Chapter <797> requires the hood to be wiped with isopropyl alcohol at the beginning and numerous times during the day to prevent contamination of sterile products.

34. Chapter 7
  a. Incorrect. Blood is not the only fluid that contains pathogens.
  b. Correct. Universal precautions should be used any time a healthcare professional might be exposed to contaminated bodily fluids, and all patient fluids are considered contaminated.
  c. Incorrect. Sterility is not the only way to prevent transfer of pathogens from one individual to another.
  d. Incorrect. This is the procedure used to make sterile products for patient use.

35. Chapter 11
  a. Incorrect. Override reports tell who is overriding DUE warnings.
  b. Incorrect. Work total reports might be useful to see who is doing the work.
  c. Correct. Usage reports help identify what drugs are used and how much.
  d. Incorrect. Diversion reports help identify control substance use and by whom.

36. Chapter 8
  a. Incorrect. This would supply the whole 20 mg.
  b. Incorrect. This would be 10 mg of Prozac.
  c. Incorrect. This would be 4 mg of Prozac.
  d. Correct. Use a proportion: x mL/1 mg = 5 mL/20 mg, x mL = 0.25 mL.

37. Chapter 10
  a. Incorrect. This is only the cost of the ingredients.
  b. Incorrect. This is the cost of ingredients and a 30% markup.

c. Incorrect. This is the cost of ingredients and the compounding fee.
d. Correct. First, calculate the markup: $8.76 × 0.3 = $2.63. Second, calculate the charge for the patient: $8.76 original price + $2.63 markup + $10.00 compounding fee = $21.39.

38. Chapter 9
a. Incorrect. Although this is what you want, the wholesaler sells the product only in quantities of 10 vials at a time.
b. Correct. Order the product that will bring you close to the inventory requirement. Do not order a strength you do not normally carry.
c. Incorrect. You need to order something so that you will not run out if you have another patient who needs Cytoxan.
c. Incorrect. You do not stock this strength, and it will not replace what you used.

39. Chapter 6
a. Incorrect. Thalidamide has a REMS called STEPS.
b. Incorrect. Clozapine has a REMS but it is a clozapine registry program.
c. Correct. Isotretinoin is teratogenic and iPLEDGE is the REMS for registry of users, prescribers, and pharmacies.
d. Incorrect. Injectable olanzapine has a REMS called Zyprexa Relprevv Patient Care Program.

40. Chapter 3
a. Incorrect. Thiazide diuretics cause potassium wasting by the kidneys.
b. Correct. Triamterene, amiloride, and spironolactone are the three potassium-sparing diuretics available.
c. Incorrect. Metolazone works similar to thiazide diuretics and leads to potassium loss.
d. Incorrect. Furosemide is a loop diuretic and causes an increase in potassium loss.

41. Chapter 3
a. Incorrect. AcipHex (rabeprazole) is a proton pump inhibitor used to treat ulcers.
b. Incorrect. Accutane (isotretinoin) is an agent used to treat acne and requires iPLEDGE enrollment (a mandatory, national registry).
c. Incorrect. Accupril (quinapril) is an ACE inhibitor used to treat hypertension.
d. Correct. Aricept (donepezil) was one of the first agents approved to slow the process of Alzheimer's disease.

42. Chapter 4
a. Incorrect. Never make a statement that requires professional judgment; always offer to have the pharmacist explain in these situations.
b. Incorrect. Never say never, we are all human, be empathetic and not confrontational.
c. Correct. A pharmacy technician should always have the pharmacist explain about drug indications and reasons for taking a particular medication, but calming the patient is also important.
d. Incorrect. Never say anyone has made a mistake. Offer to look into it, and notify the pharmacist.

43. Chapter 6
a. Incorrect. A prescription would be required.
b. Incorrect. A prescription would be required.
c. Correct. At 17 with proof of age the morning after pill can be sold without a prescription.
d. Incorrect. At 14 a prescription would be required.

44. Chapter 5
a. Incorrect. No part of the capsule is called the top.
b. Incorrect. No part of the capsule is called the bottom.
c. Correct. The body is used to punch the powder, and the cap is placed on the body to hold the powder in.
d. Incorrect. The cap covers the body once it is punched with powder.

45. Chapter 5
a. Incorrect. This is the largest capsule size.
b. Incorrect. This is the third from the largest capsule size.
c. Incorrect. This is the fourth from the largest capsule size.
d. Correct. The larger the number is, the smaller the capsule will be, with 000 being the largest.

46. Chapter 6
    a. Incorrect. This is not a necessary warning against use in pregnancy.
    b. Incorrect. If it is not approved for use in humans it will not be in the pharmacy.
    c. Correct. The black box warning is extra information to the physician or pharmacist that is critical to correct use.
    d. Incorrect. This is not a recall warning.

47. Chapter 4
    a. Incorrect. Buprenorphine is Subutex, which can be dispensed in a community pharmacy for maintenance narcotic detoxification therapy.
    b. Incorrect. Naloxone blocks opioid receptors, causing immediate withdrawal, and is therefore not used for narcotic addiction. It is used in emergency departments for overdoses.
    c. Incorrect. Butorphanol is a narcotic agonist-antagonist used to treat pain.
    d. Correct. Methadone for maintenance and detoxification from heroin or other opioids may be dispensed only at special DEA-licensed sites. If prescribed for pain, it may be dispensed in a community pharmacy.

48. Chapter 3
    a. Correct. Augmentin is a combination drug in the penicillin family.
    b. Incorrect. Tetracyclines are antibiotics like doxycycline for acne, Lyme disease, or malaria.
    c. Incorrect. Aminoglycosides are IV antibiotics like gentamicin or tobramycin for gram negative rods, particularly Pseudomonas infections.
    d. Incorrect. While a beta-lactam ring is in both penicillins and cephalosporins, Augmentin is not a cephalosporin.

49. Chapter 3
    a. Incorrect. Erythromycin is a macrolide, and gentamicin is an aminoglycoside.
    b. Correct. Biaxin (clarithromycin) is also a macrolide, similar to erythromycin, and should be avoided in this patient.
    c. Incorrect. Penicillin should be fine if erythromycin is her only allergy medication.
    d. Incorrect. Doxycycline is a tetracycline and should be fine if erythromycin is her only allergy medication.

50. Chapter 5
    a. Correct. As directed in USP Chapter <797>, working in a LAFW requires working at least 6 inches from all edges.
    b. Incorrect. You would be too close to the high-efficiency particulate air (HEPA) filter and straining your arms.
    c. Incorrect. You would be too close to the HEPA filter and straining your arms.
    d. Incorrect. You would be working too far away, which may result in contamination.

51. Chapter 9
    a. Incorrect. This is not reverse distribution.
    b. Incorrect. This is never allowed.
    c. Correct. Returning drugs for credit once expired is reverse distribution.
    d. Incorrect. This is not an example of reverse distribution.

52. Chapter 11
    a. Incorrect. Your ID badge should be worn at all times so staff and patients know who you are and what area you should be allowed into.
    b. Incorrect. BIN and PCN are used by PBMs to identify the insurer to bill.
    c. Correct. Login and password are unique to you and should not be shared.
    d. Incorrect. Override codes are used to accept and override and continue filling a prescription or medication order.

53. Chapter 4
    a. Incorrect. Only a registered pharmacist may perform this duty.
    b. Incorrect. Only a registered pharmacist may receive a verbal order.
    c. Correct. A pharmacy technician may take a written prescription from a patient for processing.
    d. Incorrect. The pharmacist is responsible for verification.

54. Chapter 10
    a. Incorrect. If you never ask you will not know about insurance coverage and have to redo your work to submit to an insurer.
    b. Correct. All new patients should be asked about insurance coverage.
    c. Incorrect. If a drug is non-formulary and rejected, you already have the insurance card information.
    d. Incorrect. Insurance does not change as often as refills so you will not need to ask every time you refill a prescription.

55. Chapter 8
    a. Incorrect. The indication does not have to be on the prescription.
    b. Correct. The date written should be on a prescription.
    c. Incorrect. The responsible party for payment is needed by the pharmacy and must be gathered from the patient, but this information is not on the prescription.
    d. Incorrect. Refill information should be included or assumed as *no refills* if not filled in.

56. Chapter 8
    a. Correct. A prescriber's DEA number must be on a prescription for a controlled substance only.
    b. Incorrect. Only written prescriptions must have the prescriber's actual signature.
    c. Incorrect. This should be on all prescriptions to help locate the prescriber in case of questions.
    d. Incorrect. The date written should be on all prescriptions.

57. Chapter 11
    a. Incorrect. Class I recalls require the pharmacy to notify patients who received the recalled drug lot.
    b. Correct. A usage report narrowed down to just the drug recalled will give you a list of patients to notify.
    c. Incorrect. Memory will not recall all patients receiving a drug.
    d. Incorrect. This method is labor intensive and may miss patients.

58. Chapter 9
    a. Correct. Proper storage of medication is necessary to guarantee the safety and efficacy of a drug.
    b. Incorrect. Checking the refrigerator temperature is a quality assurance step that ensures drugs are stored at the appropriate temperature and that the inventory is not being wasted by improper storage.
    c. Incorrect. Although a repackaged product may need to be refrigerated, the temperature is checked for quality assurance.
    d. Incorrect. The five rights are patient, drug, strength, route, and time.

59. Chapter 5
    a. Incorrect. The LAFW should be running at all times. If it is turned off, it should run for 30 minutes before being used.
    b. Correct. An LAFW must be cleaned at the beginning of the day and repeatedly throughout the day to ensure a clean environment in which to prepare sterile products.
    c. Incorrect. Air currents may contaminate the hood working area.
    d. Incorrect. Necessary materials to mix should be wiped with alcohol and placed in the hood so you do not have to leave the hood once you start mixing.

60. Chapter 3
    a. Incorrect. This is a medicine for insomnia and would not be used in the morning.
    b. Incorrect. This medication is taken once a day at bedtime.
    c. Incorrect. This medication is taken once a day at bedtime.
    d. Correct. Ambien (zolpidem) is a hypnotic and is given to induce sleep.

61. Chapter 11
    a. Correct. DUR would check all these problems.
    b. Incorrect. These are not examples of insurance plan limitations.
    c. Incorrect. These are not mediation adherence program notifications.
    d. Incorrect. An override report will identify who overrode all these warnings but is not an example of these.

62. Chapter 6
    a. Incorrect. ISMP and the Joint Commission have banned the use of trailing zeros.
    b. Correct. Do not include any trailing zeros, unnecessary decimal points, or leading zeros that may confuse the order.
    c. Incorrect. This is one half of 1 milligram.
    d. Incorrect. Although this is another way of writing 5 mg, it is not the best answer to this question.

63. Chapter 11
    a. Incorrect. While it may do this it is not the most important reason to e-prescribe.
    b. Incorrect. If it is a new patient, the prescription may not be ready.
    c. Correct. Hand writing is a major cause of medication errors, and e-prescribing eliminates this problem.
    d. Incorrect. This is not necessarily true.

64. Chapter 6
    a. Incorrect. This risk level means no risk in pregnancy.
    b. Incorrect. This risk level means caution is advised.
    c. Incorrect. A pregnancy risk of D indicates that human or animal studies have identified a definite risk.
    d. Correct. This risk level means these drugs, like the drug lisinopril, are not to be used in pregnancy.

65. Chapter 7
    a. Correct. NDC numbers and barcode scanning are critical to drug selection.
    b. Incorrect. While used in inventory, this is not a safety issue.
    c. Incorrect. Storage is done by name not NDC number.
    d. Incorrect. NDC is used in claim reconciliation but is not a safety issue.

66. Chapter 8
    a. Incorrect. Dairy products do not affect the absorption of tramadol.
    b. Correct. Tramadol does cause drowsiness.
    c. Incorrect. You do not have to avoid sunlight while taking tramadol.
    d. Incorrect. You do not have to take tramadol on an empty stomach.

67. Chapter 7
    a. Correct. A nosocomial infection is acquired while a patient is in a medical facility.
    b. Incorrect. Empiric therapy means treating without knowing the causative agent.
    c. Incorrect. This is a term for a bacterium that needs oxygen to survive.
    d. Incorrect. This is a new infection that complicates the course of therapy for an existing infection.

68. Chapter 4
    a. Incorrect. The FDA enforces manufacturing regulations.
    b. Incorrect. This group enforces the Poison Prevention Act.
    c. Correct. Under the Controlled Substance Act, the DEA is responsible for enforcing the law pertaining to controlled substances, like Vyvanse for ADHD.
    d. Incorrect. HIPAA violations can be reported to this group.

69. Chapter 3
    a. Incorrect. Although gout is painful and acetaminophen (Tylenol) is a pain reliever, it does not treat gout.
    b. Incorrect. Amlodipine (Norvasc) is a calcium channel blocker that is used to decrease blood pressure.
    c. Incorrect. Atenolol (Tenormin) is a beta blocker used to treat high blood pressure and tachycardia.
    d. Correct. Allopurinol (Zyloprim) is one of the agents used to manage gout.

70. Chapter 10
    a. Incorrect. Turnover is how often you sell the value of your inventory.
    b. Correct. More receipts means more money was taken in (income) than was paid out (expenses); also known as profit.
    c. Incorrect. This is the difference between an item's cost to the pharmacy and its selling price to patients.
    d. Incorrect. This is a charge to the patient that takes into account overhead and professional costs of dispensing the prescription.

71. Chapter 9
   a. Incorrect. You did remove the stock from the shelves.
   b. Incorrect. You may not sell a drug with a Class II recall.
   c. Correct. You must remove the stock from sale and follow the return instructions with the recall.
   d. Incorrect. Do not throw out as you can get credit for the product recalled.

72. Chapter 9
   a. Incorrect. The idea is to place short-dated products where they will be used first; therefore, placing the item other stock is not ideal.
   b. Incorrect. This will only clutter the work space.
   c. Correct. When stocking shelves, always rotate the stock and make sure product with the shortest date is in front so it will be used first.
   d. Incorrect. This will not allow easy identification of stock that should be used first.

73. Chapter 10
   a. Incorrect. Insurance companies no longer bill by a patient's social security number.
   b. Incorrect. DOB is not on an insurance card.
   c. Correct. BIN is used by PBM's to identify who to bill and process a claim.
   d. Incorrect. The employer phone number is not on the insurance card. The processing company is.

74. Chapter 8
   a. Incorrect. This is not a reason to take a drug off formulary.
   b. Correct. Many products are not available in unit doses, therefore the technician will have to repackage the drug in the appropriate unit dose packaging.
   c. Incorrect. To prevent medication errors, bulk packages are not sent to the patient care area.
   d. Incorrect. Only the P&T committee can make a therapeutic change to formulary.

75. Chapter 8
   a. Correct. Cephalexin pediatric suspension should be refrigerated and shaken before use.
   b. Incorrect. This formulation does not need to be refrigerated.
   c. Incorrect. This formulation does not need to be refrigerated.
   d. Incorrect. This formulation does not need to be refrigerated.

76. Chapter 7
   a. Incorrect. This book would contain information on products that are extemporaneously compounded.
   b. Incorrect. This log is a list of products that have been unit dosed.
   c. Correct. Always check the policy and procedure manual for information on the appropriate handling of drug products.
   d. Incorrect. This manual usually contains job descriptions, hiring information, and similar information in which human resources might be involved.

77. Chapter 7
   a. Incorrect. This is a process of collecting names on a list with a commonality.
   b. Incorrect. Licensure is a process required to practice a profession.
   c. Incorrect. Voluntarily taking an examination to demonstrate proficiency is certification, like a pharmacy technician certification exam.
   d. Correct. Institutions such as hospitals undergo inspection for accreditation to prove that they meet a certain level of care.

78. Chapter 8
   a. Incorrect. This is the number of days the patient will be on the therapy.
   b. Incorrect. This number is correct if the patient were on each daily schedule for 4 days. However, after 8 days, the daily schedule drops to 2 days of therapy.
   c. Correct. Add up the total number of doses $(16 + 12 + 4 + 2 + 1 = 35)$.
   d. Incorrect. If you do not split the tablet on the last 2 days and save the half tablet, you might need an extra tablet, but pharmacies do not usually give extras this way.

79. Chapter 8
   a. Incorrect. This is the abbreviation for eyedrops, and Patanol is used to treat allergic eye symptoms.
   b. Correct. Although *OU* is not an acceptable abbreviation, many prescribers still write it, so you need to know it means *both eyes*.
   c. Incorrect. The abbreviation for the right eye is *OD*.
   d. Incorrect. The abbreviation for the right ear is *AD*.

80. Chapters 6 and 8
   a. Incorrect. Hormone replacement therapy is not exempt from child-resistant packaging.
   b. Correct. Given that these are dispensed in the manufacturer-provided monthly packets, they need not be in child-resistant containers.
   c. Incorrect. ISDN sublingual and chewable is exempt, but isosorbide mononitrate is not.
   d. Incorrect. Unit dose forms of potassium chloride are available in packets of powder or effervescent tablets but not oral tablets.

81. Chapter 9
   a. Incorrect. While it may be at body temperature during use, before use it should be refrigerated.
   b. Incorrect. Freezing may alter the drug.
   c. Incorrect. This is not a controlled substance.
   d. Correct. The package label on NuvaRing indicates that it should be refrigerated until dispensed, then relabeled with a four-month expiration date.

82. Chapter 11
   a. Incorrect. If your computer is filling too often, you have to reprogram the refill program.
   b. Correct. You can have little control over compliance by the patient.
   c. Incorrect. Duplicate labels should be noticed by the fillings staff.
   d. Incorrect. If your automatic filling machine is not working correctly, it should be fixed.

83. Chapter 10
   a. Incorrect. This is not related to the pharmacy.
   b. Correct. The PBM is the company responsible for managing the payment for an insurance company.
   c. Incorrect. This is not the patient's human resource company.
   d. Incorrect. Pharmacies do not usually help patients locate insurance coverage.

84. Chapter 10
   a. Incorrect. The pharmacist is not allowed to get the PA coverage of a prescription.
   b. Incorrect. The patient does not get the PA, but can call the insurer to start the process for reconsideration if the PA is refused.
   c. Incorrect. The pharmacy technician can contact the prescriber but not the insurer for a PA.
   d. Correct. The prescriber or his office staff are responsible for getting prior authorization for a drug.

85. Chapter 4
   a. Correct. The federal government requires pseudoephedrine to be sold only by pharmacies with special recording documentation of each purchaser because of the drug's use in making methamphetamine.
   b. Incorrect. Each state controls the sale of syringes, as they may be used by IV drug abusers.
   c. Incorrect. Only sales of Plan B to women under 17 years of age are restricted to behind-the-counter sales.
   d. Incorrect. Dextromethorphan is abused by teenagers, but sale is not restricted by the federal government.

86. Chapters 4 and 8
   a. Incorrect. Although a date is required on a prescription, the lack of one does not indicate a forgery.
   b. Incorrect. Although the DEA number is needed, the lack of one does not mean it is forged.

- **c. Correct.** Any time a quantity change is made on a Vicodin prescription, it should not be filled.
- d. Incorrect. The patient's nervousness is not a definite reason to consider a prescription tampered or forged.

87. Chapter 7
    - a. Incorrect. Even a prescription checked by a pharmacist may be filled incorrectly, so if you notice a problem bring it to the attention of the pharmacist.
    - **b. Correct.** Returning it to the filling area for a triple-check will prevent a medication error.
    - c. Incorrect. That would be wasteful and not teach anyone anything about the causes of a misfill.
    - d. Incorrect. If this medication is wrong the patient might take it anyway and have an adverse drug event.

88. Chapter 7
    - **a. Correct.** The barcode can be scanned by the filling pharmacist or technician or administering nurse to make sure the drug matches the order.
    - b. Incorrect. Though the barcode might be used for the inventory, this is not its main purpose.
    - c. Incorrect. Patients have no use for the barcode.
    - d. Incorrect. Barcode or some type of scanner can be used for OTC products to prevent theft but not for the prescription products.

89. Chapter 10
    - **a. Correct.** The donut hole happens when a senior with Medicaid Plan D depletes the initial value set by the government to help cover prescription expenses.
    - b. Incorrect. Most Plan D premiums are taken automatically from social security.
    - c. Incorrect. Your records will indicate she has insurance and it has paid in the past.
    - d. Incorrect. Usually the formulary does not change without notification.

90. Chapter 10
    - a. Incorrect. Atenolol is a heart medication that must be taken daily.
    - **b. Correct.** Sumatriptan is for migraine headaches and the manufacturer does not recommend daily use.
    - c. Incorrect. Gemfibrozil is taken daily for high triglycerides.
    - d. Incorrect. Metformin is for diabetes and must be taken daily.

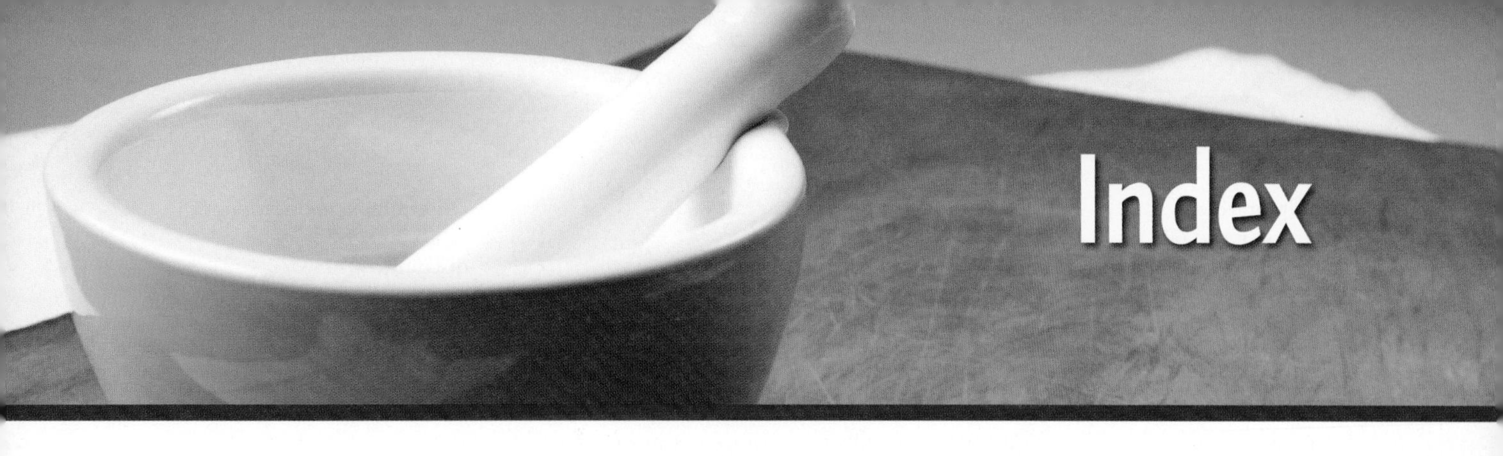

Index

f. following a page number refers to a figure; i. following a page number refers to an illustration; t. following a page number refers to a table.

B

C

D

E

I

J

K

L

N

O

P

Q

R

S